Clinical Practice in Urology
Series Editor: Geoffrey D. Chisholm

Titles in the series already published

Urinary Diversion
Edited by Michael Handley Ashken

Chemotherapy and Urological Malignancy
Edited by A. S. D. Spiers

Urodynamics
Paul Abrams, Roger Feneley and Michael Torrens

Male Infertility
Edited by T. B. Hargreave

The Pharmacology of the Urinary Tract
Edited by M. Caine

Bladder Cancer
Edited by E. J. Zingg and D. M. A. Wallace

Forthcoming titles in the series

Adenocarcinoma of the Prostate
Edited by Andrew W. Bruce and John Trachtenberg

Controversies and Innovations in Urological Surgery
Edited by J. C. Gingell and Paul Abrams

Urological Prostheses, Appliances and Catheters
Edited by J. P. Pryor

Percutaneous and Interventional Urology and Radiology

Edited by
Erich K. Lang

With 223 Figures

Springer-Verlag
Berlin Heidelberg New York Tokyo

Erich K. Lang, MD

Professor and Chairman, Department of Radiology, School of
Medicine in New Orleans, Louisiana State University Medical
Center, 1542 Tulane Avenue, New Orleans, LA 70112-2822, U.S.A.

Series Editor

Geoffrey D. Chisholm, ChM, FRCS, FRCSEd Professor of Surgery,
University of Edinburgh; and Consultant Urological Surgeon,
Western General Hospital, Edinburgh, Scotland

ISBN-13: 978-1-4471-1388-1   e-ISBN-13: 978-1-4471-1386-7
DOI: 10.1007/978-1-4471-1386-7

Library of Congress Cataloging in Publication Data
Main entry under title:
Percutaneous and interventional urology and radiology
(Clinical practice in urology)
Includes bibliographies and index.
1. Urinary organs—Radiography. 2. Radiology, Interventional. 3.
Kidneys—Radiography. I. Lang, Erich K. (Erich Karl), 1929– . Series. [DNLM: 1.
Technology, Radiologic. 2. Urography. 3. Urologic Diseases—therapy. WJ 166 P429]
RC874.P47 1986 616.6′0757 85–22166

Filmset by Latimer Trend & Company Ltd, Plymouth
Printed by Page Bros (Norwich) Ltd, Mile Cross Lane, Norwich, England.

2128/3916–543210

Series Editor's Foreword

Any book with the words percutaneous and interventional is immediately identified as one that brings to its readers a distillation of a number of new and exciting techniques. Percutaneous is not exactly a new word but it has come to take on an entirely new meaning in recent years. Interventional is a recent acquisition to medical language indicating an entirely new approach to many aspects of medical management. Exactly when is the right time to make a distillation of new thoughts and expertise requires something of the art of a master brewer. First the ingredients must be prepared, the recipe must be just right, there must be excellent quality control as well as the master brewer's touch to produce the product when the time is right. Dr. Lang has assembled just the right ingredients in the form of a very impressive team of experts in these new fields of uroradiology and urological management.

Ventures into percutaneous urology may date back 30 years but the main growth in the range of procedures and the development of the technology has occurred only in the last 10 years. Relieving upper tract obstruction seemed a natural sequel to renal biopsy but the imagination to develop an effective treatment for stones was an impressive extension of the concept of minimally invasive surgery. In the face of ever-changing technology, the exact place of these methods in the treatment of stones is certainly not finally defined but they have, for the present, an important cost-effectiveness. More changes in the management of renal stones are on the horizon but the art of percutaneous stone extraction will remain for a long time to come. A range of other chapters in this book covering other percutaneous techniques adds to the completion of the ingredients for this part of the book.

The development of interventional radiology has added an entirely new dimension to the management of a wide range of medical conditions, and in urology—from renal artery stenosis to the management of a varicocele. The contributions on interventional radiology in this book indicate both the extent and the success of the advances made by those with this expertise.

To return to the analogy of the master brewer, Dr. Lang has selected his contributors and has monitored their contributions to give a final product which will have a wide appeal and will be greatly appreciated by urologists and radiologists.

Edinburgh, November 1985   Geoffrey D. Chisholm

Preface

Interventional uroradiology epitomizes the evolution of new disciplines from such classical clinical disciplines as urologic surgery and diagnostic radiology.

The last 25 years have witnessed a spectacular growth in the application of so-called invasive diagnostic procedures. In the last 15 years many of these procedures have been modified to serve therapeutic purposes. Initially the development was in line with customary concepts and based upon the established body of knowledge of urology and diagnostic radiology. In the last 10 years, however, a successful integration of the body of knowledge of urologic surgery, diagnostic, vascular, and interventional radiology has taken place, leading to the emergence of a new subspecialty concerned with percutaneous and interventional urology and radiology. The growth rate of this new subspecialty has been exponential, and its scope and boundaries expand literally with the appearance of new publications in our specialty journals. Interest from urologists and radiologists in learning about interventional techniques has paralleled the spectacular rise of these procedures as principal treatment modalities.

It is the intent of this book to offer an up-to-date presentation and review of percutaneous and interventional uroradiologic procedures. As with any surgical procedure, the effectiveness and safety of interventional methods depend on operator technique. For this reason technique, pitfalls, complications, and results are discussed in detail. The merits of different technical approaches and results in attaining a given goal are analyzed and, if warranted by statistical information, an editorial opinion is expressed.

In several chapters updated concepts of diagnostic assessment are reviewed for those conditions most often proposed for interventional uroradiologic management. Since the diagnosis of conditions treated by percutaneous interventional uroradiology is no longer confirmed by surgical exploration, the level of diagnostic confidence and accuracy must be improved by other means. Fortunately this is possible using constellations of criteria provided by a plethora of new diagnostic modalities such as dynamic computed tomography, magnetic resonance imaging, and above all invasive diagnostic tests employing guided needle biopsies.

The reader is guided through the mental deliberations aimed at achieving a diagnosis with a confidence level that will permit institution of definitive treatment by percutaneous and interventional urology and radiology.

The text is intended to unfold seemingly complex diagnostic and management considerations in a stepwise development that the reader will be able to apply to his own case material.

Finally, I would like to acknowledge gratefully the enthusiasm, support, and energy of the many contributors to this volume. The final product is a recognition of their toil.

New Orleans, January 1986   Erich K. Lang

Contents

Contributors

P. Alken
Urologische Abteilung, Universitätsspital, Mainz, Federal Republic of Germany

Klemens H. Barth
Professor of Radiology, Georgetown University School of Medicine, 3900 Reservoir Road, N.W., Washington, D.C. 20007, U.S.A.

Bruce R. Baumgartner
Department of Radiology, Emory University, Atlanta, Georgia, U.S.A.

Michael E. Bernardino
Associate Professor of Radiology, Emory University, Atlanta, Georgia, U.S.A.

Lawrence R. Bigongiari
Veteran's Administration Medical Center, 4801 Linwood Boulevard, Kansas City, Missouri 64128, U.S.A.

Jean deKernion
Professor of Urology, Division of Urology, University of California Los Angeles, 10833 LeConte 66128, Los Angeles, California 90024, U.S.A.

N. Reed Dunnick
Professor of Radiology, Box 3808, Department of Radiology, Duke University Medical Center, Durham, North Carolina 27710, U.S.A.

Leif Ekelund
Department of Diagnostic Radiology, University Hospital, 221 85 Lund, Sweden

Milton Elkin
Professor and Chairman Department of Radiology, Albert Einstein Medical College, Bronx, New York, U.S.A.

Peggy J. Fritzsche
Director Outpatients Services, Department of Radiology, Loma Linda
Medical Center, Loma Linda, CA 92354, U.S.A.

Stanford M. Goldman
Department of Radiology, Baltimore City Hospital, 4940 Eastern
Avenue, Baltimore, Maryland 21224, U.S.A.

William G. Guerriero
Associate Professor of Urology, Baylor University College of Medicine, 1200 Moursund Avenue, Houston, Texas 77030, U.S.A.

Rolf W. Günther
Röntgen-Institut, Universitätsspital, Mainz, Federal Republic of Germany

Erich K. Lang
Professor and Chairman, Department of Radiology, School of Medi-
cine in New Orleans, Louisiana State University Medical Center, 1542
Tulane Avenue, New Orleans, LA 70112-2882, U.S.A.

John D. Maldazys, Major, U.S.A.F., M.C.
Department of Urology, Wilford Hall, U.S.A.F. Medical Center,
Lackland Air Force Base, Texas, U.S.A. 78236

Helen T. Morehouse
Associate Professor of Radiology, Department of Radiology, Albert
Einstein Medical College, Bronx, New York, U.S.A.

Richard C. Pfister
Associate Professor of Radiology, Massachusetts General Hospital,
Boston, Massachusetts U.S.A.

Janet C. Hoffman-Tretin
Associate Professor of Radiology, Department of Radiology, Section
of Ultrasound, Albert Einstein Medical College, Bronx, New York,
U.S.A.

E. Zeitler
Radiologisches Zentrum, Abt. Diagnostik-Klinikum, Flurstrasse 17,
Nürnberg, Federal Republic of Germany

Chapter 1

Percutaneous Nephrostomy

Richard C. Pfister

Introduction

Percutaneous nephrostomy (PCN) was first described 30 years ago [57] as a method to obtain relief of obstruction in marked hydronephrosis when retrograde drainage was technically impossible or inappropriate and surgical nephrostomy was not indicated or feasible. After a slow beginning in the 1960s, its use exploded in the 1970s with improved imaging systems (image intensified fluoroscopy, ultrasonography, computed tomography) and technical innovations such as thin needle antegrade pyelography and Seldinger guide wire and catheter techniques which made guided percutaneous catheter insertion a practical clinical procedure [1–12, 14, 15, 17–55, 57–67, 69–91, 93–120, 122–140].

Percutaneous nephrostomy has today been accepted as the procedure of choice, in adults and children [41, 102, 133], in almost all cases of urinary obstruction requiring temporary drainage of the urinary tract. Further experience has led to its use in several situations for permanent drainage by extended nephrostomy or antegrade stents.

With the realization that needles and catheters could be safely and quickly used on the kidney, the method of PCN became the window into this organ for a variety of interventional uroradiologic and endourologic procedures, and its use has now been extended to situations of nondilated pyelocalyceal systems. The favorable experience with PCN has opened the door to a variety of new diagnostic and more often definitive therapeutic interventions [60, 73, 85, 97, 99, 105, 136]. The resulting improved patient care has been associated with reduced morbidity, minimal mortality, and cost reduction compared with previous, usually surgical approaches [98].

This chapter will cover those aspects relating mainly to PCN per se, leaving the details of its offspring procedures to other contributing authors.

Table 1.1. Indications for percutaneous nephrostomy

Diagnostic
   Split renal function
   Brush biopsy
   Nephroscopy/nephroureteroscopy

Therapeutic
   Urinary diversion
      Obstruction
      Leaks or fistulas
   Stricture dilatation (ureteroplasty)
   Antegrade stent
   Chemotherapy irrigation urothelial tumor
   Stone management
      Displacement
      Dissolution
      Extraction
      Disintegration (lithotripsy)
   Removal of foreign bodies

Indications

The overall and specific indications for PCN are outlined in Table 1.1. In general, the procedure is used as an alternative to surgery, as a temporary measure until definitive operative correction can be carried out or as a means of gaining initial access to the urinary tract for secondary therapeutic percutaneous procedures. Critically ill patients can be rapidly managed by PCN with minimal morbidity and mortality; contributing factors to poor surgical risk of many patients include metabolic instability and limited cardiopulmonary reserve, as well as local tissue disruption with or without infection.

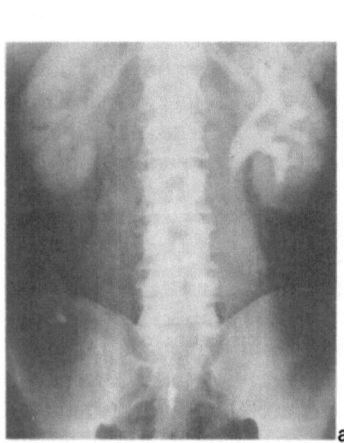 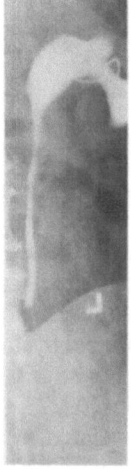

a   b

Fig. 1.1a,b. Young man with total anuria and severe bilateral flank pain of 2 days' duration. **a** Urogram showing both kidneys obstructed and **b** left percutaneous nephrostomy demonstrating multiple uric acid calculi in the ureter; similar findings on other side during simultaneous tube placement.

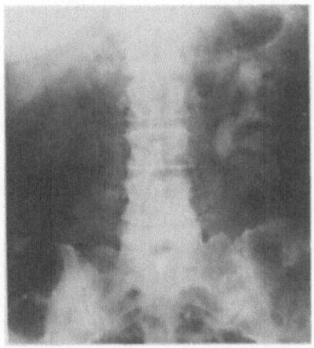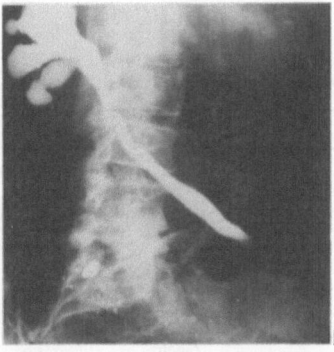

a   b

Fig. 1.2a,b. Middle-aged women with ileal loop diversion for neurogenic bladder. a Urography showing poorly functioning right kidney. b The obstructed ureteroileal junction was due to severe fibrosis which did not respond to percutaneous balloon dilatation following initial nephrostomy drainage.

Obstruction/Pyonephrosis

Urinary diversion for simple obstruction and for pyonephrosis is the most frequent indication for PCN [3, 8, 9, 15, 19, 26, 39, 40, 43, 48, 51, 52, 60, 61, 65, 67, 71, 73, 78, 85, 88, 95–99, 105, 112, 116–118, 132, 138]. In the sterile kidney, high-grade obstruction may be tolerated for up to 1 week before irreversible nephron damage begins; in most cases of ureteral calculi, either small stones will pass in this time or the obstruction is incomplete. Conversely, obstructions with little likelihood of early reversal will require drainage. The obstructed kidney(s) complicated by azotemia or infection ordinarily require prompt relief. While drainage can be obtained by either the retrograde or percutaneous route, the former method may be technically difficult or impossible, as in the obliterated ureteral orifice or ileal conduit. In other cases where other secondary manipulations are feasible, as in stricture dilatation or stone removal, the percutaneous approach is the desirable choice.

Common causes of benign obstructions requiring temporary PCN, besides stones (Fig. 1.1), are postsurgical ureteral anastomotic stenoses (Fig. 1.2), vascular reconstruction with ureteral obstruction, gynecologic repairs with ureteral entrapment, and idiopathic retroperitoneal fibrosis.

Percutaneous nephrostomy is also useful when the functional reserve capacity of an obstructed kidney is uncertain [73, 98, 104]. Benign congenital lesions such as severe ureteropelvic junction and primary megaureter are common candidates for assessment of individual renal function determination (Fig. 1.3).

Frequently, malignancy from the bladder, prostate (Fig. 1.4), uterus, colon, breast, and lung will result in renal obstruction. With the exception of lymphoma, many malignant obstructions have little expectation of response to further therapy. While palliative percutaneous drainage can be utilized, the technique should not be used merely to prolong life if intractable pain is likely in the end [68, 92, 121]. In situations of malignant obstruction, long-term nursing care is simplified by converting simple PCN to an external-type antegrade stent or, if this is not possible, to one of the extended nephrostomy catheter arrangements.

Regardless of the etiology, patients with urinary tract obstruction are at high risk for *pyohydronephrosis*, which carries a high morbidity and mortality [56].

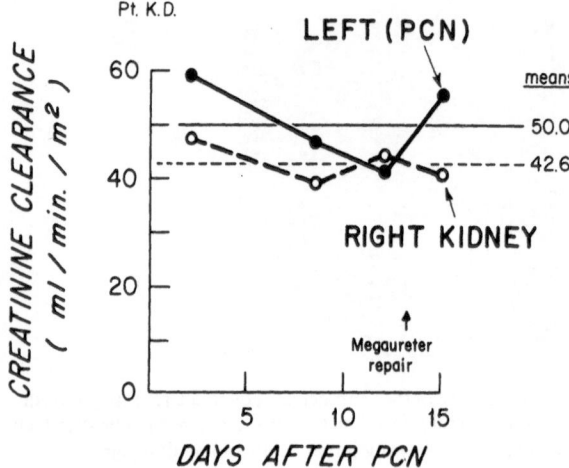

Pt. K.D.

Fig. 1.3. Split renal function determinations on first the right and then the left kidney were performed prior to final approach to surgical correction.

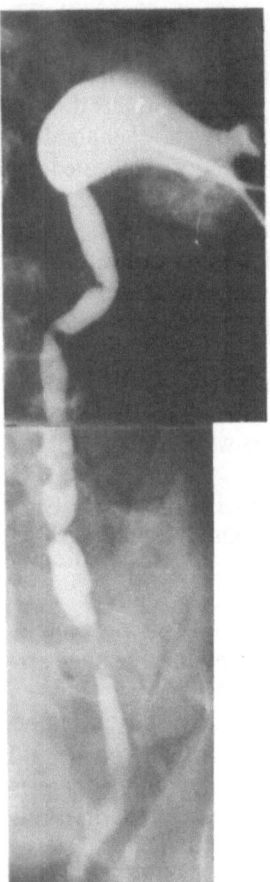

Fig. 1.4. Composite view of kidney and lower ureter following percutaneous nephrostomy for azotemia; carcinoma of the prostate was subsequently documented.

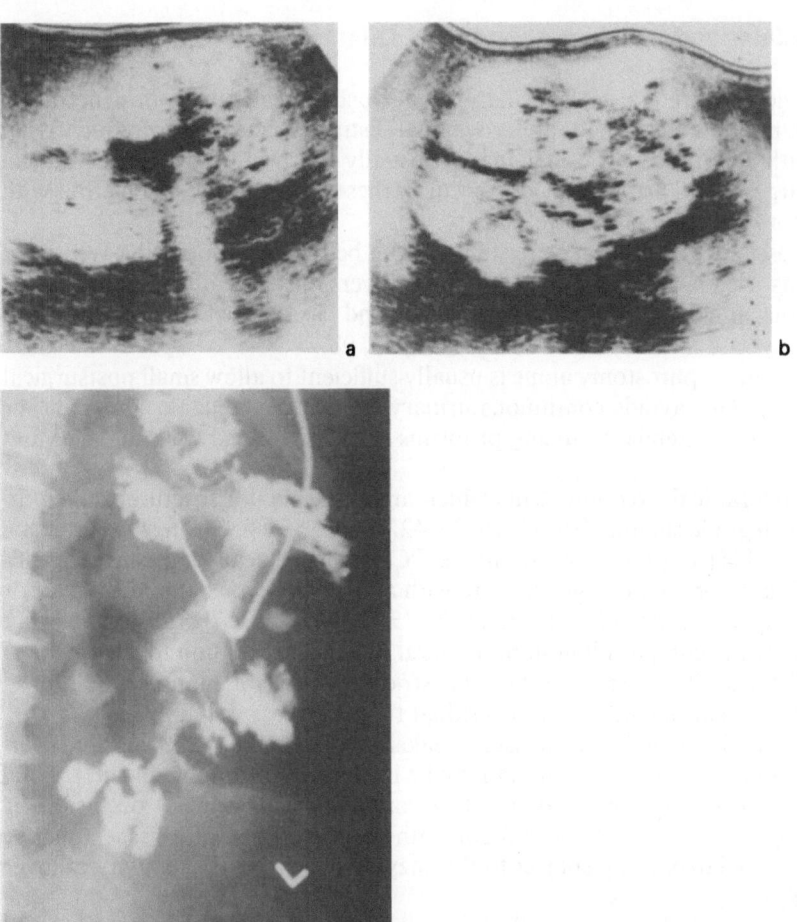

Fig. 1.5a–c. Obtunded woman with fever and uremia. **a** Medial and **b** lateral parasagittal renal sonograms demonstrating large staghorn calculus and hydrocalyces containing low level internal echoes. **c** Flank pus aspirated and PCN with 12-F catheter performed. Note characteristic distribution of contrast media in viscous fluid of pyonephrosis.

Percutaneous intervention in these febrile patients is safer than the operative approach; suspected pyonephrosis can be diagnosed by direct sampling of the urine from the kidney(s) [9, 26, 98, 138]. If infected urine is present, PCN provides rapid decompression (Fig. 1.5). However, despite antibiotic coverage, exacerbation of sepsis can occur even in the absence of diagnostic pyeloureterography; careful monitoring of the blood pressure and other vital signs is necessary during the first 12 h [97, 132]. Nephrostomy drainage affords a temporary benefit while the septic episode subsides; additionally, many of these kidneys will demonstrate surprising functional recovery [138]. Subsequently, the obstructing lesion can be treated surgically or percutaneously where feasible. In cases in which malignant disease has caused obstruction, PCN frequently provides the final definitive treatment.

Leaks/Fistulas and Strictures: Stents and Dilatation

Renal pelvic and ureteral leaks usually result postsurgically or from penetrating trauma. Ureteral-enteric and ureterovaginal fistulas occur most frequently in women with advanced pelvic malignancy, usually following radiation or radical surgery; large vesical fistulas can also occur in these settings or in association with inflammatory or malignant bowel disease.

When possible, ureteral leaks are stented from below cystoscopically. When not possible, as well as in patients with loop diversions and anastomotic leaks, percutaneous management is effective and safe and has reduced the morbidity and nephrectomy rate in many situations [14, 72, 75, 98].

Percutaneous nephrostomy alone is usually sufficient to allow small postsurgical leaks to heal. This avoids continuous urinary soilage of the flank, abdomen, or perineum and its attendant nursing problems of skin care and wet bandages and bedding.

Large ureteral leaks require stents which are desirable if a stricture is likely to develop. Antegrade stenting [10, 15, 16, 36, 42, 46, 49, 55, 60, 71, 76, 79, 81, 83, 85, 91, 98, 103, 115] is preferable to simple PCN when a leak is associated with stenosis. Dilatation of a benign stricture with a Gruntzig-type balloon catheter or graduated tapered catheter [6, 31, 53, 69, 70, 75, 80, 98, 111, 137] prior to final stent placement may accomplish long-term ureteral patency in addition to treatment of the leak/fistulas. However, longstanding strictures (several months) and those associated with chronic infection or residual tumor do less well [6].

In larger unobstructed (low pressure) leaks/fistulas simple PCN will not divert urine flow and even ureteral stenting may be inadequate or impossible [97]. Total urine diversion can be obtained by PCN combined with ureteral occlusion by either a Fogarty or a detachable balloon catheter; deposition of a tissue adhesive has been less reliable, being subject to the enzymatic degradation activity of urine [62, 97, 98].

If direct manipulative access to the ureter is anticipated in the management of a leak/fistula, the intrarenal access route should be one that allows easy catheterization of the ureteropelvic junction. Conversely, if only simple PCN drainage is required then catheter entry and position in the kidney are not critical.

Biopsy and Nephroscopy

In many cases standard urine cytology is positive for transitional cell tumors of the kidney. Occasionally, however, after ultrasonography and/or computed tomographic exclusion of a nonopaque stone, it is necessary to separate a malignant urothelial tumor from other benign disorders such as pyelitis cystica, malacoplakia, intramural or luminal hemorrhage, sloughed papilla, and ectopic papilla. If visualization and/or biopsy with a retrograde ureteroscope cannot be accomplished, the percutaneous approach can be employed (Fig. 1.6).

In the antegrade technique [74, 97], a PCN is done and the tract dilated to accept a steerable catheter or flexible nephroscope; either can be introduced over a guide wire or more easily advanced through an outer working sheath. The steerable

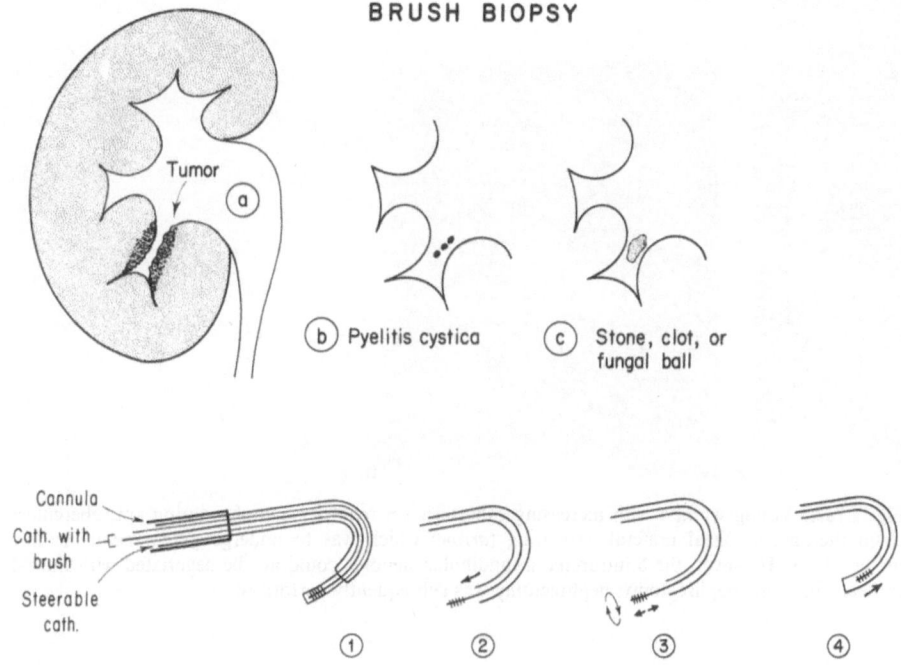

Fig. 1.6. Schema of guided percutaneous brush biopsy with flexible instrumentation. (From Pfister and Newhouse [98], with permission)

catheter (Medi-Tech, Inc., Watertown, Massachusetts) is guided by fluoroscopic control while the flexible fiberoptic nephroscope (Olympus Corp., 4 Nevada Drive, New Hyde Park, New York) has a direct straight ahead viewing lens but requires some experience in its use [18, 25, 107].

Nylon brushes and small grasping or biopsy forceps can be passed through these instruments, to obtain a tissue sample of various depths where indicated. Available in 9–16 F size and various lengths, they can be directed into the ureter as well, particularly when it is mildly dilated.

Stone Management

Mechanical advancement of small 3–5 mm ureteral stones into the bladder may be accomplished percutaneously with long stent catheters of 7–10 F size during PCN for obstruction [97, 128, 134]. Similar caliber nephrostomy tubes can be used for chemolysis of calculi of struvite, apatite, carbonate, cystine, and uric acid composition [32–35, 87, 89, 122, 124, 127].

Carefully positioned larger nephrostomy tracts of 22–30 F size are needed to directly extract intact 7- to 10-mm stones or to accommodate the popular 22–26 F rigid right-angled nephroscopes for ultrasonic lithotripsy [1, 2, 5, 20, 23, 24, 44, 45, 47, 60, 89, 119, 123, 125, 136].

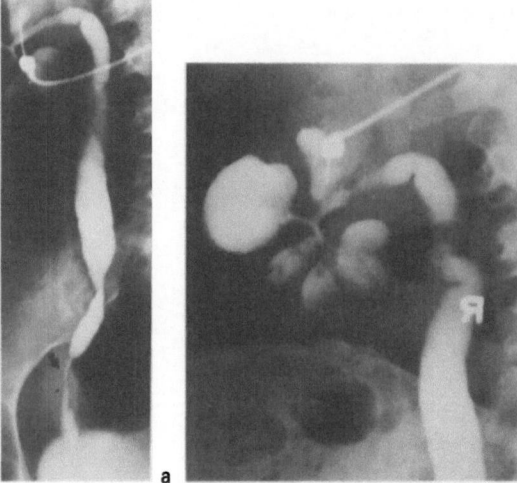

Fig. 1.7a,b. Young woman with increasing caliectasis on renal sonography during antituberculosis chemotherapy. **a** Distal ureteral narrowing (*arrow*) which was to undergo percutaneous balloon ureteroplasty. However, the **b** intrarenal infundibular stenoses could not be negotiated with the 8-F catheter following nephrostomy; nephrectomy was subsequently performed.

Contraindications

While no absolute contraindication exists, bleeding disorders constitute a strong relative contraindication to PCN [97, 129, 132]. In the setting of urosepsis and disseminated intravascular coagulopathy, PCN may be the only hope for management however [97]. Renal tuberculosis (Fig. 1.7) and urothelial neoplasm are no longer considered contraindications to PCN, although it may be argued that one should avoid it unless absolutely necessary.

General Considerations

Clinical and Radiologic Aspects

In preparation for nephrostomy, consultation with a urologic surgeon is advisable since most disorders requiring PCN are within their domain and any untoward complication may require urgent surgical exploration.

The procedure should be explained to the patient or his relatives so that informed consent can be obtained. The coagulation profile (prothrombin time, partial thromboplastin, platelet count, or others) is usually obtained; in its absence, careful inquiry is made into any drugs which may affect bleeding parameters. Appropriate antibiotics and analgesics or sedatives are obtained for administration as needed.

Assessment of splenic size should be made since an enlarged spleen may produce anterior and medial displacement of the left kidney so that the usual percutaneous route may be compromised.

Computed tomography and renal sonography can provide helpful information on renal depth. In the absence of recent urography an abdominal radiograph clearly demonstrating renal position is necessary and should be supplemented by sonography when possible.

Placement of a peripheral intravenous line to simplify administration of medication or contrast media is desirable; intramuscular analgesics and vasopressors may be inconsistent in their effectiveness.

Antibiotics

Aseptic technique in PCN performance should not cause bacteremia or urinary infection [97, 102, 132]. However, deep or malpositioned needle passes may enter the colon and subsequently contaminate the urine. All patients with pyonephrosis are not febrile, and cloudy urine is always suspect of being currently infected. Extensive manipulations of stone removal, stenting, and ureteroplasty may also result at times in bacteremia from surface bacteria or infected stones. While there is no absolute reason to give antibiotics routinely for simple PCN, their purpose is to decrease the chance of septicemia and hypotension.

A useful prophylactic antibiotic regime is ampicillin (1 g IV) combined with an aminoglycoside such as gentamicin or tobramycin (80 mg IV or IM) in a single dose 1 h prior to the procedure. The former is effective against enterococcus and most proteus bacteria while the latter is effective against all gram-negative organisms but not enterococcus.

Premedication

Analgesic premedication such as Phenergan and morphine or meperidine (0.5 ml/lb) is very valuable, but those with severe azotemia often require less, being sedated by their disease. Small doses of intravenous diazepam (5 mg) and meperidine (25 mg) or fentanyl can be administered as needed during more painful aspects of a procedure, such as rapid dilatation of the nephrostomy tract to large caliber. Intravenous analgesic and sedative injection is more reliable than intramuscular and should be done with blood pressure monitoring.

In infants and children premedication with one of various pediatric-mix cocktails can be employed, the dose per body weight being more critical than it is in the usual adult (Table 1.2).

Table 1.2. Pedi-mix for sedation of infants and children

Meperidine	25 mg	⎫
Chlorpromazine	8 mg	⎬ in 1 ml
Promethazine	5 mg	⎭

Dose: 1 ml/kg, not to exceed 2 ml

Approach

Imaging Guidance

Thin needle renal puncture can be performed with fluoroscopy, ultrasonography, or computed tomography control. However, catheter placement and all guide wire–catheter–dilator manipulations and tube positioning are best done with fluoroscopic control for safety purposes [97, 139]. Computed tomography [63] is cumbersome and expensive and requires subsequent patient movement to a fluoroscopic suite; its use is seldom necessary or desirable.

Sonography allows accurate assessment of depth and is useful in pregnant women, in those at risk from intravenous contrast media, and in nonopacifying kidneys or at the bedside [4, 12, 37, 66, 93, 94, 114, 130, 135, 139]. Many use real-time sonography with or without an aspiration transducer to guide the 22-gauge antegrade pyelogram needle into the collecting system; only a few carry out the entire procedure with ultrasonic guidance.

Most workers perform the entire procedure of PCN under fluoroscopic guidance. Once one is experienced, skinny needle antegrade pyelography can be rapidly performed without administering intravenous contrast media in all but the nondilated or mildly dilated collecting system; the location of the kidney beforehand must be known or demonstrable on abdominal radiography or visible under fluoroscopy [97, 98].

Patient Position: Tract Selection

Antegrade pyelography and subsequent percutaneous nephrostomy is best performed under fluoroscopic guidance with the patient in the prone or the prone oblique position with the side to be punctured elevated 30°. The choice is dependent on the operator's preference and experience as well as on individual patient considerations of physical limitations (e.g., scoliosis) and renal position. In either approach the tube tract is posterolateral through the renal parenchyma rather than directly into the free wall of the renal pelvis.

In the prone position, a posterolateral entry approach for PCN (Fig. 1.8) allows visualization of the needle or trocar course as it is advanced without including the operator's fingers in the coned beam. The patient can roll slightly into the obliquity necessary for the needle to be seen in the third dimension if desired. Alternatively, calculation of depth can be made by triangulation. If the depth from an initial vertically introduced antegrade needle is known and the distance from this entry to the posterolateral PCN puncture site is calculated, the third side of triangulation can be ascertained or even physically laid out on the sterile field itself, using the second needle for direct comparison.

An initial prone oblique position allows an essentially vertical needle or trocar passage; access is easiest if the fluoroscopic beam, the puncture site, and the target are aligned vertically. Intermittent coned beam fluoroscopy avoids exposure to the fingers. Alternatively, a commercial needle holder or a simple 9- to 12-in. length obstetric sponge forceps can be employed to grasp the needle during fluoroscopic advancement into the collecting system; such critical small target entries are usually limited to PCN for subsequent stone removal rather than simple drainage of the dilated obstructed kidney.

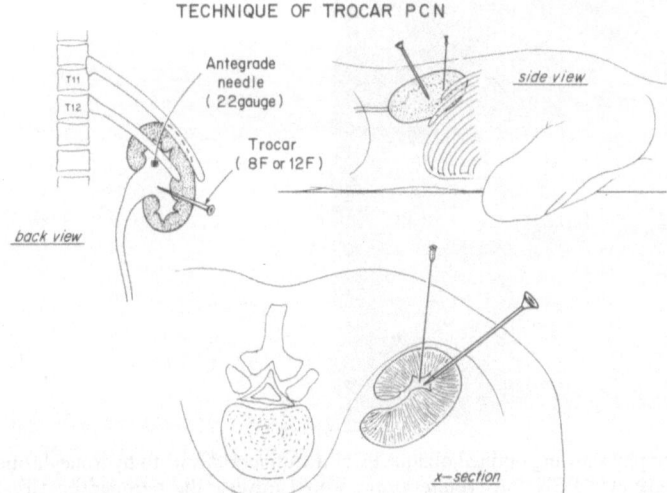

Fig. 1.8. Schema for two-step puncture nephrostomy technique by either the trocar–cannula, the Seldinger, or the needle/trocar–catheter method. Initial subcostal antegrade pyelography is followed by PCN. (From Pfister and Newhouse [98], with permission)

The transparenchymal renal PCN tract ensures entry into the relative avascular zone (Brodel's line) of the kidney and provides a tight seal around the nephrostomy catheter. A transpelvic approach reduces intrarenal catheter length and increases the possibility of tearing the pelvis or lacerating a major vessel in the renal hilum. Most urinomas and significant renal bleeding would appear to be related to entry attempts into the renal pelvis rather than into the calyx or infundibulum.

It is not necessary or desirable to utilize more than a 30° prone oblique position since in some patients the colon or spleen lie deep and adjacent to the perirenal fossa and would be within any 45° skin entry trajectory path to the kidney (Fig. 1.9). However, a direct posterior nephrostomy position should be avoided when possible since it does not allow the patient to lie supine in bed comfortably.

Exceptions to the posterior axillary line approach are malrotated and pelvic kidneys. In simple malrotation and in the horseshoe kidney the renal pelvis lies anterior, and in these cases the PCN tract is placed more vertical to enter the proper portion of the collecting system.

In ectopic pelvic kidneys and renal transplants the approach is anterolateral [7, 47, 54]. In the latter situation it should be lateral to the incision to avoid traversing the peritoneal cavity, while in the former, CT guidance is helpful to document avoidance of bowel loops.

In all other situations, however, the puncture site should be below the 12th rib to eliminate the potential for pneumothorax and for damage to intercostal vessels, which are capable of significant bleeding, particularly during placement of large nephrostomy tracts [113].

For simple drainage, the point where the nephrostomy catheter enters the kidney is of limited concern; pressure is equivalent throughout the system and the catheter will drain providing it is not wedged into the tip of a calyx or the obstructed segment of the ureter. In stone disease, however, intrarenal entry

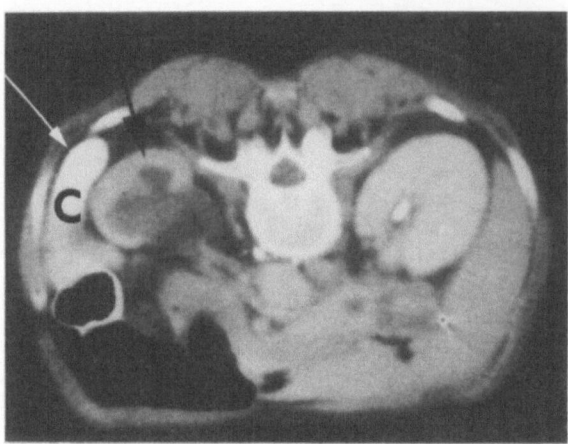

Fig. 1.9. Computed tomography showing optimal oblique PCN tract (*black arrow*) to hydronephrotic kidney. Note that an exaggerated PCN tract (*white arrow*) would traverse the retroperitonealized portion of the contrast-filled colon (*C*).

location is critical for percutaneous treatment. Since the upper pole of the kidney is usually above the 12th rib, an approach through the lower pole is most often used for stones in the lower calyx, upper calyx, pelvis, or ureter. When accessible, a lower lateral or middle calyx allows an easier approach to upper ureteral calculi. In low-lying kidneys, PCN access can also be established through an upper pole calyx for calculi in the pelvis, ureter, or lower pole calyces. Similarly, if PCN is a prelude to antegrade stent placement, a more cephalad renal entry site is helpful.

Techniques and Equipment

A great range of needles, guide wires, trocars, cannulas, sheaths, and catheters have been described and are available commercially. The choice of equipment has evolved as the personal preferences of individual workers have grown. The many techniques of PCN are variations on two principles and three techniques for instrumentation and two resulting methods of application. Whichever technique, instrument, or approach is used, patient positioning and skin puncture site with nephrostomy tract course are the same.

Catheter insertion into the kidney can be performed by going "over" (a guide wire or needle) or "under" (an outer cannula or sheath); while simplistic in principle, the resulting instruments, manipulations, and types of catheter employed are different [15, 19, 21, 22, 27, 29, 39, 40, 43, 48, 52, 57, 61, 77, 88, 90, 97, 100, 105, 116–118, 126, 132].

The three basic techniques for PCN are (a) angiographic (Seldinger), (b) trocar–cannula, and (c) needle/trocar–catheter. These can be variously utilized with the single or dual puncture methods of approach. All the instruments, techniques, and methods of catheter placement have their advantages and limitations.

Antegrade Pyelography

A 22-gauge Chiba or spinal needle is guided by ultrasound or fluoroscopy into the kidney. Under local anesthesia, the needle is advanced in gradual increments with frequent intermittent aspirations and deposition of anesthetic. Since urine may not flow spontaneously through the needle, a small attached syringe is used. A sample of urine is inspected and sent for culture. If infection is suspected, contrast media should be injected only after an equivalent volume of urine has been removed; this prevents overdistention and the increased risk of bacteremia. The antegrade needle provides anatomic definition of the collecting system and determines the depth of the kidney from the skin (Fig. 1.7b). If urine is not obtained, the needle is redirected to a slightly different position and advanced again [61, 67, 97, 105].

Single Puncture Seldinger Method

A 21- or 22-gauge needle is used to enter the collecting system [29, 61, 105]. One method has a shorter, wider 18-gauge needle preloaded coaxially on a longer thin 22-gauge needle. Once the thin needle is in place the shorter one is advanced over the top into the collecting system, the thin needle removed, and an 0.038-in. (0.97-mm) J-tipped guide wire advanced inside the kidney [Cook, Inc. (Gunther) (Mitty-Pollack), PO Box 489, Bloomington, Indiana 47402; Surgitek, Medical Engineering Corp., 3037 Mt. Pleasant St., Racine, Wisconsin 53404]. The larger needle is then withdrawn, leaving the guide wire in place, preferably down the ureter or at the opposite end of the kidney from its entry site or partially coiled in the renal pelvis.

Another system utilizes a 21-gauge needle which accepts an 0.018-in. (0.46-mm) stiff guide wire with a gentle curved flexible tip. After needle removal, a clever reinforced 6.3-F conversion catheter is advanced into the kidney and the small guide and reinforcer are removed. Passage of an 0.038-in. J-tipped guide wire through the larger back portion of the catheter permits its exit through a distal side hole [Cook, Inc., (Cope), PO Box 489, Bloomington, Indiana 47402]; after removal of the conversion catheter the J-tipped guide can be exchanged for a straight torque guide wire for manipulation into the ureter if desired (Fig. 1.10).

The thin 21- and 22-gauge needle nephrostomy techniques permit safe exploration with only the fine needle. They allow performance of antegrade pyelography simultaneously prior to further manipulation. If the initial needle position is not desirable, the needle can be redirected to a more suitable location. Each method requires some experience to master the finer details of its application.

Two Puncture Seldinger Method

One technique incorporates a closely fitted external Teflon sheath over a 19-gauge needle [Cook, Inc., (Rutner), PO Box 489, Bloomington, Indiana 47402; UMI Corp., (Spataro), Box 100, Ballston Spa, New York 12020; Becton-Dickinson (Longdwel), Rutherford, New Jersey]. After puncture with the tandem unit the needle is removed, an 0.038-in. J-tipped guide wire advanced into the collecting system, and the sheath removed. Alternatively, the unit can be advanced slightly beyond the desired location, the needle withdrawn, and the sheath placed on gentle aspiration while it is slowly withdrawn until fluid is aspirated. Following this a guide wire is advanced into the kidney and the sheath removed.

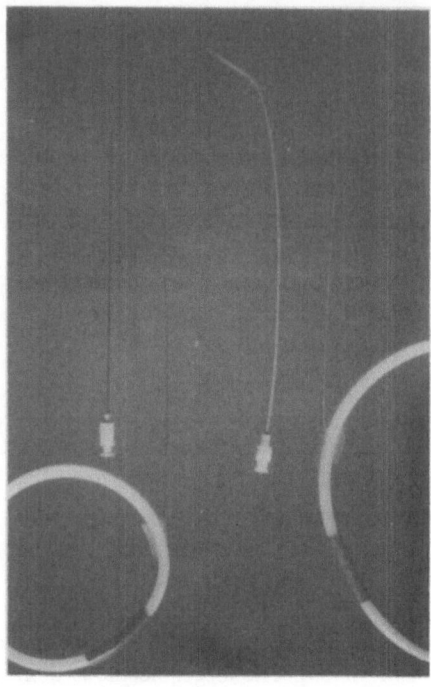

Fig. 1.10. One-step puncture equipment (Cope system). *From left to right*: 21-gauge needle, 0.018-in. guide wire, 6.3-F converting catheter, and 0.038-in. torque guide wire (substituted for J tip) for positioning into the ureter.

Another method uses a simple 18-gauge needle alone. Once advanced into the kidney, the stylet is removed, an 0.038-in. J-tipped guide wire passed, and the needle removed [Cook, Inc., (Rutner), PO Box 489, Bloomington, Indiana 47402].

Since both the 18-gauge needle and the 19-gauge sheathed needle have larger cutting edged bevels to the needle tips, they are not ideally suited as exploring needles; most workers use the larger needle nephrostomy technique following antegrade pyelography with a fine 21- or 22-gauge needle.

Once an 0.038-in. guide wire is in position with either the single or double puncture Seldinger methods the tract is dilated with one or more dilators to a size approximating the nephrostomy catheter [113].

Straight, pigtail, or loop-type nephrostomy catheters of 7–10 F are then introduced over the guide wire [17, 27, 40, 60, 90, 116]. During dilator and nephrostomy catheter passage the guide wire should be held straight in its normal trajectory path and steady traction applied as the catheter is advanced in short firm thrusts. Intermittent fluoroscopy allows frequent checking for any buckling of the catheter, angulation of the guide wire, or withdrawal of the guide wire.

In general, the usual J-tipped 0.038-in. guide wire is relatively soft; it has little directional control by the operator and a tendency to buckle. Heavy duty 0.038-in. torque control wires overcome both of these problems to a large extent. Also available is an extra stiff stainless steel "coat-hanger" type guide wire (Lundequist) of similar size; this is useful in fibrotic perinephric tissues which have resulted from previous surgery but ideally should only be used when it can be passed down the ureter, which secures a long purchase. If this guide wire can only be positioned inside the kidney, one must be careful of any further advancement of it during dilator or catheter passage since it can easily perforate and tear the wall of the renal pelvis or even renal parenchyma.

Alternatively, a tear-away sheath-dilator system [Cook Inc., (Pfister), PO Box 489, Bloomington, Indiana 47402; USCI, (Cope), CR Bard Inc., PO Box 566, Billerica, MA 01821] can be used over an 0.038-in. guide wire. Following removal of the plastic dilator, this method allows for easy passage of a silicone catheter [Dow-Corning Corp., (Cystocath), Med. Products, Hemlock, Michigan], which has the advantage of being extremely pliable. Problems of catheter buckling during Seldinger exchange are thus completely obviated with these catheter passage assemblies. Once the catheter is in the desired position, the outer Teflon sheath is simply stripped away from the nephrostomy tube.

Two Puncture Trocar–Cannula Method

As in the dual puncture Seldinger technique, a preliminary antegrade pyelogram is done to delineate the intrarenal collecting system; patient positioning, selection of skin and renal entrance sites, and imaging guidance are also similar (Fig. 1.8).

This technique utilizes a pencil point hollow metal trocar with a distal side hole. The trocar fits into a thin-walled tear-away Teflon sheath cannula [Cook, Inc., (Pfister), PO Box 489, Bloomington, Indiana 47402]. The coned end of the trocar is noncutting and displaces tissue rather than incising or lacerating it (Fig. 1.11).

After making a small skin incision, the trocar–cannula unit is advanced stepwise toward the calyceal target [88, 97, 98, 100]. The trocar should be advanced on a straight trajectory rather than redirecting its course while it is in the soft tissues. By ensuring a direct tissue–kidney course the catheter will lie in a straight plane which allows easier catheter exchange over a guide wire at some later juncture. Once fluid

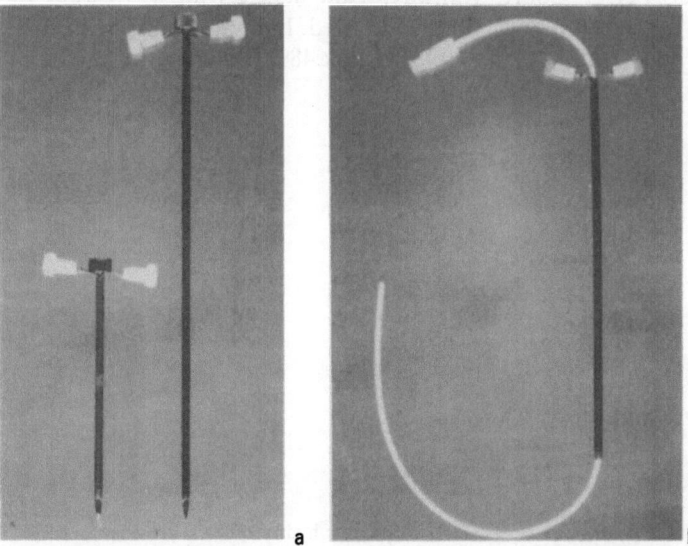

a   b

Fig. 1.11. a Short pediatric and longer adult fluid returning metal trocar units with overlying tear-away sheath cannulas. **b** A catheter of any type or pliability may be introduced through the sheath.

is returned out of the end of the trocar, the latter should be quickly capped with a finger to prevent decompression of the collecting system. The unit is advanced a few more millimeters to ensure that the cannula remains in the collecting system during trocar removal and the rapid insertion of the catheter (Fig. 1.11b). A soft silicone 8-F catheter is passed with ample catheter length coiled in the renal pelvis or down the ureter to minimize the likelihood of dislodgement. If exact catheter position is critical, a torque control guide wire can be placed through the catheter.

As alternatives to the pliable straight silicone catheter, polyethylene pigtail [Cook, Inc. (Rutner) (Amplatz-Stamey) (Cope), PO Box 489, Bloomington, Indiana 47402], Malecot [Cook, Inc. (Rutner) (Amplatz-Stamey) (Cope), PO Box 489, Bloomington, Indiana 47402], or loop-type [Cook, Inc. (Rutner) (Amplatz-Stamey) (Cope), PO Box 489, Bloomington, Indiana 47402; USCI (Cope), CR Bard, Inc., PO Box 566, Billerica, Massachusetts 01821] catheters as well as antegrade stent tubes [Cook, Inc. (Rutner) (Amplatz-Stamey) (Cope), PO Box 489, Bloomington, Indiana 47402; Surgitek, MEC, 3037 Mt. Pleasant St., Racine, Wisconsin 53404] can be inserted through the cannula. After desired catheter positioning, the cannula is removed by pulling on the small handles, which splits the sheath. While most radiologists are dedicated to the Seldinger approach, the major advantages of trocar nephrostomy are its speed and elimination of guide wire problems.

Two Puncture Needle/Trocar–Catheter Method

These instruments can be used for PCN after initial thin needle antegrade pyelography as in the dual puncture Seldinger and trocar–cannula methods.

The principle is a single or one-step insertion of a catheter over a needle/trocar assembly. Following placement into the collecting system, the catheter is simultaneously advanced off the introducer while the latter is withdrawn, leaving the catheter in place. The catheter tip is available in pigtail [Electro-Catheter Corp. (Elecath-Sacks), 2100 Felver Court, Rahway, New Jersey 07065], balloon or straight tip [Argyle (Ingram) (Gerzof), Sherwood Med. Ind., St. Louis, Missouri], and Malecot [Cook, Inc. (Amplatz-Stamey), PO Box 489, Bloomington, Indiana]

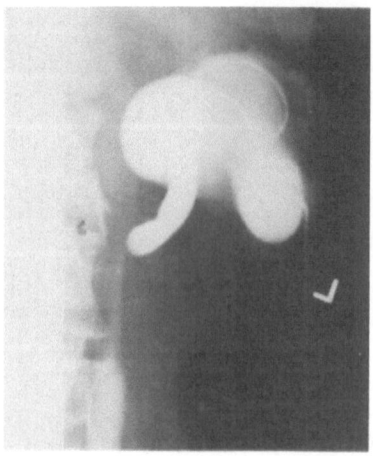

Fig. 1.12. Moderate hydronephrosis provides an easy target; calyceal entry is followed by an adequate length of the intrarenal catheter.

configurations; the last unit can also be inserted by the modified Seldinger technique [21, 22, 51, 126].

One undesirable feature of some of these assemblies is their large cutting bevel edge to the needle tip. Other units have a solid trocar introducer which does not allow for a fluid return to signal entry into the collecting system.

Calyceal Size: Intrarenal Access

In marked and moderately dilated collecting systems, percutaneous transparenchymal entry is usually easy (Fig. 1.12). All the previously described nephrostomy systems can be utilized successfully, although those with cutting tips would appear less safe to the wall of an artery. With decreasing calyceal size, entry into the kidney becomes more difficult. However, the mildly or nondilated but obstructed kidney still provides a reasonable target providing the 12th rib leaves an unimpeded pass into the lower pole of the kidney.

In nondilated and unobstructed low pressure collecting systems, intrarenal access becomes technically more difficult (Fig. 1.13). In this situation, a high-riding kidney and large body girth can further compound the difficulty of successful PCN, and knowledge of and experience with the various instruments and their technical use becomes imperative.

The use of short equipment is helpful. Long (20 cm) and thin (21- to 22-gauge) needles are difficult to position since they are easily deflected by minimal resistance, with resulting malposition of the needle tip. Intrarenal entry is often prolonged because their inherent flexibility requires nearly complete withdrawal for any realignment of the track. On the other hand they cannot torque the perirenal tissue planes as can heavier 18-gauge needles and the trocar systems. Straight tracks from the skin to the collecting system are necessary to prevent guide wire buckling in the retroperitoneum.

In the near normal sized collecting system, the smaller the instrument the greater the success. With larger coaxial/sheathed needles and trocar–cannula units the tip of the needle, sheath, or cannula often lies partially in and partially out of the

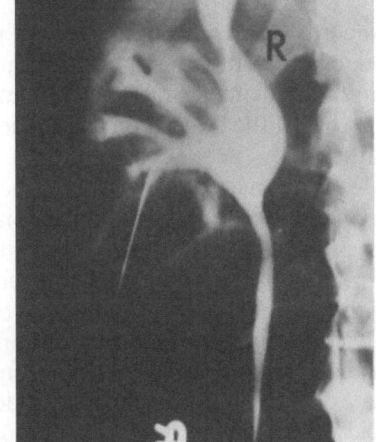

Fig. 1.13. Unobstructed normal sized collecting system containing pelvic calculus. Two-step Seldinger puncture method with lower pole calyceal entry angulated upward under the 12th rib (*R*). The 0.038-in. torque guide wire has been manipulated down the ureter for stability during the subsequent tract dilation and placement of a 24-F nephrostomy tube.

calyx. Contrast injection or guide wire or catheter passage out of the tip of these units will often be or result in a pericalyceal or sinus position. In mildly dilated or larger collecting systems this is not a problem since their tips are proportionately smaller than the calyx and contrast, guide wire, or catheter will easily advance down the infundibulum and into the pelvis.

In the moderately hydronephrotic kidney all the instruments for percutaneous nephrostomy are easily utilized in either the one- or the two-step puncture approach. However, in the minimally dilated obstructed system and the undilated nonobstructed collecting system their successful application is progressively more difficult; for the inexperienced or the occasional user each has its particular nuances, and the more complex the manipulative maneuvers required the greater is the probability of failure. It may be that the simplest method of a plain 18-gauge needle with small J-tipped 0.035–0.038 in. guide wire provides the most dependable access instrument; the needle's short tip and nondeflecting shaft, the absence of a sheath or coaxial needle, and the acceptance of a firm nonperforating guide wire make this an unsophisticated but reliable technique.

As previously indicated, for simple nephrostomy drainage the position of the tube tip is relatively unimportant but adequate intrarenal catheter length is necessary (Fig. 1.12). In Seldinger-type nephrostomy and any other procedure (such as percutaneous stone removal) where a guide wire is used, the wire guide should be advanced as soon as possible to a stable position. This is accomplished by advancing the guide wire and catheter through the ureteropelvic junction (UPJ) and down the midureter (Fig. 1.13). In this position they are well tolerated, do not dislodge, and are stable for subsequent dilatation of the nephrostomy tract or ureteral stenosis dilatation and stenting. While a more cephalad entry site into the kidney (upper pole, middle calyx) is helpful to negotiate the UPJ, the 12th rib usually dictates entry into the lower pole; with use of a memory retentive torque guide wire and/or preformed curved angiographic catheter one should be able to advance into the ureter in nearly all cases. Situations where it may not be possible to negotiate the ureter are the presence of staghorn stones, impacted UPJ or upper ureteral stones, high take-off congenital UPJ obstruction, and operative stenosis or extreme tortuosity of the proximal ureter.

Catheters and Anchorage

Nephrostomy catheters come in a great variety of materials, configurations, and flexibility. Additionally, wall thickness greatly affects outer diameter (French size) and inner diameter or effective lumen size. As a result, the French size of a tube may have little bearing on its functional capability, as in the situation of Foley-type catheters.

Catheter material also affects the pliability of the tubes. Pure silicone catheters are the softest (Fig. 1.14) but can only be introduced through an outer sheath or in an established mature tract over a guide wire. Stiffer catheters are easily introduced through a sheath or over a guide wire in a fresh tract but have a tendency to kink, with resulting partial or complete obstruction.

Crystal aggregation (encrustation) on tubing occurs to varying degrees in both acid and alkaline urine. Inherent inner surfaces of catheters are smooth except for Latex and PVC (polyvinyl-chloride), as determined by electron microscopy. In acid urine, heavy crystallization occurs on Latex, while PVC, polyurethane, and

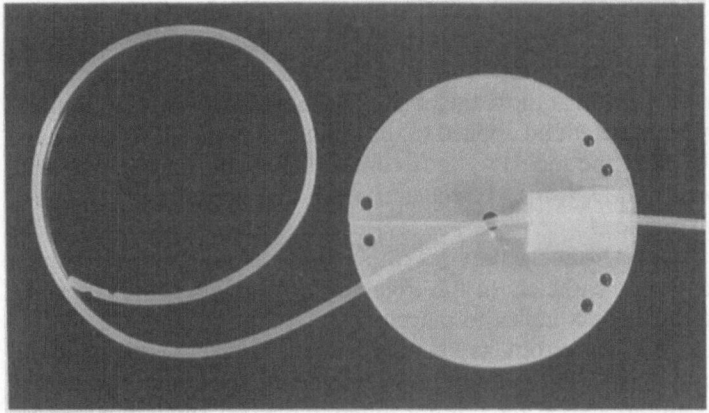

Fig. 1.14. Pure silicone catheters are extremely pliable, nonabrasive to the urothelium, and most resistant to encrustation. Modified silcone disc (Cystocath) for catheter fixation to the skin requires sutures for definitive anchorage.

polyethylene show moderate crystal deposits and silicone the least. In alkaline urine, crystallization is heavy with Latex, PVC, polyethylene, and polypropylene and least with Teflon (polytetrafluoroethylene), polyurethane, and silicone. Silicone and polyurethane appear to be the most suitable and Latex and PVC the least desirable materials for nephrostomy catheter drainage [13].

Straight catheters require skin fixation to prevent accidental dislodgement. Pigtail and Malecot catheters have some retentive capabilities but also require fixation. It appears that the Cope loop catheter [27] provides the best intrarenal retention of the small caliber catheters; in this tube, a distal loop is formed within the renal pelvis by pulling on an anchoring suture exiting the proximal end of the tube. However, release of the loop may be a problem, requiring its removal through an outer Teflon sheath [28].

There are several approaches to fixing the catheter to the skin. Usually, the tube is sutured to the skin. Alternatively, the skin can be protected by swabbing the area with tincture of benzoin and tape or a disc applied and sutured in place. In the former a strip of adhesive tape is wrapped around the catheter, the tape sutured, and slit gauze squares inserted between the catheter and skin to prevent kinking; Elastoplast can then be used for a covering. Plastic discs of the Molnar, Cystocath

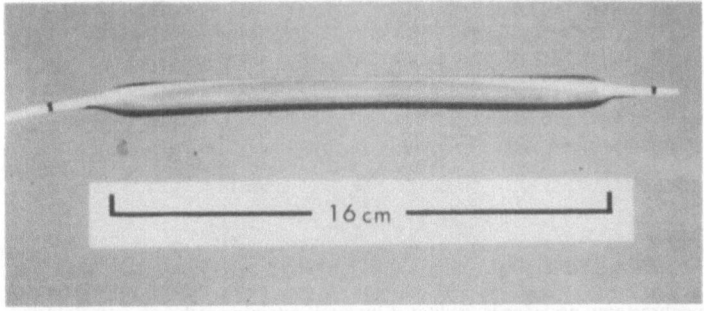

Fig. 1.15. Medi-Tech balloons (24, 30, 36 F) of sufficient length to rapidly dilate the entire nephrostomy tract with one inflation of 5 min duration.

(Fig. 1.14), and Stomadhesive types are also most satisfactory for temporary fixation [16, 98]. Most discs require skin sutures for definitive anchorage. Synthetic suture material is preferable to silk as it causes less irritation. Betadine ointment is useful when applied to the skin at the catheter site. A Stomadhesive wafer (Squibb) can be slipped over the catheter and applied to the molnar disc and skin. The wafer responds to the body heat and molds to body contours. Patients may shower and wash with the wafer in place; it may be replaced every 2–3 weeks by the patient following proper instructions.

Long-term nephrostomy drainage requires careful skin care. This is more easily facilitated by self-retaining catheters of the Foley or U-tube types; the latter are more reliable but technically complex to place [77, 109]. Silicone Foley catheters [Dow-Corning Corp., Medical Products Plant, Hemlock, Michigan] are available which have reliable integrity. The balloon must be carefully positioned so that it does not obstruct draining calyces, and it is not suited to the very small renal pelvis. Current techniques allow it to be placed with a fresh nephrostomy tract. Following rapid tract dilatation with a dedicated Gruntzig balloon (Fig. 1.15) and insertion of an 18-F sheathed dilator unit [Cook, Inc. (Pfister), PO Box 489, Bloomington, Indiana] over an 0.038-in. guide wire, a 14–16 F Foley catheter with its tip removed is advanced through the sheath, the balloon inflated, and the sheath torn away (Fig. 1.16). This method circumvents the older difficult passage of a Foley balloon catheter with a rod introducer for extended nephrostomy drainage.

Ideally, if the ureter is negotiable, an internal stent catheter can be placed but this requires cystoscopic replacement every 2–3 months. An externalized stent still requires skin care but is easily exchanged and does not need the drainage bag of the nephrostomy catheter.

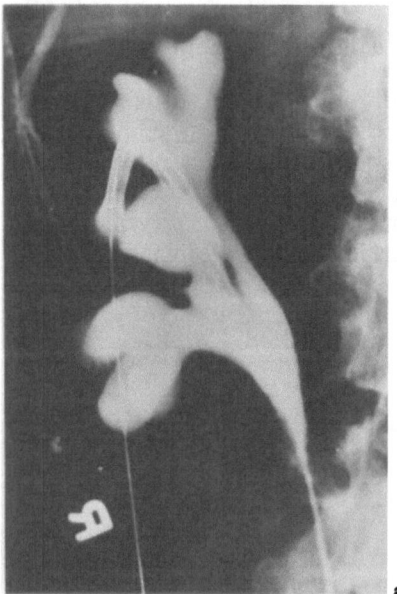 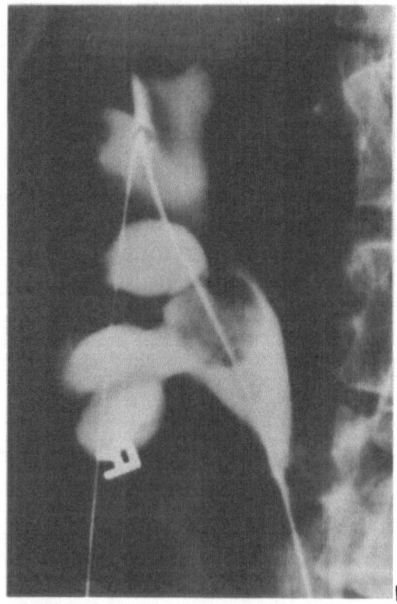

a   b

Fig. 1.16a,b. Extended nephrostomy drainage is facilitated by a self-retaining catheter. **a** 18-F dilator with outer tear-away sheath over an 0.038-in. guide wire in the ureter. The soft Foley catheter is passed through the sheath and **b** inflated in the renal pelvis.

Results and Complications

With some experience, PCN should be successful in 95%–98% of adult [60, 67, 98, 132] and pediatric [41, 102, 133] cases. A lower initial success rate of 80%–90% will occur in nondilated collecting systems or when the target calyx or entire pyelocalyceal system is filled with calculus. In such situations the collecting system must be distended by a separate antegrade needle, a retrograde ureteral catheter, or intravenous contrast combined with a ureteral compression device.

Minor complications such as postnephrostomy transient bleeding or local transient extravasation (Fig. 1.17) are to be expected [67, 98, 102, 129, 132]. Similarly, inadvertent catheter dislodgement will occasionally occur from a variety of causes; in fresh PCN tracts a new puncture into the parenchyma is usually required since the tract closes rapidly in the absence of the tube. Nephrostomy tracts require a longer time to mature when silicone catheters are utilized compared with other materials [98]. Several approaches to probing the tract are available after initially opacifying the tract with dilute contrast media to reduce tissue irritation [58, 59, 84]. The steerable catheter may be used, as can 5–7 F pediatric nasogastric feeding tubing. Such small catheters may be used in conjunction with an 0.035–0.038 guide wire of floppy-tip or tight J configuration. A straight dilator may also be tried, but in general the stiffer instruments result in a false tract.

Temporary catheter obstruction from fresh clots, debris, or pus may require gentle irrigation to restore patency to the nephrostomy tube. If irrigation fails, insertion of a stiff guide wire will usually clear the tube. If this also fails, the end of the catheter should be cut off and an outer closely fitting sheath advanced over the occluded catheter and into the kidney [11, 28, 106]. The old catheter is replaced with a new one and following a nephrostogram to check its position, the sheath is removed (Fig. 1.18).

Significant complications from PCN are relatively infrequent and substantially less than from surgical nephrostomy; in the latter the mortality ranges from 6%–8%, while in the presence of septicemia it approaches 12% [56]. Complications requiring specific therapy or prolonged hospitalization occur in 3%–5% of PCNs

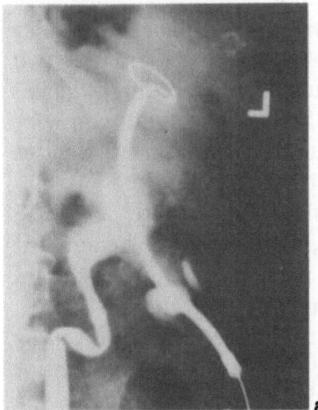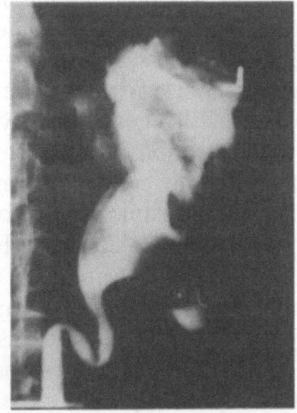

Fig. 1.17. a Stiff dilator and guide wire inadvertently advanced through the upper renal pole with **b** local transient extravasation of no subsequent consequence in a sterile collecting system.

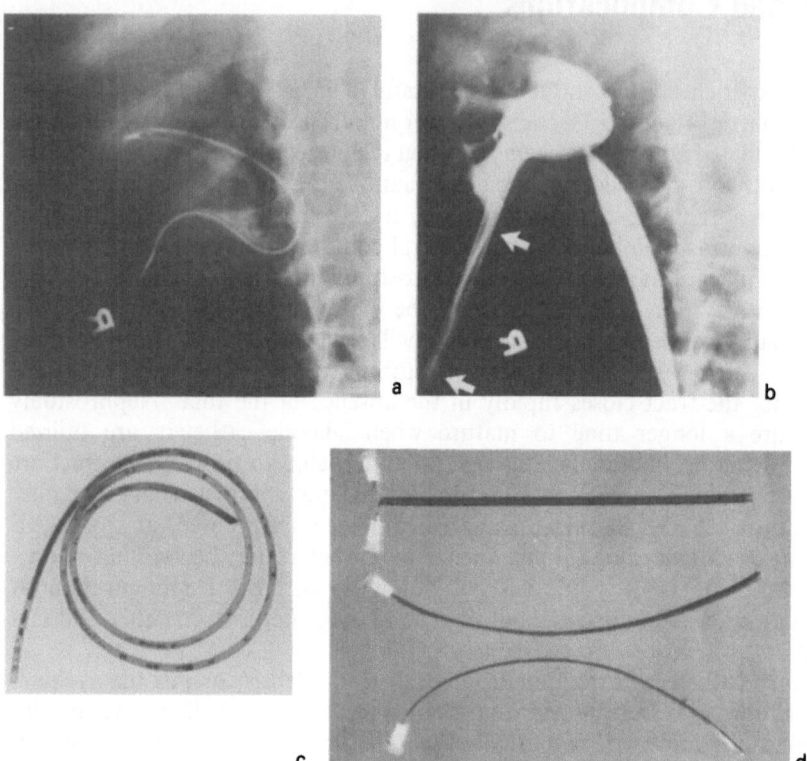

Fig. 1.18a–d. Replacement of obstructed 8-F nephrostomy catheter. **a** Partial filling of the PCN tube which also resisted passage of a wire guide. **b** Sheath advanced into the kidney over the top of the old catheter and a new tube inserted. **c** Inspissated uric acid crystals occluding old catheter; patient was receiving radiation therapy for bladder cancer. **d** 10-F sheath when intact (*top*) and after separation by pulling away on the handles.

compared with 25% of surgical nephrostomies [61]. More serious complications of PCN such as pneumothorax [110, 132] and urinoma [108, 129] formation are avoidable while many of those involving bleeding are not.

The most frequent severe complication is hemorrhage; significant vascular trauma may occur in 1%–2% of patients. In a review of 1207 PCNs there were two deaths (0.2%) [132]. Of the four reported deaths all resulted from bleeding, which is more pronounced in the patient with a coagulopathy. Significant bleeding may be immediate, delayed with the formation of pseudoaneurysms and arteriovenous fistulas, or late when the nephrostomy catheter is removed or exchanged [30, 50].

Early arterial injury is manifested clinically by continued hematuria after 3–5 days and by the formation of new clots. Alternatively, if a drop in the hematocrit occurs, out of proportion to the observed hematuria, a perirenal hematoma should be suspected and investigated by ultrasound or computed tomography [64].

Although psuedoaneurysms and arteriovenous fistulas have been reported as complications of renal biopsy [38], they generally close spontaneously and are not commonly seen in PCN; this is probably due to the displacement of renal tissue during PCN rather than to the removal of a tissue core as occurs with standard renal biopsy. If, however, bleeding persists or spontaneously recurs after PCN, a renal arteriogram is indicated for diagnostic and therapeutic reasons since selective embolic occlusion of the involved segmental renal artery can be performed while preserving most of the remaining renal parenchyma [30, 50, 120].

About 15% of patients undergoing PCN will have pyonephrosis; 1%–28% of them may have some exacerbation of their illness from tube placement; shaking chills, increased temperature, and transient hypotension are not infrequent, while septic shock can occur in 7% of cases [138]. Elevation of intrarenal pressure from contrast injection during PCN increases the risk of bacteremia and/or fungemia and should be avoided. Perinephric abscess may occur concomitantly with this disease and should be drained simultaneously with another percutaneous catheter. The development of perinephric abscess as a complication of PCN should only result in a previously infected patient; computed tomography or sonography is a useful adjunct for evaluating the extrarenal tissues in these patients. Blood pressure monitoring with intravenous antibiotic administration should be done before, during, and following percutaneous catheter placement for pyonephrosis and perinephric abscess management.

Several types of foreign bodies within the upper urinary tract may occur following percutaneous, cystoscopic, or operative procedures. Migrated stents and broken guide wires or catheter tips may be retrieved percutaneously with a variety of techniques after an initial PCN. A steerable catheter with a grasping instrument (basket, forceps, deflectable guide wire) is a safe and effective approach to their removal [60, 82, 101, 140].

References

1. Alken P, Hutschenreiter G, Gunther R, Marberger M (1981) Percutaneous stone manipulation. J Urol 125:463–466
2. Alken P, Hutschenreiter G, Gunther R (1982) Percutaneous kidney stone removal. Eur Urol 8:304–311
3. Almgard LE, Fernstrom I (1974) Percutaneous nephropyelostomy. Acta Radiol [Diagn] (Stockh) 15:288–294
4. Babcock JR, Skolnik A. Cook WA (1979) Ultrasound-guided percutaneous nephrostomy in the pediatric patient. J Urol 121:327–329
5. Banner MP, Pollack HM (1982) Percutaneous extraction of renal and ureteral calculi. Radiology 144:753–758
6. Banner MP, Pollack HM, Ring EJ, Wein AJ (1983) Catheter dilatation of benign ureteral strictures. Radiology 147:427–433
7. Barbaric ZL, Thomson KR (1978) Percutaneous nephropyelostomy in the management of obstructed renal transplants. Radiology 126:639–642
8. Barbaric ZL, Wood BP (1977) Emergency percutaneous nephropyelostomy: experience with 34 patients and review of the literature. AJR 128:453–458
9. Barbaric ZL, Davis RS, Frank IN et al. (1976) Percutaneous nephropyelostomy in the management of acute pyohydronephrosis. Radiology 118:567–573
10. Barbaric ZL, Gothlin JH, Davies RS (1977) Transluminal dilatation and stent placement in obstructed ureters in dogs through the use of percutaneous nephropyelostomy. Invest Radiol 12:534–536
11. Baron RL, McClennan BL (1981) Replacing the occluded percutaneous nephrostomy catheter. Radiology 141:824
12. Baron RL, Lee JKT, McClennan BL, Melson GL (1981) Percutaneous nephrostomy using real-time sonographic guidance. AJR 136:1018–1019
13. Bastian HP, Weissbach, Lunow R, Gebhardt M (1979) An experimental study of crystal aggregation on catheters of various materials. Urol Res 7:32 (abstr)

14. Bettmann MÁ, Murray PD, Perlmutt LM, Whitmore WF III, Richie JP (1983) Ureteroileal anastomotic leaks: percutaneous treatment. Radiology 148:95–100
15. Bigongiari LR (1981) The Seldinger approach to percutaneous nephrostomy and ureteral stent placement. Urol Radiol 2:141–145
16. Bigongiari LR, Dixon GD (1979) Use of the Molnar disk to secure an angiographic catheter for a percutaneous nephrostomy. Radiology 180:804
17. Bigongiari LR, Lee KR, Moffat RE et al. (1979) Percutaneous ureteral stent placement for stricture management and internal urinary drainage. AJR 133:865–868
18. Burchardt P (1982) The flexible panendoscope. J Urol 127:479–481
19. Burnett LL, Correa RJ, Bush WH (1976) A new method for percutaneous nephrostomy. Radiology 120:557–561
20. Bush WH, Crane RE, Brannen GE (1984) Steerable loop snare for percutaneous retrieval of renal calix calculi. AJR 142:367–368
21. Castaneda-Zuniga WR, Amplatz K (1982) Percutaneous nephrostomy with the Stamey catheter: a new introducing technique. Urol Clin North Am 9:65–67
22. Castaneda-Zuniga WR, Smith A, Tadavarthy SM et al. (1981) A flexible trocar for percutaneous nephrostomy. AJR 136:434
23. Castaneda-Zuniga WR, Miller RP, Amplatz K (1982) Percutaneous removal of kidney stones. Urol Clin North Am 9:113–119
24. Castaneda-Zuniga WR, Clayman R, Smith A et al. (1982) Nephrostolithotomy: percutaneous techniques for urinary calculus removal. AJR 139:721–726
25. Clayman RV, Miller RP, Reinke DB, Lange PH (1982) Nephroscopy: advances and adjuncts. Urol Clin North Am 9(1):51–60
26. Coleman BG, Arger PH, Mulhern CB Jr, Pollack HM, Banner MP (1981) Pyonephrosis: sonography in the diagnosis and management. AJR 137:939–943
27. Cope C (1980) Improved anchoring of nephrostomy catheters: loop technique. AJR 135:402–403
28. Cope C (1982) Replacement of obstructed loop and pigtail nephrostomy and biliary drains. AJR 139:1022
29. Cope C (1982) Conversion from small (0.018 inch) to large (0.038 inch) guide wires in percutaneous drainage procedures. AJR 138:170–171
30. Cope C, Zeit RM (1982) Pseudoaneurysms after nephrostomy. AJR 139:255–261
31. Dixon GD, Moore JD, Stockton R (1982) Successful dilatation of ureteroilial anastomotic stenosis using Gruntzig catheter. Urology 19:555–558
32. Dretler SP, Pfister RC (1983) Percutaneous dissolution of renal calculi. Ann Rev Med 34:359–366
33. Dretler SP, Pfister RC (1984) Primary dissolution therapy of struvite calculi. J Urol
34. Dretler SP, Pfister RC, Newhouse JH (1979) Renal-stone dissolution via percutaneous nephrostomy. N Engl J Med 300:341–343
35. Dretler SP, Pfister RC, Newhouse JH, Prien EL Jr (1984) Percutaneous dissolution of cystine calculi. J Urol 131:216–219
36. Druy EM, Gharib M, Finder CA (1983). Percutaneous nephroureteral drainage and stenting for postsurgical ureteral leaks. AJR 141: 389–394
37. Dubuisson RL, Eichelberger RP, Jones TB (1983) A simple modification of real-time sector sonography to monitor percutaneous nephrostomy. Radiology 146:232
38. Ekelund L (1982) Arteriovenous fistulae secondary to renal biopsy, an experimental study in the rabbit. Acta Radiol [Diagn] (Stockh) 10:255–261
39. Ekelund L, Karp W, Klefsgard O (1980) Percutaneous nephrostomy—indicational and technical considerations. Urol Radiol 1:227–231
40. Elyaderani MK, Dorn JS, Gabriele OF (1979) Percutaneous nephrostomy utilizing a pigtail catheter: a new technique. Radiology 132:750
41. Elyaderani MK, Kalinowski D, Gabriele OF (1981) Percutaneous nephrostomy by pigtail catheter in children. South Med J 74:421–423
42. Elyaderani MK, Belis JA, Kandzari SJ, Gabriele OF (1982) Facilitation of difficult percutaneous ureteral stent insertion. J Urol 128:1173–1176
43. Fernstrom I, Andersson L (1977) Percutaneous puncture nephrostomy. In: Diagnostic Radiology, vol 5/1 (Suppl). Springer, Berlin Heidelberg New York
44. Fernstrom I, Johansson B (1976) Percutaneous pyelolithotomy. A new extraction technique. Scand J Urol Nephrol 10:257–259
45. Fernstrom I, Johansson B (1982) Percutaneous extraction of renal calculi. In: Baert AL et al. (eds) Frontiers in European radiology, vol 1. Springer, Berlin Heidelberg New York
46. Finney RP (1982) Double-J and diversion stents. Urol Clin North Am 9(1):89–94
47. Fisher MF, Haaga JR, Persky L et al. (1982) Renal stone extraction through a percutaneous nephrostomy in a renal transplant patient. Radiology 144:95–96

48. Fowler JE Jr, Meares EM Jr, Goldin AR (1975) Percutaneous nephrostomy: techniques, indications, and results. Urology 6:428–434
49. Fowler JE Jr, Raife MJ, Sennott R (1980) A method for placement of a ureteral stent following supravesical intestinal diversion. J Urol 124:547–549
50. Gavant ML, Gold RE, Church JC (1982) Delayed rupture of renal pseudoaneurysm: complication of percutaneous nephrostomy. AJR 138:948–949
51. Gerber WL (1982) Use of the Argyle catheter for nephrostomy drainage. Urol Clin North Am 9:61–63
52. Gerber WL, Brown RC, Culp DA (1981) Percutaneous nephrostomy with immediate dilation. J Urol 125:169–171
53. Glanz S, Gordon DH, Butt K, Rubin B, Hong J, Sclafani SJA (1983) Percutaneous transrenal balloon dilatation of the ureter. Radiology 149:101–104
54. Glass NR, Crummy AB, Fisher R et al. (1982) Management of ureteral obstruction after transplantation by percutaneous antegrade pyelography and pyeloureterostomy. Urology 20:15–19
55. Goldin AR (1977) Percutaneous ureteral splinting. Urology 10:165–168
56. Gonzalez-Serva L, Weinerth JL, Glenn JF (1977) Minimal mortality of renal surgery. Urology 9:253–255
57. Goodwin WE, Casey WC, Woolf W (1955) Percutaneous trocar (needle) nephrostomy in hydronephrosis. JAMA 157:891–894
58. Gordon RL, Oleaga JA, Ring EJ et al. (1980) Replacing the "fallen out" catheter. Radiology 134:537
59. Greenfield AJ (1982) Percutaneous biliary drainage. In: Athanasoulis CA, Pfister RC, Greene RE, Roberson GH (eds) Interventional radiology. WB Saunders, Philadelphia, pp 535–556
60. Gunther R, Alken P (1982) Percutaneous nephropyelostomy and endourological manipulations. In: Baert AL et al. (eds) Frontiers in European radiology, vol 1. Springer, Berlin Heidelberg New York, pp 25–50
61. Gunther R, Alken P, Altwein JE (1979) Percutaneous nephropyelostomy using a fine-needle puncture set. Radiology 132:228–230
62. Gunther R, Marberger M, Klose K (1979) Transrenal ureteral embolization. Radiology 132:317–319
63. Haaga JR, Zelch MG, Alfidi RJ et al. (1977) CT-guided antegrade pyelography and percutaneous nephrostomy. AJR 128:621–624
64. Harris RD, Walter PC (1984) Renal arterial-injury associated with percutaneous nephrostomy. Urology 23:215–217
65. Harris RD, McCullough DL, Talner LB (1976) Percutaneous nephrostomy. J Urol 115:628–631
66. Heckemann R, Meyer-Schwickerath M, Hezel J, Eickenberg HU (1981) Percutaneous nephropyelostomy under continuous real-time ultrasound guidance. Urol Radiol 3:171–175
67. Ho PC, Talner LB, Parsons CL, Schmidt JD (1980) Percutaneous nephrostomy: experience in 107 kidneys. Urology 16:532–535
68. Holden S, McPhee M, Grabstald H: The rationale of urinary diversion in cancer patients. J Urol 121:19–21
69. Kadir S, White RI Jr, Engel R (1982) Balloon dilatation of a ureteropelvic junction obstruction. Radiology 143:263–264
70. Kaplan JO, Winslow OP Jr, Sneider SE, Pryor TH, Caplan LH, Messinger NH (1982) Dilatation of a surgically ligated ureter through a percutaneous nephrostomy. AJR 139:188–189
71. Kaufman JJ, Ehrlich RM (1982) Prophylactic and therapeutic use of abdominal drains and percutaneous nephrostomies and stents for treatment of precarious ureteroileal anastomosis. Urology 20:118–120
72. Lang EK (1981) Diagnosis and management of ureteral fistulas by percutaneous nephrostomy and antegrade stent catheter. Radiology 138:311–317
73. Lang EK, Price ET (1983) Redefinitions of indications for percutaneous nephrostomy. Radiology 147:419–426
74. Lang EK, Alexander R, Barnett T, Palomar J, Hamway S (1978) Brush biopsy of pyelocalyceal lesions via a percutaneous translumbar approach. Radiology 129:623–627
75. Lang EK, Lanasa JA, Garrett J et al. (1979) The management of urinary fistulas and strictures with percutaneous ureteral stent catheters. J Urol 122:736–740
76. Levine RS, Pollack HM, Banner MP (1982) Transient ureteral obstruction after ureteral stenting. AJR 138:323–327
77. Levy JM, Potter WM, Stegman CJ (1979) A new catheter system for permanent percutaneous nephrostomy. J Urol 122:442–443

78. Link D, Leff RG, Hildel J, Drago JR (1979) The use of percutaneous nephrostomy in 42 patients. J Urol 122:9–10 ·
79. Mardis HK, Kroeger RM, Hepperlen TW et al. (1982) Polyethylene double-pigtail ureteral stents. Urol Clin North Am 9:95–101
80. Martin EC, Frankuchen EI, Casarella WJ (1982) Percutaneous dilatation of ureteroenteric strictures of occlusions in ileal conduits. Urol Radiol 4:19–21
81. Mazer MJ, LeVeen RF, Call JE, Wolf G, Baltaxe HA (1979) Permanent percutaneous antegrade ureteral stent placement without transurethral assistance. Urology 14(4):413–419
82. Meranze SG, Pollack HM, Banner MP (1982) The use of grasping forceps in the upper urinary tract: technique and radiologic implications. Radiology 144:171–173
83. Miller RP, Reinke DB, Clayman RV, Lange PH (1982) Percutaneous approach to the ureter. Urol Clin North Am 9:31–40
84. Miller RP, Reinke DB, Clayman RV, Lange PH (1982) Reestablishment of a nephrostomy tract. Urol Clin North Am 9:75–78
85. Mitty HA, Gribetz ME (1982) The status of interventional uroradiology. J Urol 127:2–9
86. Mitty HA, Train JS, Dan SJ (1983) Antegrade ureteral stenting in the management of fistulas, strictures and calculi. Radiology 149:433–438
87. Mulvaney WP (1960) The clinical use of Renacidin in urinary calcifications. J Urol 84:206–212
88. Newhouse JH, Pfister RC (1981) Percutaneous catheterization of the kidney and perinephric space: trocar technique. Urol Radiol 2:157–164
89. Newhouse JH, Pfister RC (1981) Therapy for renal calculi via percutaneous nephrostomy: dissolution and extraction. Urol Radiol 2: 165–170
90. Oosterlinck W, DeSy WA (1983) A percutaneous nephrostomy set. J Urol 129:466–467
91. Oppenheimer RO, Himnam F Jr (1956) The effect of urinary flow upon ureteral regeneration in the absence of splint. Surg Gynecol Obstet 416–422
92. Ortlip SA, Fraley EE (1982) Indications for palliative urinary diversion in patients with cancer. Urol Clin North Am 9:79–84
93. Pedersen JF (1974) Percutaneous nephrostomy guided by ultrasound. J Urol 112:157–159
94. Pedersen JF, Cowan DF, Kristensen JK, Holm HH, Hancke S, Jensen F (1976) Ultrasonically-guided percutaneous nephrostomy. Radiology 119:429–431
95. Perinetti E, Catalona WJ, Manley CB et al. (1978) Percutaneous nephrostomy: indications, complications and clinical usefulness. J Urol 120:156–158
96. Pfister RC (1982) The role of percutaneous nephrostomy. In: O'Reilly PH, Gosling JA (eds) Idiopathic hydronephrosis. Springer, New York, pp 102–114
97. Pfister RC, Newhouse JH (1979) Interventional percutaneous pyeloureteral techniques. II. Percutaneous nephrostomy and other procedures. Radiol Clin North Am 17:351–363
98. Pfister RC, Newhouse JH (1982) Percutaneous nephrostomy: types of catheters for drainage, occlusion, and dilatation, and fiber-optics for endoscopy. In: Athanasoulis CA, Pfister RC, Greene RE, Roberson GH (eds) Interventional radiology. WB Saunders, Philadelphia, pp 467–496
99. Pfister RC, Yoder IC, Newhouse JH (1981) Percutaneous uroradiologic procedures. Semin Roentgenol 16:135–151
100. Pfister RC, Yoder IC, Newhouse JH (1983) A trocar–cannula unit for percutaneous procedures. Br J Urol (Suppl) 64–68
101. Pfister RC, Johnson RD, Pollack HM, Banner MP et al. (1983) Removal of pyeloureteral foreign bodies using a percutaneous approach. Br J Urol (Suppl) 75–78
102. Pfister RC, Newhouse JH, Yoder IC, Hendren WH et al. (1983) Complications of pediatric percutaneous renal procedures: incidence and observations. Urol Clin North Am 10:563–571
103. Pingoud EG, Bagley DH, Zeman RK, Glancy KE, Pais OS (1980) Percutaneous antegrade bilateral ureteral dilatation and stent placement for internal drainage. Radiology 134:780
104. Pode D, Shapiro A, Gordon R, Lebesart P (1982) Percutaneous nephrostomy for assessment of functional recovery of obstructed kidneys. Urology 19:482–485
105. Pollack HM, Banner MP (1981) Percutaneous nephrostomy and related pyeloureteral manipulative techniques. Urol Radiol 2:147–154
106. Pollack HM, Banner MP (1982) Replacing blocked or dislodged percutaneous nephrostomy and ureteral stent catheters. Radiology 145:203–205
107. Pollack HM, Banner MP (1982) Work in progress: percutaneous fiber-optic endoscopy of the upper urinary tract. Radiology 145:651–654
108. Portela LA, Patel SK, Callahan DH (1979) Pararenal pseudocyst (urinoma) as complication of percutaneous nephrostomy. Urology 13:570–571
109. Reddy P, Smith AD (1982) Circle tube nephrostomy and nephroureterostomy. Urol Clin North Am 9:69–73

110. Redman JF, Arnold WC, Smith PL, Seibert JJ (1982) Hypertension and urino-thorax following an attempted percutaneous nephrostomy. J Urol 128:1307–1308
111. Reimer DE, Oswalt C Jr (1981) Iatrogenic ureteral obstruction treated with balloon dilation. J Urol 126:689–690
112. Rosen RJ, McLean GK, Freiman DB et al. (1980) Obstructed ureteroileal conduits: antegrade catheter drainage. AJR 135:1201–1204
113. Rusnak B, Castaneda-Zuniga WR, Kotula F et al. (1982) An improved dilator system for percutaneous nephrostomies. Radiology 144:174
114. Sadlowski RW, Finney RP, Branch WT et al. (1979) New technique for percutaneous nephrostomy under ultrasound guidance. J Urol 121:559–561
115. Salazar JE, Johnson JB, Scott R, Pinstein M (1983) A simplified method for placement of internal ureteral stents. AJR 140:611–612
116. Saxton HM (1981) Percutaneous nephrostomy—technique. Urol Radiol 2:131–139
117. Schilling A, Goettinger H, Marx FJ et al. (1981) A new technique for percutaneous nephropyelostomy. J Urol 125:475–476
118. Segal AJ, Spitzer RM (1981) Simplified procedure for percutaneous nephrostomy. AJR 137:1078–1079
119. Segura JW, Patterson DE, LeRoy AJ et al. (1983) Percutaneous lithotripsy. J Urol 130:1051–1054
120. Selman SH, Zelch JV, Kursh ED (1979) Successful treatment of a renal arteriovenous fistula with a Fogarty catheter. J Urol 122:387–388
121. Sharer W, Grayhack JT, Graham J (1978) Palliative urinary diversion for malignant ureteral obstruction. J Urol 120:162–164
122. Sheldon CA, Smith AD (1982) Chemolysis of calculi. Urol Clin North Am 9:121–130
123. Smith AD, Lange PH, Reinke DB, Miller RP (1978) Extraction of ureteral calculi from patients with ileal loops: a new technique. J Urol 120:623–625
124. Smith AD, Lange PH, Miller RP, Reinke DB (1979) Dissolution of cystine calculi by irrigation with acetylcysteine through percutaneous nephrostomy. Urology 13:422–423
125. Smith AD, Reinke DB, Miller RP, Lange PH (1979) Percutaneous nephrostomy in the management of ureteral and renal calculi. Radiology 133:49–54
126. Smith AD, Castaneda-Zuniga WR, Tadavarthy SM, Amplatz K (1981) A modified Stamey catheter kit for long-term percutaneous nephrostomy drainage. Radiology 139:230–231
127. Spataro RF, Linke CA, Barbaric ZL (1978) The use of percutaneous nephrostomy and urinary alkalinization in the dissolution of obstructing uric acid stones. Radiology 129:629–632
128. Spataro RF, McLachlan MSF, Davis RS et al. (1981) Percutaneous antegrade extrusion of ureteral stones. Radiology 139:725–728
129. Stables DP (1982) Percutaneous nephrostomy: techniques, indications and results. Urol Clin North Am 9:15–29
130. Stables DP, Johnson ML (1979) Percutaneous nephrostomy: the role of ultrasound. Clin Diagn Ultrasound 2:73–86
131. Stables DP, Holt SA, Sheridan HM, Donohue RE (1975) Permanent nephrostomy via percutaneous puncture. J Urol 114:684–687
132. Stables DP, Ginsberg NJ, Johnson ML (1978) Percutaneous nephrostomy: a series and review of the literature. AJR 130:75–82
133. Stanley P, Bear JW, Reid BS (1983) Percutaneous nephrostomy in infants and children. AJR 141:473–477
134. Twomey BP, Wilkins RA (1983) Ureteric stone displacement using a new technique. Radiology 146:832
135. Weinstein BJ, Skolnick ML (1978) Ultrasonically guided antegrade pyelography. J Urol 120:323–327
136. Wickham JEA, Kellett MJ, Miller RA (1983) Elective percutaneous nephrolithotomy in 50 patients: an analysis of the technique, results and complications. J Urol 129:904–906
137. Witherington R, Shelor WC (1980) Treatment of postoperative ureteral stricture by catheter dilation: a forgotten procedure. Urology 16:592–595
138. Yoder IC, Pfister RC, Lindfors KK, Newhouse JH (1983) Pyonephrosis: imaging and intervention. AJR 141:735–740
139. Zegel HG, Pollack HM, Banner MP et al. (1981) Percutaneous nephrostomy: comparison of sonographic and fluoroscopic guidance. AJR 137:925–927
140. Zegel HG, Teplick SK, Khanna OP (1981) Removal of a dislodged ureteral stent through a percutaneous nephrostomy. AJR 137:629–630

Chapter 2

Obstruction and Percutaneous Ureteral Urodynamics: The Whitaker Test

Richard C. Pfister

Introduction

Considerable knowledge has been acquired in recent years, experimentally and in man, toward the further understanding of the urodynamics of the upper urinary tract in the normal and altered or diseased state [1–63]. This information is crucial in determining the optimal type of management (surgical or medical) to preserve and/or improve function of the hydronephrotic kidney.

Dilatation of the nonrefluxing upper urinary tract may exist in the presence or absence of obstruction [1, 4, 6, 9, 12–15, 18, 30, 35, 36, 48, 51]. Some enormously dilated systems are not obstructed while others with a minor degree of dilatation are. When renal function is compromised or deteriorating because of ureteral obstruction, prompt intervention is necessary; conversely, it is inappropriate to operate on a dilated upper urinary tract without objective evidence that it is obstructed and whether the bladder has any role in its pathogenesis.

Pathophysiology of Obstruction

Upper Tract

The degree to which the kidney is damaged by pyeloureteral obstruction depends upon the completeness and the duration of the obstruction (Fig. 2.1). Obstruction results in a reduction of renal blood flow with a subsequent relative ischemia; it may be absolute as well, since renin production may be stimulated during obstructive nephropathy.

Increases in intrapelvic pressure are transmitted to the renal tubules. Because filtration pressure between the capillary blood pressure and the intraluminal tubular pressure is reduced, there is a resultant fall in glomerular filtration rate. With time, the number of functional nephrons will progressively decrease also.

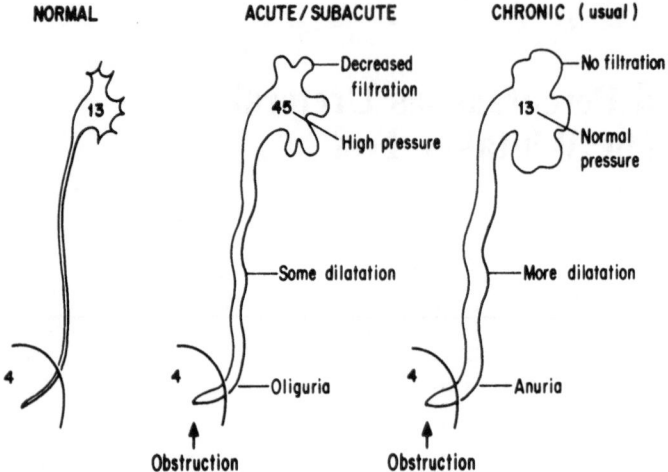

Fig. 2.1. Effect of resistance on renal pressures. With a similar bladder pressure of 4 cm water, the opening, resting, or baseline pressure in the normal kidney (13 cm H_2O) may be similar to that of chronic high grade obstruction (13 cm H_2O). High pressure encountered in acute obstruction (45 cm H_2O or more) results from continued renal function. (From Pfister et al. [40], with permission)

Since obstruction reduces glomerular filtration rate to a lesser degree than it affects blood flow, more filtrate reaches the distal nephron; the damaged renal tubules are unable to concentrate and acidify urine.

In acute obstruction both ureteral pressure and ureteral diameter increase. In acute severe obstruction, intrapelvic pressures in excess of 55 cm water are common in the healthy kidney. Initially, peristalsis may be more frequent as the tension on the ureteral wall stimulates the stretch initiation of the contraction waves. As obstruction continues toward a chronic state, a further increase in ureteral radius and volume occur and tortuosity ensues but peristaltic waves decrease in amplitude. As the ureter decompensates, peristalsis becomes ineffective as it does not coapt or approximate the ureteral walls [20, 36, 48].

The usual normal resting pressure in the pyeloureteral unit is 7 (± 5) cm water. With peristalsis, a bolus of urine is created ahead of each contraction wave. The amplitude of these waves produces pressures of 2 cm water in the renal pelvis, 14 cm water in the upper ureter, 19 cm water in the middle ureter, and 26 cm water in the distal ureter. Pressures reaching 45–70 cm water in the lower ureter have been recorded, depending on the method and size of the recording ureteral catheter used [36].

Lower Tract

When there is obstruction to the bladder outlet (bladder neck or urethra) intravesical pressure will rise. Initially, urine flow rates are maintained because the bladder wall detrusor muscle hypertrophies. With progression of obstruction, in time or severity, further hypertrophy can no longer occur and urine flow then decreases; increased residual volumes, bladder dilatation, and eventual retention may result.

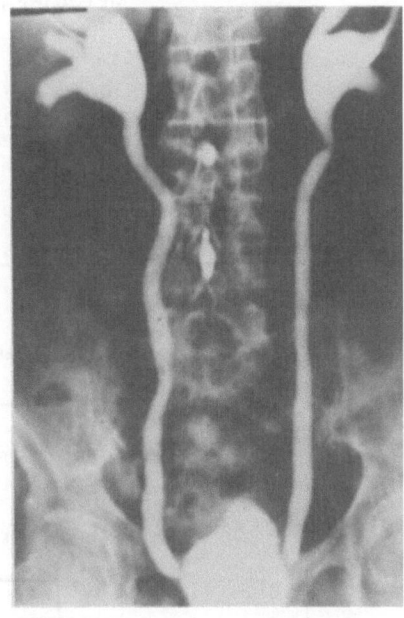

Fig. 2.2. Effect of high pressure bladder on the upper urinary track. Sixty-four year old woman with catheter drainage of neurogenic bladder and recurrent urinary infections with sepsis. Bilateral perfusion studies at 10 ml/min flow rate. Renal pressures of 16 and 35 cm H_2O with empty and full bladder pressures of 19 and 55 cm H_2O. Distended ureters and calyces in the absence of ureteral reflux or obstruction but elevated pressure when the bladder fills necessitate continual diversion to maintain low renal pressures.

In the normal situation, the mean pressure of the nearly empty bladder is 5 cm water. When full, its pressure rises another 7 cm water, while during voiding higher intravesical pressures normally occur.

With outlet obstruction, abnormally elevated intravesical pressures at rest (30 ± 10 cm water) are encountered and these may approach or exceed ureteral peristaltic bolus pressures. In this situation and in the hypertonic neurogenic bladder, the ureter(s) cannot effectively overcome bladder pressure and incomplete ureteral emptying occurs. Increased ureteral fluid volumes with elevated renal pelvic and ureteral pressures and pyeloureterectasis result [13, 36, 40, 41] (Fig. 2.2).

The effects of high absolute renal pelvic pressures are responsible for the progressive azotemia of obstructive nephropathy; other complications of large stagnant urine pools are infection, pyonephrosis, and struvite (triple phosphate) stone disease.

Sites and Causes of Obstruction

Obstruction may occur at any site distal to the glomerulus [36]. Diffuse intrarenal obstruction may result from tubular blockage by Tamm-Horsfall proteinuria and uric acid crystals. Focal intrarenal obstruction most frequently involves the infundibulum of a calyx, as from a calculus, tuberculosis, or tumor.

Diffuse dilatation of the intrarenal collecting system may result from a parapelvic mass (cyst or tumor) compressing the renal pelvis or any narrowing of the ureter at or below the ureteropelvic junction (UPJ).

Generalized ureteral dilatation or megaureter (Fig. 2.3) indicates an abnormality at or near the ureterovesical junction in the form of ureteral reflux or

MEGAURETER   STATES

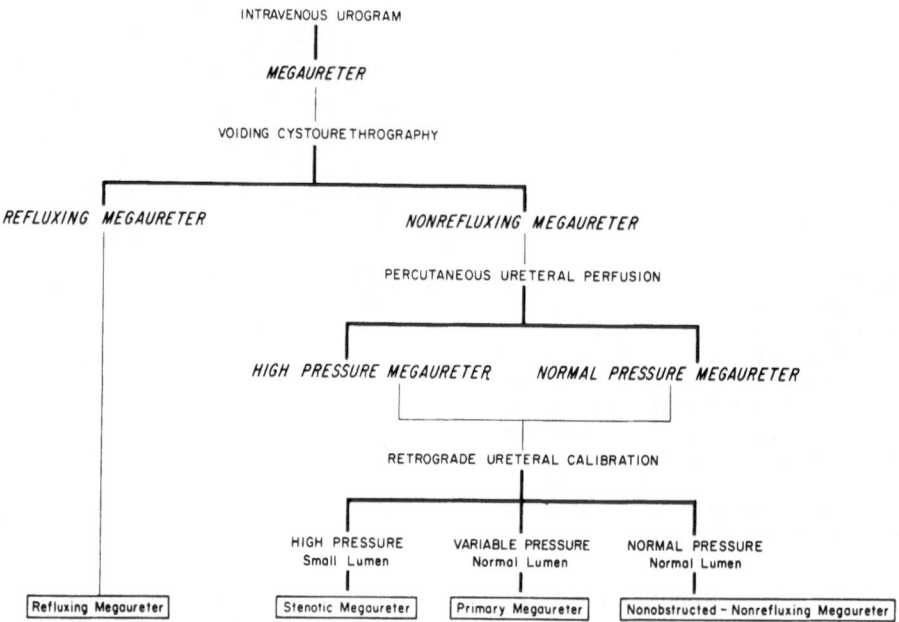

Fig. 2.3. Flow chart for evaluation and classification of various types of megaureters. (From Pfister and Hendren [35], with permission)

obstruction. Alternatively, it may imply a loss of ureteral tone, either ongoing (prune-belly syndrome, bacterial endotoxin paralysis) or remote (past chronic reflux or obstruction) which has been relieved [18, 35, 36] (Table 2.1).

Limited ureterectasis may involve the proximal, middle, or distal thirds of the ureter. Localized areas of lower ureteral dilatation can occur in the form of a ureterocele or the milder form of primary megaureter. Many lesions resulting in ureteral dilatation are associated with deviation in the course of the ureter either medially or laterally and at all levels of the ureter. Most deviated and obstructed ureters are the result of extrinsic processes.

Localized intraluminal defects reduce ureteral caliber from within and are the commonest cause of obstruction in the adult. Opaque ureteral stones head the list of easily diagnosed obstruction. Apparent nonopaque filling defects may be intraluminal or extraluminal in location but can be difficult to differentiate when small without computed tomography, owing to the narrow caliber of the tube being affected.

Intramural abnormalities of the ureteral wall may occur either developmentally or on an acquired basis. Since the peristaltic contraction wave propagates by excitation of action potentials from one muscle cell to another (nexus), any process which results in deficient and/or disorganized musculature or any excess of collagen will not transmit normal peristalsis. Proximally, in congenital ureteropelvic junction obstruction and distally, in primary megaureter (Fig. 2.4) a functionally obstructing defect is usually encountered without any anatomic narrowing demonstrable by catheterization or at histologic examination [4, 5, 24, 35, 48].

Table 2.1. Ureteral dilatation (from Pfister and Newhouse [36], with permission)

1. Distal third (only)
    Ureterocele
    Primary megaureter (grade 1)
    Vesicoureteral reflux (grade 1–2)
    Tumor (primary)

2. Middle third (only)
    Suprailiac ureteral spindle
    Tumor (primary)
    Congenitally defective musculature

3. Proximal third (only)
    Stone
    Postcaval ureter
    Retroperitoneal fibrosis
    Tumor (primary)
    Metastasis
    Retroperitoneal mass (abscess, tumor, hematoma, urinoma)
    Trauma (operative, penetrating)

4. Upper two-thirds
    Stone
    Retroperitoneal fibrosis
    Tumor (primary)
    Metastasis
    Pelvic/retroperitoneal mass (abscess, tumor, hematoma, urinoma)
    Pregnancy and postpartum (right side predominantly)
    Ovarian vein (±)
    Tuberculous stenosis
    Trauma (operative, penetrating)
    Retroiliac ureter

5. Entire ureter
    Stone
    Tumor infiltration:
        Cervix, prostate, bladder, etc.
    Vesicoureteral reflux (grade 3–4)
    Primary megaureter (grade 2–3)
    Ectopic obstructed ureter
    Tuberculous stenosis
    Bacterial infection (endotoxin paralysis)
    Orifice obstruction (bladder tumor, reimplantation)
    Pelvic mass (abscess, tumor, hematoma, urinoma, lymphocele, endometrioma)
    Outlet obstruction lower urinary tract
        Posterior urethral valves, BPH, urethral stricture
    Prune belly (triad syndrome)
    Past chronic obstruction/reflux now relieved

In the lower tract, neurogenic bladder and urethral sphincter spasm are common problems in all age groups. In children, posterior and anterior urethral valves may be severely obstructing. In the adult, traumatic and inflammatory urethral strictures and prostatic encroachment on the urethral lumen due to benign hypertrophy, carcinoma, or prostatitis are common. Deep pelvic masses due to lipomatosis or genital tract cysts (müllerian, seminal vesicle) may affect the bladder base or ureters.

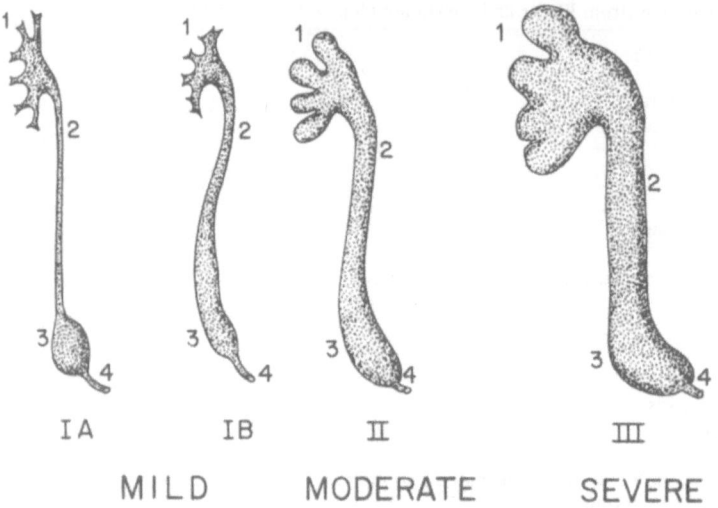

IA   IB   II   III

MILD   MODERATE   SEVERE

Fig. 2.4. Schema of increasing severity of primary megaureter (PM). Mild (grade I) PM is characterized by normal calyces. Moderate (grade II) PM has caliectasis and increasing ureteral dilatation throughout all portions of the ureter. Severe (grade III) PM shows significant hydroureteronephrosis and compromised renal function. The milder grades are usually encountered incidentally in the adult while the severe form presents symptomatically in the child. (From Pfister and Hendren [35], with permission)

Evaluation of Obstruction

Ultrasonography

Renal sonography is a rapid noninvasive method of evaluation for hydronephrosis. Varying degrees of separation of the central fatty echogenic sinus on ultrasonography correlates with normal fullness of the intrarenal collecting system or minimal dilatation to increasing severity of pyelocaliectasis. Infundibular continuity from calyces to the renal pelvis is necessary for ultrasonographic diagnosis (Fig. 2.5a); parapelvic cyst(s) may otherwise simulate dilatation of the collecting system. Evidence for upper ureteral dilatation in the lumbar area and lower ureterectasis in the bladder region should be obtained to complete the study.

Computed Tomography

The evaluation of hydronephrosis, particularly in the poorly or nonfunctioning kidney, is usually easy by computed tomography (CT). On plain noncontrast renal CT, multiple confluent parapelvic cysts may simulate caliectasis and both a large central single parapelvic cyst and the subcapsular hematoma may be confused with a dilated renal pelvis; attenuation values are helpful in the latter instance and contrast enhanced images are useful in both situations for definitive evaluation. Identification of the type of ureteral obstruction (nonopaque stone, retroperitoneal mass) is usually easily obtained by CT.

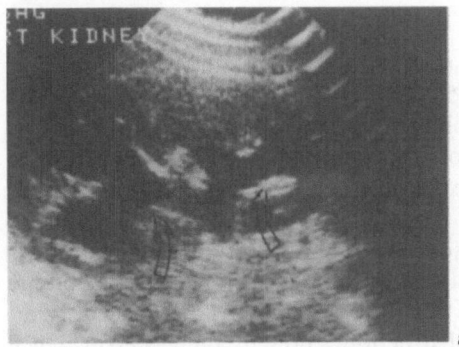

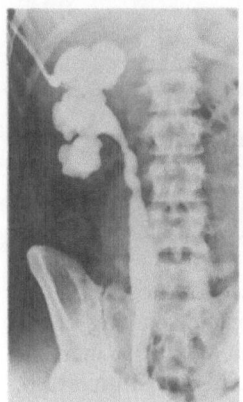
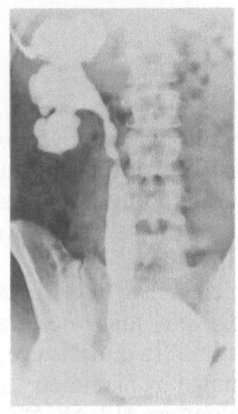

Fig. 2.5a–c. Persisting dilatation of solitary kidney in a 21-year-old man 11 years after ureteral reimplantation for reflux; no current reflux. **a** Parasagittal renal sonography demonstrates moderate intrarenal dilatation of collecting system with upper and lower pole infundibuli (*arrows*). **b** Empty and **c** full bladder perfusion runs at 10 ml per min: maximal renal absolute pressure of 20 cm H_2O and differential pressure of 10 cm H_2O excludes obstruction.

Voiding Cystourethrography

Voiding cystographic studies may be performed by urethral catheter or suprapubic puncture techniques. Voiding cystourethrography (VCUG) is almost always necessary to complement urography or renography for complete evaluation of the urinary tract in children since vesicoureteral reflux is a common cause of the megaureter (Fig. 2.3) in this and occasionally in the adult age groups. Bladder and urethral morphology, bladder volume, sensation, and emptying are easily obtained. In more complex functional disturbances of the lower tract (e.g., sphincter dyskinesia), urodynamic evaluation in conjunction with the VCUG may be necessary.

In lesions affecting the anterior urethra, retrograde urethrography may be particularly useful; at times combined VCUG and urethrography is advantageous in severely obstructive disease at sites within the posterior and anterior urethral segments.

Retrograde Pyelography

Useful in delineating the anatomy of the upper urinary tract, this procedure has a 4% incidence of introducing infection [35].

Delayed radiography at 5–30 min following retrograde pyelography is frequently obtained, as with intravenous urography and radionuclide renography, to aid in determining the presence or absence of obstruction in the dilated nonrefluxing ureter.

However, persistence of contrast or isotope within a reservoir or renal pelvis may not always indicate obstruction. Contrast washout is prolonged if the volume of the reservoir or pelvis is large or if the flow rate through it is diminished. In an experimental situation in which outflow obstruction is present, there is no evidence of persistence of contrast, provided flow and volume are not altered [30].

Intravenous Urography

Intravenous urography is the most commonly employed examination once upper tract obstruction is clinically suspected or known from ultrasonography or CT (Fig. 2.5a). Intravenous urography during an attack of pain and upright, prone, and delayed films are important aids in the diagnosis and evaluation of obstruction (Fig. 2.6).

The shell nephrogram and tubular crescents of advanced hydronephrosis are definitive in appearance; nephrotomography and intestinal gas-displacing prone films are often necessary for clear definition. In diuretic urography, a 20% increase in the area of the renal pelvis, as determined by planimetry, after Lasix stimulation, has been interpreted as an obstructive pattern [12, 56, 58].

Delayed visualization, prolonged nephrogram, and persistent ureteral filling are well known signs of obstruction. However, at times when renal function is poor, the ureter is markedly dilated, or operative correction of a previously dilated upper tract exists, the evaluation of obstruction may be difficult or equivocal.

Dynamic and Diuretic Renography

Radionuclide renography is a more sensitive means of evaluating the poorly functioning obstructed kidney. As with intravenous urography, delayed imaging and upright views are employed but may lead to erroneous conclusions.

Diuretic renography (DR) can serve a role in defining significantly obstructive upper urinary tracts from dilatation that is nonobstructive [3, 7, 17, 21–24, 26, 32, 33, 44, 56, 57, 59]. Following Lasix diuresis, the isotope will clear more slowly from the high pressure obstructed system than from the nonobstructed but dilated one.

The gamma camera renogram is performed using ^{99m}Tc-DTPA, a glomerular agent, or [123–131]I-Hippuran, which is eliminated by tubular secretion and glomerular filtration. A standard technique should be used employing intravenous hydration, a weight-adjusted dose of an isotope, and catheter drainage of the bladder.

Once the entire collecting system is filled with the tracer, Lasix (0.5–1.0 mg/kg up to 40 mg maximum) is administered. Sequential images are obtained, the regions of interest in the kidney and/or ureter are defined, a time–activity curve is generated, and a calculated half-time clearance is computed.

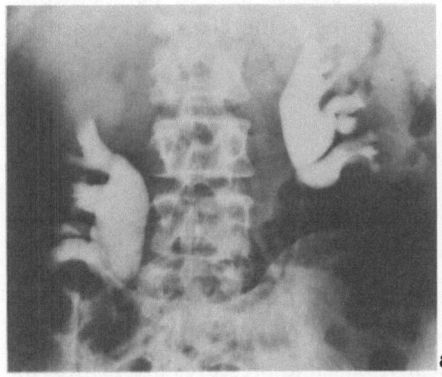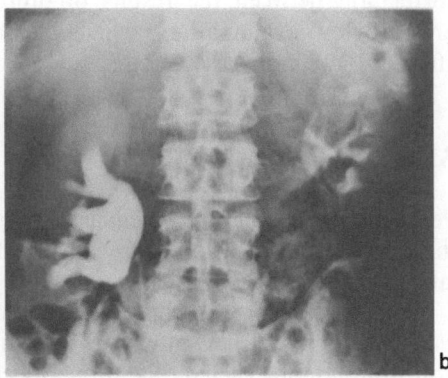

Fig. 2.6. Middle-aged man with intermittent right back discomfort. Infusion urography in **a** supine and **b** upright positions reveals prompt emptying of left collecting system. Note apparent symmetric extrarenal pelves in recumbent position.

A calculated half-time of less than 15 min is felt to be nonobstructive, one of between 15 and 20 min indeterminate, and one in excess of 20 min obstructive. Flow rates of 15–25 ml/min may be obtained under diuresis; the rising curve in the dilated obstructed tract continues to rise, while in the nonobstructed system there is prompt washout of the tracer. While the slope may reflect the effect of obstruction on the kidney, it should not be used to assess the degree of obstruction; specifically, slow elimination should not be misinterpreted as obstruction.

Finally, by means of deconvolution analysis, both parenchyma and whole kidney isotope transit times can be assessed quantitatively. The renal parenchymal curve is derived by subtracting the pelvic curve from the whole kidney curve. Prolonged parenchymal isotope transit times are encountered in significant obstruction [59].

A number of conditions may make the DR test inaccurate. Neonates and children less than 1 year of age may not respond well to diuresis because of depressed levels of renal function. Renal function below 30% of normal in any age group is the most significant limitation with DR, as it is with intravenous urography; not enough isotope is cleared to produce an accurate DR.

In the absence of a bladder catheter, bladder activity may overlap and obscure the lower ureter, particularly in small children, and lead to a false-positive result. Bladder distention with elevated intravesical pressure may lead to a false-positive renal obstructive curve itself. Failure to obtain ureteral histograms can lead to a false-negative renal obstructive pattern when the obstruction is at or near the ureterovesical junction and associated with a large compliant ureter; in these cases the renal curve may show a nonobstructive washout pattern. Parenchymal transit times are difficult to obtain and interpret in grossly dilated systems and thin parenchyma.

Little experience has evolved with the solitary kidney where elevated pressure may be present yet the system empties because of its high total output. The role of diuretic studies in evaluation of obstruction at sites in the ureter other than the ureteropelvic junction is not clear. Many reports do not indicate whether previous corrective surgery has been performed, or the level or apparent degree of obstruction. Most importantly, they usually do not monitor bladder filling or measure its pressure or its effect on the dilated kidney. Currently there is a lack of correlation between the results of diuretic renal studies and of percutaneous pressure-flow examinations which directly measure pyeloureteral resistance in 10%–30% or more of cases.

Antegrade Pyelography

Percutaneous pyelography is invasive but provides unexcelled anatomic display of the upper urinary tract; additionally, urine can be obtained for culture and other laboratory studies [36, 37].

While baseline or resting pyeloureteral pressures can be performed with a simple water manometer, they may be grossly misleading in differentiating true obstruction from nonobstructed dilatation. Specifically, baseline pressures are helpful in the diagnosis of obstruction only when they are elevated; pressures above 20 cm water are suspect but require further evaluation to avoid diagnostic errors [37, 41].

Resting pressures in the presence of obstruction may be high or low depending on the state of hydration, the degree and duration of the obstruction, and the compliance of the system. Following the onset of obstruction, urine retention results in increased fluid volume, increased pressure, and increased ureteral size. Within a short time, intraluminal pressure reaches a peak, then declines due to (1) decreased renal blood flow and glomerular filtration rate, (2) reabsorption of fluid into venous and lymphatic channels (renal backflow), and (3) changes in wall tension (elastic properties) of the pelvis or ureter. The pressure then falls to relatively low levels even though continued ureteral distention may occur [36, 40, 41].

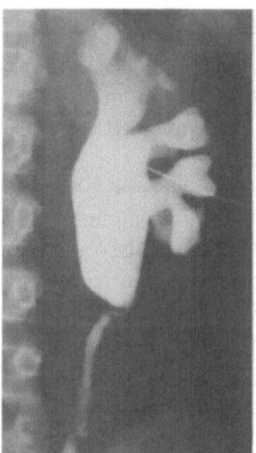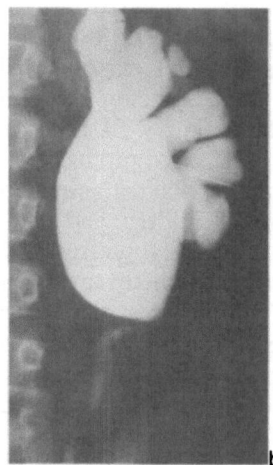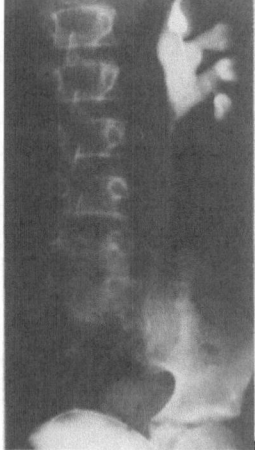

Fig. 2.7a–c. Effect of varying and increased flow rates during ureteral perfusion on the ureteropelvic junction in an 11-year-old girl with recurrent left flank pain. Perfusion rates of **a** 10 ml/min and **b** 15 ml/min resulted in renal pressures of 14 and 18 cm H_2O and differential pressures of 10 and 14 cm H_2O respectively: at a 20 ml/min perfusion rate the ureteropelvic junction decompensated with a differential pressure of 21 cm H_2O and simulation of her flank pain. **c** Three months after pyeloplasty, the step-off pressure was 6 cm H_2O at 10 ml/min and remained normal at higher flow rates. (Reproduced in part from Pfister et al. [41], with permission)

The degree of compliance of various pyeloureteral units may vary. A low compliant system reaching its maximum volume and wall tension quickly would rapidly produce elevated intrarenal pressure. Conversely, a highly compliant system would take longer to reach maximum tension and provide a buffering mechanism for intermittent episodes of diuresis, increased flow, and pressure (Fig. 2.7). In general, acquired obstruction in a previously normal upper urinary tract behaves in the former fashion and some congenitally dilated systems appear to reflect the latter [42].

Percutaneous Ureteral Perfusion

With continuing advances in surgery of the ureter, evaluation of ureteral function has become an important task. Ideally, a test for upper tract obstruction should be noninvasive, provide good anatomic detail and urodynamic information, and estimate overall and differential renal function. No single test exists which can accomplish these ends.

Since the urinary tract is a nonstatic system it is fortunate that serial urography and renography are not the only methods available to make the decision as to the existence, progression, or regression of obstruction.

Since its introduction in 1973, percutaneous renal puncture for the assessment of pyeloureteral dynamics has been extensively evaluated and, as suggested by Whitaker [49–54, 60, 61], the technique has proven to be invaluable [15, 29, 41].

Percutaneous puncture of the renal pelvis following catheterization of the bladder permits definitive pyeloureteral urodynamic evaluation. It measures directly the resistance to various known flow rates of diluted contrast along the course of the ureter with controlled bladder volumes and pressures. Bladder pressures are needed so that upper urinary tract pressure can be interpreted accurately; this is particularly important in the high pressure bladder (Fig. 2.2) due to outlet obstruction or neurogenic disease and after ureteral reimplantation (Figs. 2.8, 2.9) or any form of urinary diversion.

The Whitaker test is objective, reproducible, and unaffected by the kidney's individual glomerular filtration rate; thus in addition to defining the presence or absence of obstruction in renal insufficiency, it provides unexcelled anatomic definition of the dilated urinary tract.

Physiologic information on the ability of the ureter to transport or conduct urine to a reservoir (bladder, loop, intact colon, skin) may be obtained by percutaneous renal puncture [1, 2, 4, 7–11, 13, 15, 19, 21, 24, 25, 27–31, 34–39, 41, 43, 45–47, 49–56, 60–63]. Precise quantitation of resistance is possible with pressure-flow studies, and the exact values of differential pressure in centimeters of water between the kidney and reservoir in the normal and in varying degrees of obstruction have been investigated.

Indications

Obstruction constitutes an important cause of renal failure. At times, the diagnosis is apparently obvious from standard and modified (diuretic) urography and

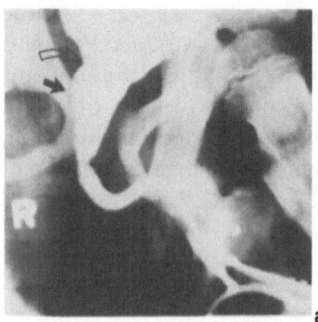

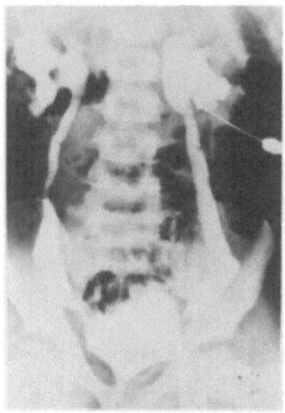
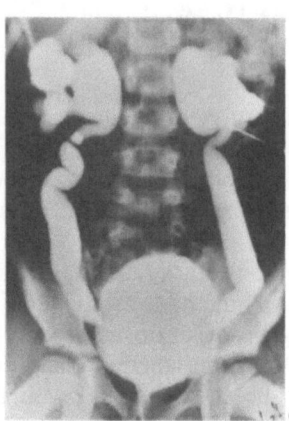

Fig. 2.8a–c. Value of perfusion studies with the bladder empty and full. This 6-year-old boy had his posterior urethral valves removed and ureteral reimplants as newborn elsewhere. At the time of these studies he was being treated with anticholinergics for supposed hypertonic bladder. The external sphincter was normal by EMG, and the urethral profile unremarkable, with pressures of 65 cm H$_2$O. **a** Cystourethrogram reveals patulous bladder neck (*open arrow*) and mildly dilated prostatic urethra (*solid arrow*); no voiding residual or ureteral reflux. **b** Simultaneous bilateral perfusions with semi-empty and **c** distended bladder. Bladder pressures of 7 and 16 cm H$_2$O during 15 ml/min flow rate resulted in renal pressures of 16 and 38 cm H$_2$O respectively; abnormal differential pressures of 24 cm H$_2$O in each kidney reflecting obstructed ureters only when bladder is full. Pressures returned to normal following repeat ureteral surgery.

radionuclide studies. In other cases the diagnosis of obstruction is questionable or uncertain and percutaneous perfusion studies are particularly useful.

Dilatation of the upper urinary tract may be encountered in high urinary outflow states [6, 10, 14, 18, 36, 48] or in association with bladder disease [13]; in both situations, elevated renal pressures may exist in the absence of ureteral obstruction and only differential pressures between the kidney and bladder can prove this [41, 51].

In other conditions, such as congenital megacalicosis, extrarenal pelves, milder forms of primary megaureter, and small adult type ureteroceles, only localized alterations are present and the diagnosis of elevated renal pressure may be uncertain (Fig. 2.10). Postprocedural dilatation of the urinary tract following pyeloplasty (Fig. 2.11), ureterolithotomy, balloon or stent dilatation of ureteral stenosis, ureteroneocystostomy, ureteroureterostomy, and other types of diversion [63] or undiversion [1] may give patterns where genuine obstruction and non-

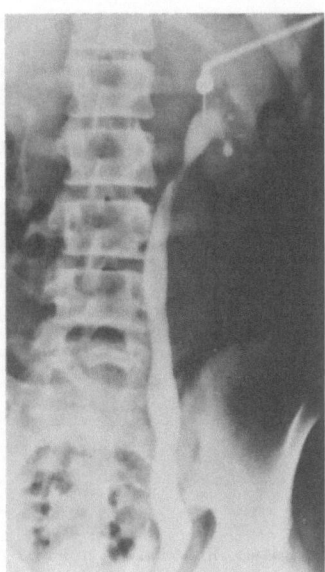

Fig. 2.9. Persisting ureterectasis 2 years following ureteral reimplantation for reflux in a 14-year-old patient; no current reflux. Perfusion runs at 10, 15, and 20 ml/min produced renal pressures of 12, 14, and 16 cm H_2O with differential pressures of 9, 11, and 13 cm H_2O, which excluded obstruction.

obstructive hypotonic dilatation cannot be differentiated with certainty by studies employing glomerular filtration agents. In the final analysis, whenever the diagnosis of obstruction is equivocal a pressure flow study is indicated [41, 53].

Contraindications

Bleeding is the most serious complication of percutaneous ureteral perfusion (PUP), and a blood coagulation disorder is a contraindication to the procedure. In

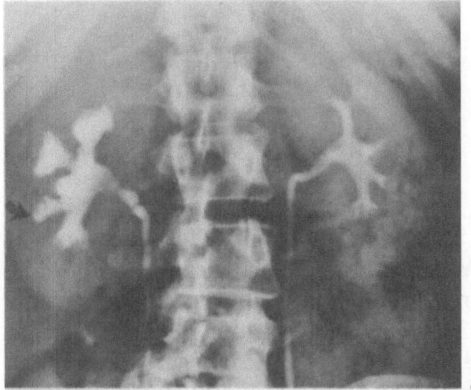
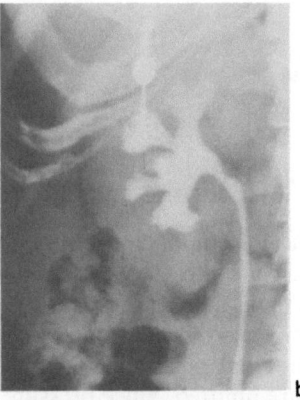

a   b

Fig. 2.10. a Urography and **b** right Whitaker test on a 40-year-old woman with a long history of urinary tract infections and analgesic intake for arthralgia; note papillary necrosis (*arrow*). Renal pressures of 12 and 19 cm H_2O at 10 and 15 ml/min flow rates and low differential pressures exclude an obstructive component from irregularity at the ureteropelvic junction.

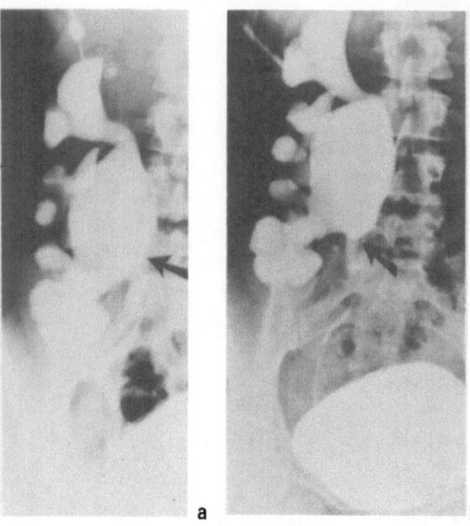

a   b

Fig. 2.11a,b. Reliability of ureterodynamics in solitary kidney. No change in renal function, lower abdominal pain, pyelocaliectasis, or normal perfusion studies after **a** pyeloplasty or **b** repeat pyeloplasty in which the UPJ (*arrow*) was moved to a dependent position. Renal pressures of 4 and 13 cm H_2O with step-off values of 3 and 11 cm H_2O for the two studies respectively at a 10 ml/min flow rate. (From Pfister et al. [40], with permission)

clinical practice, only those patients known or suspected to have such a disorder undergo blood clotting studies. Table 2.2 lists other situations where PUP is avoided.

Table 2.2. Contraindications to ureteral perfusion

1. Bleeding diathesis
2. Active urinary infection
3. High grade or complete obstruction
4. Vesicoureteral reflux without trapping (ipsilateral)

Technique

Equipment

A basic list of equipment required for performance of the study is provided in Table 2.3. The method as described by Whitaker has been significantly modified to minimize renal damage, decrease instrumentation complexity, and reduce examination time in a busy clinical practice [34, 37–39]. Thus, a thin flexible 22-gauge needle for renal perfusion is employed and the pressure transducer and chart recorder are omitted. Since pressure transducers must be calibrated with a simple water manometer at each examination, their use is required only if a permanent paper recording of renal pelvis and bladder pressures during different flow rate perfusion runs is desired. A pen or strip recorder serves no significant purpose and

Table 2.3. Equipment for perfusion studies

Hardware:
    Infusion pump (Sigmamotor; double head, 4004)
    Intravenous stands (2), movable (6')
    Table, movable (24" × 36")

Sterile disposables:
    Infusion pump tubing (Sigmamotor, 8403)
    Manometers (2), plastic 56 cm (Medex, MX2694:04170-12)
    Three-way stopcocks (2), plastic (Pharmaseal) ·
    Thin flexible 22-gauge needle; 4, 9, and 15 cm (Sherwood)
    Urethral Catheter, 5- and 10-F feeding tube, 15" (Argyle)
    168-cm needle extension line (Pharmaseal, K50L)
    168-cm urethral extension line (Pharmaseal, K50L)
    84-cm manometer extension lines (2) (Pharmaseal)
    Diluted (20%) contrast medium bottles (2) (500 ml)
    230-cm positive pressure extension line, bottle (McGaw)
    250-ml bowl; urethral catheter (Superior, 610)

only accumulates reams of paper. In addition, the cost of these items is considerable, particularly when personnel and physician time are included for their care and calibration.

Renal and bladder pressure are obtained during each perfusion sequence and immediately recorded; this includes (1) pressure readings, (2) perfusion rate and time, (3) bladder volume, and (4) frequency and percent of coaptation of ureteral

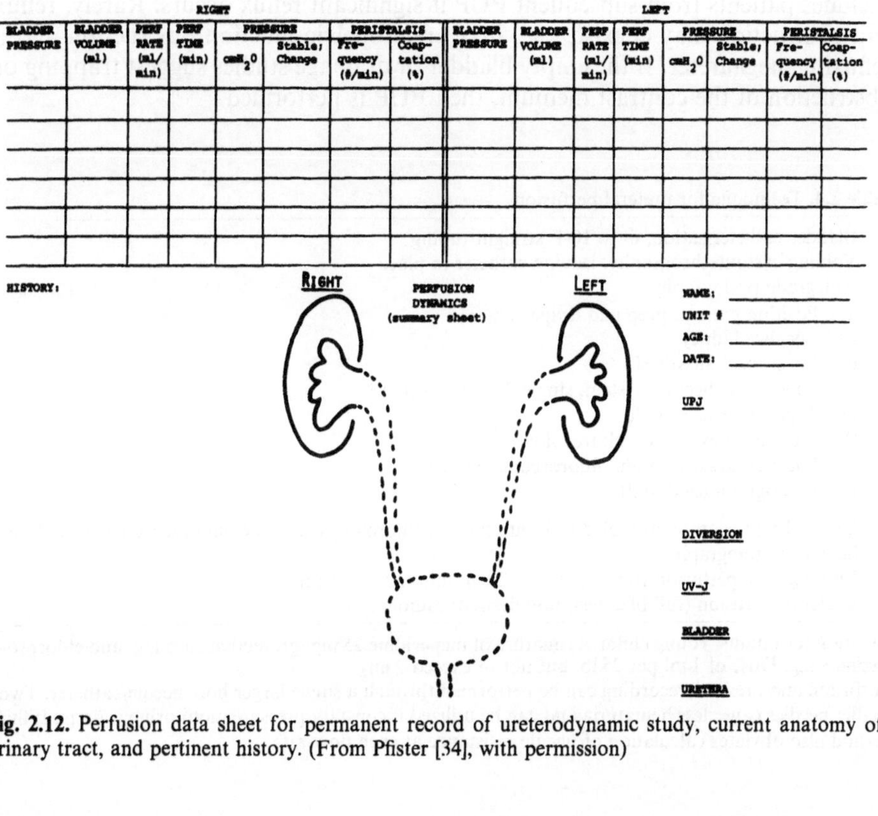

Fig. 2.12. Perfusion data sheet for permanent record of ureterodynamic study, current anatomy of urinary tract, and pertinent history. (From Pfister [34], with permission)

peristalsis on a predesigned perfusion data sheet. Space for pertinent history and details of the study (needle length, performance of perfusion, etc.) are provided alongside a dotted-line drawing of a normal urinary tract. The latter permits a heavy solid-line drawing of the current anatomic situation; this is valuable in quick review perusal of complex congenital or operative arrangements. The size of the perfusion data sheet ($8\frac{1}{2}'' \times 11''$) allows for easy incorporation of a given perfusion study into permanent office or hospital records; the patient's name and age, the hospital number, and the date of examination are listed (Fig. 2.12).

Conduct

The basic steps in performing a simplified percutaneous ureteral perfusion study are listed in Table 2.4.

In everyday practice, all PUPs are done under local anesthesia; general anesthesia is not necessary [34, 37]. Infants and young children may be sedated but heavy sedation is not desirable since severe pain or a major complication might be masked. Older children will cooperate if the study is explained, surprises are avoided during the conduct of the examination, and adequate rapport with the child and parents is established.

Cystourethrography is performed immediately prior to PUP. In the infant and young child the bladder is catheterized with a 5- or 6-F pediatric feeding tube and anchored in place with paper tape; in the older child and adult, larger similar catheters may be used. If a retrograde catheter cannot be passed through the urethra, a suprapubic tube is placed using an 18-gauge catheter sheathed needle; the catheter is then taped to the lower anterior abdominal wall. This initial study excludes patients from subsequent PUP if significant reflux occurs. Rarely, reflux and obstruction may coexist, e.g., in a ureteropelvic junction obstruction and a refluxing megaureter. If the empty bladder or drainage studies suggest trapping or obstruction of the contrast medium, then PUP is performed.

Table 2.4. Technique for ureteral perfusion

1. Bladder catheterization, 6- to 10-F straight tubing
2. Voiding cystourethrography, leaving catheter in place
3. Antegrade pyelography[a]
   - a) Position patient, prep and drape skin
   - b) Localize kidney
   - c) Inject local anesthesia
   - d) Puncture collecting system, single 22-gauge needle[b]
   - e) Aspirate urine sample
   - f) Measure pressure, check free flow
   - g) Inject contrast medium, fluoroscopic control
   - h) Radiograph (optional)
4. Ureteral perfusion (empty bladder); intermittent fluoroscopy and pressure recordings (renal and bladder); radiograph
5. Variable rate perfusion runs (5, 10, 15, 20 ml/min) as desired/needed
6. Ureteral perfusion (full bladder); rate desired; radiograph

[a]Sedation for infants, young children (mixture of meperidine 25 mg, promethazine 5 mg, and chlorpromazine 8 mg. Dose of 1 ml per 25 lb. but not to exceed 2 ml).
[b]Perfusion and pressure recording can be performed through a single larger bore needle/catheter. Two smaller needles cause less hematuria and can be utilized if constant pressure monitoring is desired; this method also obviates calculation of needle resistance at each flow rate.

Following the voiding cystourethrogram, with the bladder catheter still in place, the patient is turned prone for needle puncture of the kidney.

A prone radiograph of the abdomen is obtained and the kidney is localized by reference to it; previous urography, ultrasonography, CT, or, rarely, isotopic studies may also be of help. In over 90% of cases the kidney lies beneath the 12th rib and this site is prepped and draped. In other cases the kidney may be higher (totally under the rib cage) or lower. If the kidney is very low, e.g., an ectopic pelvic kidney, then an anterior abdominal wall approach is used and the patient remains in a supine position [37, 43].

Needle puncture may be directed by ultrasonography, or in other instances the palpable 12th rib and fluoroscopically visible landmarks (ribs, transverse processes) are used to localize the kidney. With good quality image-intensified fluoroscopy the kidney itself is often visible. Infrequently, intravenous contrast medium is used; when employed it is in nondilated or minimally dilated collecting systems. The target should be a calyx rather than the renal pelvis since a good parenchymal seal about the needle is desirable.

The needle site is anesthetized with 1% xylocaine. In over 90% of cases, this location is 1–2 cm below the 12th rib and in a posterior midclavicular line. A thin 22-gauge needle of length (4, 9, or 15 cm) appropriate to patient size is chosen for puncture; the shortest needle is used in infants and the longest in stocky and/or obese patients.

A small 10-ml syringe containing 3–4 ml of local anesthetic agent is attached to the needle. This combination is used for further anesthesia and for puncture of the pyelocalyceal system. The needle is advanced from a direct posterior (vertical) direction, taking care that arching of the needle is avoided to prevent false tracking. Intermittent injections of small amounts of xylocaine during needle advancement prevent plugging of the lumen. An alternative injection–aspiration sequence is used during needle passage; free urine return signals entry within the pyelocalyceal system. Entry of the needle tip into the posterior renal cortex can be verified fluoroscopically, since the needle will flex synchronously with renal respiratory motion. If the appropriate depth has been reached but no urine obtained, the needle is slowly retracted with continuous aspiration to the skin and then readvanced using a slightly different trajectory path. In the usual case one to three needle passes will be required for successful placement.

The first 2–4 ml of aspirated urine is saved for culture or other determinations. A saline-flushed water manometer with a three-way stopcock and extension tubing are then attached to the needle. Opening or resting pressure is obtained with the zero point of the manometer at the level of the needle tip.

Free flow of fluid through the needle tip is verified by raising and/or lowering the manometer; a fixed pressure indicates absence of free flow and requires adjustment of the needle tip. Injection of contrast medium without readjustment is fruitlesss since extravasation outside the pyelocalyceal system to some degree is inevitable.

Once free flow of urine has been obtained, contrast medium can be injected by hand under fluoroscopic control and spot films obtained.

Alternatively, after attaching the renal manometer to an IV stand (base of manometer at level of needle tip), the infusion pump tubing may be attached to the three-way stopcock of the renal manometer and a formal ureteral perfusion run obtained.

Perfusion is performed by a double-head infusion pump. Each head is capable of constant speed delivery rates of 1-ml increments up to 20 ml/min. Syringe-delivery

PERCUTANEOUS PERFUSION TECHNIQUE

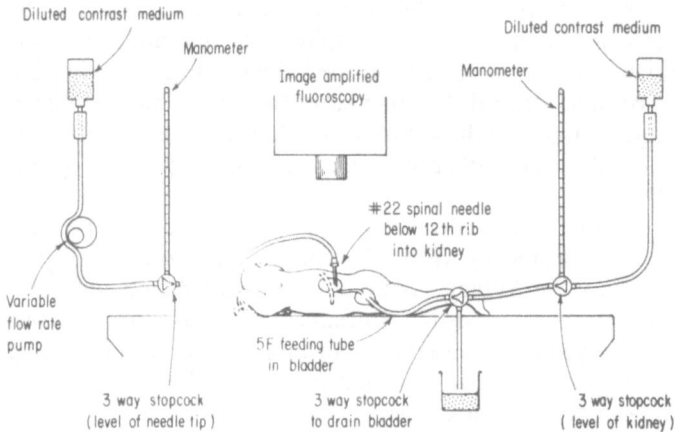

Fig. 2.13. Schema for simplified percutaneous ureteral urodynamic study. Disposable water manometers are interfaced with the renal needle and bladder catheter for simultaneous pressure measurements during each perfusion sequence. (From Pfister et al. [41], with permission)

type pumps are unable to deliver fluid at high flow rates through the small 22-gauge needle employed. Bottles up to 500 ml volume containing the infusion fluid are suspended above each pump head (Fig. 2.13).

The infusion fluid is contrast medium diluted to 20% concentration. Saline should be avoided as a perfusate since it is invisible fluoroscopically and on radiographs; extravasation with or without pain is not detectable without opaque contrast medium.

Usually, a flow rate of 5–10 ml/min is initially delivered under intermittent fluoroscopic control with intermittent pressure readings until steady-state perfusion exists [43]. Such steady-state equilibrium is present when the entire upper tract is opacified and pressure is unchanging after several minutes of perfusion at a given flow rate [38] (Figs. 2.7, 2.9, 2.10).

In the presence of significant obstruction, perfusion time and/or rate of delivery should be lower to avoid excessively high intrapelvic pressures. Maximal renal pressure during perfusion should be limited to 40–50 cm water since intrarenal and intravascular reflux may occur with intracalyceal pressures of 30–50 cm water. In very dilated upper urinary systems, perfusion time and/or delivery rate need to be increased to reach steady-state perfusion.

Because of the small caliber of the renal needle, the viscosity of the infusion fluid, and the flow rates employed, the pressure response to perfusion is obtained immediately after the pump is turned off by switching the stopcock on the manometer. By alternately turning the pump on and off and obtaining intermittent pressures, the effect of a given flow rate can be monitored. When satisfied that steady-state response has been obtained at a given flow rate, with the bladder empty and full, the pressure data of the kidney and bladder, the bladder volume, the perfusion time, and the effect of peristalsis are entered on the permanent record perfusion sheet.

URETERAL PERFUSION
INSTRUMENTATION

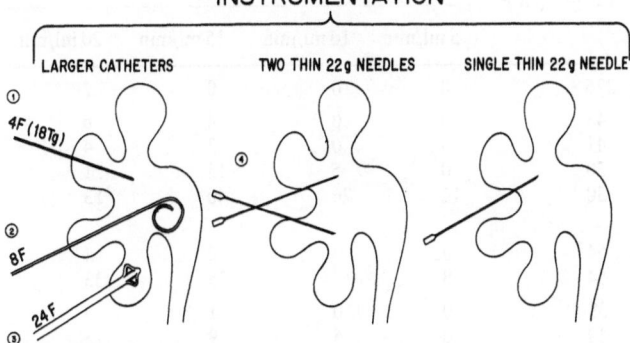

Fig. 2.14. Various renal perfusion instruments that may be employed. All single instruments require calibration of their resistance unless an intermittent perfusion-pressure recording technique is used. Continuous pressure monitoring without calibration can be obtained by dual instruments.

The interval pressure values obtained by this perfusion modification are exactly similar to the data obtained with constant pressure recording and larger bore needles or catheters that require pre- or postperfusion calibration for the pressure drops produced by various flow rates [2, 45] (Fig. 2.14). Continuous pressure monitoring, with subtraction of renal instrumental baseline values, can only be performed with large-bore instruments (internal diameter of 1.7–2.7 mm depending on their length), as these will not produce a pressure rise in the perfusion system (extension tubing and renal puncture instrument) at flow rates up to 10 ml/min. At higher flow rates of 15–20 ml/min, most instruments, including the 14-gauge needle and 12-F catheter, exhibit resistances which affect pressure readings (Table 2.5).

One alternative technique which allows continuous pressure recording without using large needles or precalibration of equipment, is the insertion of two thin 22-gauge needles into the kidney from the same anesthetic site on the skin (Fig. 2.15). Perfusion can be performed through one and constant pressure monitoring through the other [37, 39]. With this method, as with the intermittent perfusion technique through a single small needle, the resistance of the perfusion system is not relevant.

In equivocal obstruction or when differential pressures are in the "high normal, indeterminate, and low abnormal" ranges, the flow rate can be increased from the standard 10 ml/min to 15–20 ml/min [35, 38–40]. The higher flow rates maximally stress the system and may reveal a covert obstruction (Fig. 2.7). The normal pyeloureteral unit can accept these rates without an abnormal pressure rise; ureters having successful surgical correction have provided these perfusion data by acting as their own controls (Fig. 2.16).

Both the renal needle and the bladder catheter must be free flowing when pressures are obtained, or misleading differential pressures will result. Most potential problems occur with fixed bladder pressures because the bladder wall has collapsed on the catheter or a small clot occludes the catheter [37].

Following completion of the study the bladder catheter and renal needle are removed. Utilization of a thin needle for PUP permits most cases to be performed on an outpatient basis. It is not necessary to place the patient on bed rest either in

Table 2.5. Resistance pressures[a] (from Amis et al. [2], with permission)

Equipment		Length (cm)[b]	Flow rates[c]			
			5 ml/min	10 ml/min	15 ml/min	20 ml/min
Baseline tubing		275	0	0	0	2
Foley catheter	14-F	43	0	0	4	6
	12-F	41	0	0	2	4
	10-F	30	0	5	13	21
	8-F	30	12	26	40	53
Silastic catheter	12-F	54	0	0	2	4
	8-F	54	8	17	25	33
Straight catheter	10-F	39	0	0	1	3
	8-F	39	0	5	9	13
	5-F	39	22	50	55+	55+
14-gauge needle		8.75	0	0	2	4
15-gauge needle		3.75	0	1	3	5
		8.75	0	3	5	7
16-gauge needle		5.00	0	2	5	8
		20.00	0	4	11	18
18-gauge needle		5.00	2	10	18	26
		8.75	5	16	27	38
		15.00	3	9	16	23
20-gauge needle		3.75	13	31	51	55+
		8.75	25	55+	55+	55+
		15.00	31	55+	55+	55+
		20.00	55+	55+	55+	55+
22-gauge needle		8.75	55+	55+	55+	55+
		15.00	55+	55+	55+	55+

[a]Measured in cm of water.
[b]For needles, length of shaft (excluding hub) was measured.
[c]55+ = pressure in excess of manometer length.

the hospital or at home. Only postprocedural blood pressure and pulse recordings are obtained if the examination was uneventful.

In addition to the higher flow rates than those described by Whitaker, other features and modifications have been incorporated and have been found to be clinically valuable (Table 2.6).

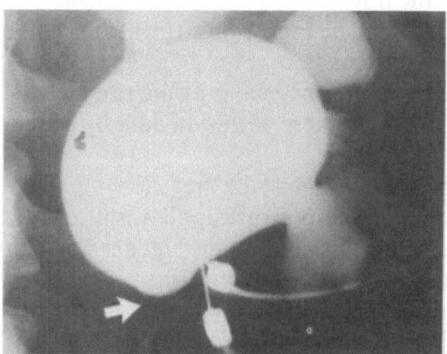

Fig. 2.15. Double thin needle (22 gauge) technique is suggested for initial percutaneous ureterodynamic studies until experience with the Whitaker test is obtained. Renal pressures of 21 and 43 cm H_2O at flow rates of 10 and 15 ml/min respectively; the ureteropelvic junction (*arrow*) is nearly totally obstructed at the higher flow rate.

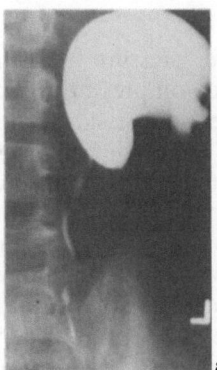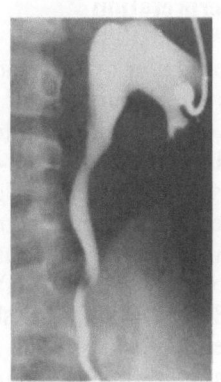

Fig. 2.16. Perfusion studies on the same ureter in a 9-year-old boy **a** before and **b** following successful pyeloplasty with wide open junction after surgery. Differential pressures of 17 and 23 cm H$_2$ fell to 10 and 11 cm H$_2$O after operation at flow rates of 10 and 15 ml/min respectively. (From Newhouse et al. [29], with permission)

a

b

Table 2.6. Comparative features of percutaneous techniques (after Pfister [34], with permission)

Item	Whitaker	MGH	Comment
Equipment:			
Pressure transducer	+	–	Requires manometer calibration
Chart recorder	+	–	Cumbersome
Water manometers	–	+	Simple, quick
Needle/catheter size	18 gT	22 g	Catheter sheathed needle (W)
Infusion pump	Single	Dual	Dual cheaper than 2 singles for bilateral studies
Conduct:			
Calculation resistance needle/catheter	+	–	Necessary with small bore unit recordings
Constant pressure monitoring	+	–	Single 22-gauge needle (MGH)
		+	Double 22-gauge needle (MGH)
Immediate preceding VCUG	–	+	Excludes intermittent significant reflux (MGH)
Fluoroscopic monitoring	+	+	Necessary
IV contrast	+	–	Only nondilated systems (MGH)
Study time	2×	1×	30 min (1 ×), average
Flow rates ml/min	2–10	2–20	Maximal stress (MGH)
Sterile urine	+	+	Necessary
Maximum renal pressure (cm water)	50–80	40–50	Intrarenal reflux 30–50
Perfusate	Saline or contrast	Contrast	Saline leak invisible, not recommended (MGH)
Patient:			
NPO	+	+	4 h
General anesthesia, young	+	–	Occasional (W)
Sedation, young	+	±	Usual (W); variable (MGH)
Hospitalization	+	–	Usual (W)
Outpatient	–	+	Over 70% (MGH)
Results:			
Permanent record	Graph	Written	Equivalent data
Induced infection from apparatus set-up	±	–	Disposable (MGH)
Morbidity	+	+	Minimal; pain, hematuria, sepsis
Renal loss	–	–	
Mortality	–	–	

Interpretation

Subtraction of the bladder pressure from the renal pelvic pressure provides the relative, differential, or step-off pressure [49–54]. At a flow rate of 10 ml/min, with the bladder empty, differential pressures below 13 cm of water are normal (Table 2.7) (Fig. 2.17). Values of 14–22 cm water suggest mild but increasing obstruction, those of 23–40 cm indicate moderate obstruction, and values above 41 cm water reflect very severe obstruction [41, 53].

As indicated previously, free-flowing pressures must be adhered to and pressure recorders (manometers) have to be set at the level of the tip of the renal needle (Fig. 2.18). Perfusion runs should be done with the bladder empty and full; in some cases, obstruction will be evident only when the bladder is distended, although most abnormal differential pressures are apparent with an empty bladder.

At higher flow rates the normal pressure-drop values with an empty bladder increase; at 15 ml/min the upper limit of normal is 18 cm water and at 20 ml/min around 21 cm water [29].

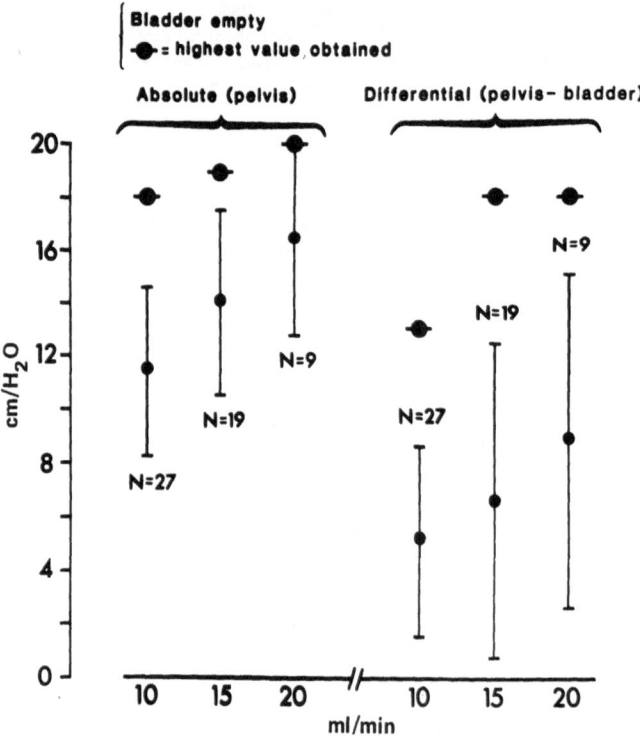

Fig. 2.17. Perfusion pressures obtained at various flow rates in 27 pyeloureteral units. Differential pressures are more reliable for clinical use since varying intra-abdominal pressure affects both the kidney and bladder. Usual perfusion rate is 10 ml/min; although higher flow rates are useful, the number of patients studied in this series with such rates was less. (From Newhouse et al. [29], with permission)

Table 2.7. Ureteral perfusion pressures following successful pyeloplasty (from Newhouse et al. [29], with permission)

Pressure (cm H$_2$0)	10 ml/min, bladder empty	15 ml/min, bladder empty	20 ml/min, bladder empty	10 ml/min, bladder full
Mean absolute	11.5 ± 3.23	14.1 ± 3.39	16.4 ± 3.46	13.5 ± 4.06
Mean differential	5.6 ± 3.71	6.6 ± 5.86	8.9 ± 6.24	2.3 ± 3.88
Mean absolute +2 SD	17.9	20.8	23.3	21.6
Mean differential +2 SD	13.0	18.3	21.4	10.1
Upper limit of range— absolute	18.0	19.0	20.0	21.0
Upper limit of range— differential	13.0	18.0	18.0	10.0

When the bladder is filled, there is a rise in intravesical pressure such that absolute renal pelvic pressure increases although the differential pressure drops [8, 11, 27, 29, 38, 62].

Results and Complications

Since percutaneous pressure-flow studies are touted as the standard to which other examinations must be compared [53] and the number of centers utilizing the technique in daily clinical practice is not extensive, it is difficult to obtain meaningful data on the predictive value of the study. Further, as with diuretic renography, some are not using similar basic techniques with measurement of bladder pressure even though this aspect has been repeatedly stressed by Whitaker.

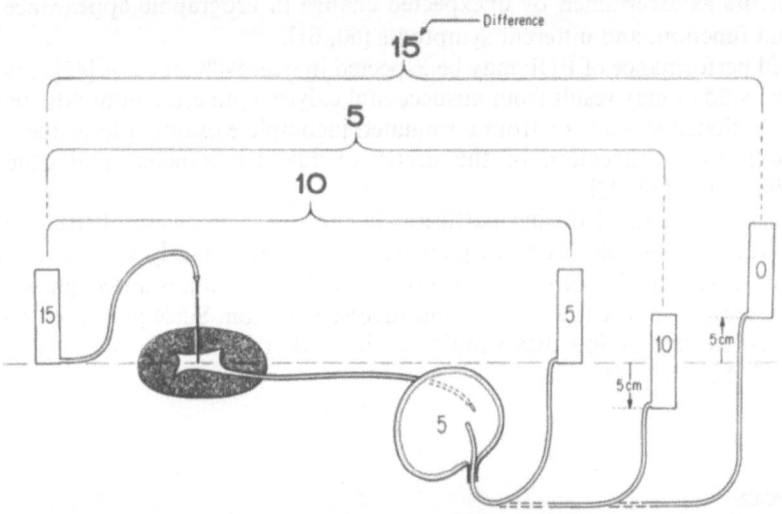

Fig. 2.18. The base (zero point) of both the renal and bladder pressure recorders (manometers) should be level with the tip of the renal needle. Spurious differential values can be avoided by careful observation of extraneous factors. (From Pfister and Newhouse [37], with permission)

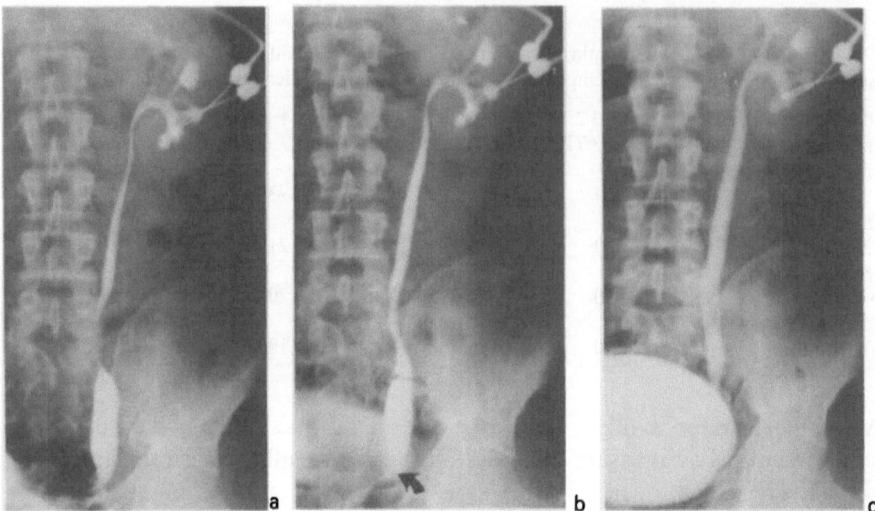

Fig. 2.19. Dual needle technique in normal perfusion study of mild (grade I) primary megaureter during **a** empty bladder, **b** partial, and **c** complete bladder filling. 28-year-old man with occasional episodes of vague abdominal pain and apparent incidental adynamic distal ureteral segment (*arrow*); absolute renal pressures of 17 cm H$_2$O or less and lower differential pressure values at flow rates of 5, 10, and 15 ml/ min. Note columning of ureter when bladder is distended and its pressure elevated normally. (From Pfister and Hendren [35], with permission)

Short-term 5-year follow-up results in 33 renal units after perfusion studies diagnosed obstruction on 16 and no obstruction in the remainder, showed no apparent errors as ascertained by unexpected change in urographic appearance, altered renal function, and different symptoms [60, 61].

Successful performance of PUP may be expected in over 94% of cases [42] (Fig. 2.19). Failed studies may result from unsuccessful calyceal puncture in nondilated or minimally dilated systems or from terminated incomplete examinations due to extravasation, clot obstruction of the ureter or bladder catheter, and other technical difficulties [37, 42].

High pressure generated during perfusion in moderate or severe obstruction should be watched carefully as flank pain may result, particularly with a rapid change in pressure. Finally, sepsis may be precipitated if infection is unrecognized; antibiotic coverage will usually prevent this adverse situation. Since pressure-flow studies are an elective option they should not be undertaken unless the urine is sterile [37, 42, 52].

References

1. Amis ES Jr, Pfister RC, Hendren WH (1981) Radiology of undiversion. Urol Radiol 3:161–169
2. Amis ES Jr, Pfister RC, Newhouse JH (1982) Resistances of various renal instruments used in ureteral perfusion. Radiology 143:267–268

3. Ash JM, Kass E, Gilday DL (1979) Diuretic renal scans in pediatric hydronephrosis (abstr.). J Nucl Med 20:623
4. Backlund L, Reuterskiold AG (1969) The abnormal ureter in children. I. Perfusion studies on the wide non-refluxing ureter. Scand J Urol Nephrol 3:219–228
5. Backlund L, Grotte G, Reuterskiold AG (1965) Functional stenosis as a cause of pelvi-ureteric obstruction and hydronephrosis. Arch Dis Child 40:203–206
6. Boyd SD, Raz S, Ehrlich RM (1980) Diabetes insipidus and nonobstructive dilation of the urinary tract. Urology 16:266–269
7. Braren V, Bauriedel JK, Jones WB, Goddard J (1982) Evaluation of normal and pathological ureteral dynamics: comparison of a radioisotope method with ureteral pressure/flow perfusion study. J Urol 127:1014–1016
8. Bratt CG, Aurell M, Erlandson BE, Nilson AE, Nilsson S (1982) Intrapelvic pressure and urinary flow rate in obstructed and nonobstructed human kidneys. J Urol 127:1136–1142
9. Coolsaet BLRA, Griffiths DJ Jr, van Mastright R et al. (1980) Urodynamic investigation of the wide ureter. J Urol 124:666–672
10. Djurhuus JC, Stage P (1976) Percutaneous intrapelvic pressure in hydronephrosis during diuresis. Acta Chir Scand (Suppl) 472:43–48
11. Djurhuus JC, Nerstrom B, Rask-Andersen H (1976) Dynamics of upper urinary tract in man. Acta Chir Scand (Suppl) 472:49–58
12. Ekelund L, Lindstedt E, Thiesen V, Jonsson MB (1980) Diuresis urography in equivocal pelvi-ureteric obstruction. Urol Radiol 1:147–150
13. Glassberg KI, Schneider M, Haller JO, Moel D, Waterhouse K (1982) Observations on persistently dilated ureter after posterior urethral valve ablation, Urology 20:20–28
14. Harrison RB, Ramchandani P, Allen JT (1979) Psychogenic polydipsia: unusual cause for hydronephrosis. AJR 133:327–328
15. Jaffe RB, Middleton AW Jr (1980) Whitaker test: differentiation of obstructive from nonobstructive uropathy. AJR 134:9–15.
16. Johnston JH (1969) The pathogenesis of hydronephrosis in children. Br J Urol 41:724–734
17. Kalika V, Bard RH, Iloreta A, Freeman LM, Heller S, Blaufox D (1981) Prediction of renal functional recovery after relief of upper urinary tract obstruction. J Urol 126:301–305
18. King LR (1980) Megaloureter: definition, diagnosis and management. J Urol 123:222–223
19. Kinn AC (1981) Pressure flow studies in hydronephrosis. Scand J Urol Nephrol 15:249–255
20. Koff SA (1981) The diagnosis of obstruction in experimental hydroureteronephrosis: mechanisms for progressive urinary tract dilation. Invest Urol 19:85–88
21. Koff SA (1982) Ureteropelvic junction obstruction: role of newer diagnostic methods. J Urol 127:898–901
22. Koff SA, Thrall JH, Keyes JW Jr (1979) Diuretic radionuclide urography: a non-invasive method for evaluating nephroureteral dilatation. J Urol 122:451–454
23. Koff SA, Thrall JH, Keyes JW Jr (1980) Assessment of hydroureteronephrosis in children using diuretic radionuclide urography. J Urol 123:531–534
24. Kreuger RP, Ash JM, Silver MM, Kass EJ, Gilmour RF, Alton DJ, Gilday DL, Churchill BM (1980) Primary hydronephrosis: Assessment of diuretic renography, pelvis perfusion pressure, operative findings and renal and ureteral histology. Urol Clin North Am 7:231–242
25. Lockhart JL, Sfakianakis GN, Al-sheikh W, Stover B, Politano VA (1982) Animal model to study megaureters non-invasively. J Urol 128:633–635
26. Lupton EW, Testa HJ, Lawson RS, Charlton Edwards E, Carroll RNP, Barnard RJ (1979) Diuresis renography and the results of pyeloplasty for idiopathic hydronephrosis. Br J Urol 51:449–453
27. Mortensen J, Djurhuus JC, Laursen H, Bisballe S (1983) The relationship between pressure and flow in the normal pig renal pelvis: An experimental study of the range of normal pressures. Scand J Urol Nephrol 17:369–372
28. Newhouse JH, Pfister RC (1981) Percutaneous upper urinary tract dynamics in equivocal obstruction (Whitaker). Urol Radiol 2:191–192
29. Newhouse JH, Pfister RC, Hendren WH, Yoder IC (1981) Whitaker test after pyeloplasty: establishment of normal ureteral perfusion pressures. AJR 137:223–226
30. Newhouse JH, Amis ES Jr, Pfister RC (1984) Pitfalls in the use of delayed contrast washout to diagnose urinary obstruction. Radiology 151:319–322
31. Odiase V, Whitaker RH (1981) Dynamic evaluation of the results of pyeloplasty using pressure-flow studies. Eur Urol 7:324–326
32. O'Reilly PH, Testa HJ, Lawson RS, Farrar DJ, Charlton Edwards E (1978) Diuresis renography in equivocal urinary tract obstruction. Br J Urol 50:76–80

33. O'Reilly PH, Lawson RS, Shields RA, Testa HJ (1979) Idiopathic hydronephrosis—the diuresis renogram: a new non-invasive method of assessing equivocal pyreloureteral junction obstruction. J Urol 121:153–155
34. Pfister RC (1982) Pressure studies II. In: O'Reilly PH, Gosling JA (eds) Idiopathic hydronephrosis. Springer, New York, pp 68–78
35. Pfister RC, Hendren WH (1978) Primary megaureter in children and adults: clinical and pathologic features of 150 ureters. Urology 12:160–176
36. Pfister RC, Newhouse JH (1978) Radiology of the ureter. Urology 12:15–39
37. Pfister RC, Newhouse JH (1979) Interventional percutaneous pyeloureteral techniques. I. Antegrade pyelography and ureteral perfusion. Radiol Clin North Am 17:341–350
38. Pfister RC, Newhouse JH, Yoder IC (1980) Effect of flow rates on ureteral perfusion results (abstr.). AJR 135:209
39. Pfister RC, Hendren WH, Newhouse JH, Yoder IC (1981) Techniques for percutaneous ureterodynamic studies (abstr.). AJR 137:196
40. Pfister RC, Yoder IC, Newhouse JH (1981) Percutaneous uroradiologic procedures. Semin Roentgenol 16:135–151
41. Pfister RC, Newhouse JH, Hendren WH (1982) Percutaneous pyeloureteral urodynamics. Urol Clin North Am 9:41–49
42. Pfister RC, Newhouse JH, Yoder IC, Hendren WH, Kim SH, Donahoe PK, Herrin JT (1983) Complications of pediatric percutaneous procedures: incidence and observations. Urol Clin North Am 10:563–571
43. Schiff M Jr, Rosenfield AT, McGuire EJ (1979) The use of percutaneous antegrade renal perfusion in kidney transplant recipients. J Urol 122:246–248
44. Thrall JH, Koff SA, Keyes JW Jr (1981) Diuretic radionuclide renography and scintigraphy in the differential diagnosis of hydroureteronephrosis. Semin Nucl Med 11:89–104
45. Toguri AG, Fournier G (1982) Factors influencing the pressure-flow-perfusion system. J Urol 127:1021–1023
46. Vela-Navarette R (1971) Percutaneous intrapelvic pressure determinations in the study of hydronephrosis. Invest Urol 8:526–533
47. Vela-Navarette R (1975) Chronic obstructive nephropathy. Urology 5:89
48. Whitaker RH (1975) Some observations and theories on the wide ureter and hydronephrosis. Br J Urol 47:377–385
49. Whitaker RH (1975) Methods of assessing obstruction in dilated ureters. Br J Urol 45:15–22
50. Whitaker RH (1976) Equivocal pelvi-ureteric obstruction. Br J Urol 47:771–779
51. Whitaker RH (1976) Investigating wide ureters with ureteral pressure flow studies. J Urol 116:81–82
52. Whitaker RH (1979) An evaluation of 170 diagnostic pressure flow studies in the upper urinary tract. J Urol 121:602–604
53. Whitaker RH (1979) Clinical application of upper urinary tract dynamics. Urol Clin North Am 6:137–141
54. Whitaker RH (1981) Percutaneous upper urinary tract dynamics in equivocal obstruction. Urol Radiol 2:187–189
55. Whitfield HN, Harrison NW, Sherwood T, Williams DI (1976) Upper urinary tract obstruction: pressure/flow studies in children. Br J Urol 48:427–430
56. Whitfield HN, Britton KE, Fry IK, Hendry WF, Nimon CC, Travers P, Wickham JEA (1977) The obstructed kidney: correlation between renal function and urodynamic assessment. Br J Urol 49:615–619
57. Whitfield HN, Britton KE, Hendry WF, Nimmon CC, Wickham JEA (1978) The distinction between obstructive uropathy and nephropathy by radioisotope transit times. Br J Urol 50:433–436
58. Whitfield HN, Britton KE, Hendry WF, Wickham JEA (1979) Fursemide intravenous urography in the diagnosis of pelviuretic junction obstruction. Br J Urol 51:445–448
59. Whitfield HN, Britton KE, Nimmon WF, Hendry WF, Wallace DMA, Wickham JEA (1981) Renal transit time measurements in the diagnosis of ureteric obstruction. Br J Urol 53:500–503
60. Witherow RON, Whitaker RH (1981) The predictive accuracy of antegrade pressure flow studies in equivocal upper tract obstruction. Br J Urol 53:496–499
61. Wolk FN, Whitaker RH (1982) Late follow-up of dynamic evaluation of upper urinary tract obstruction. J Urol 128:346–347
62. Woodside JR, Borden TA (1980) The pressure-flow relationship of the normal ureter. Invest Urol 18:82–83
63. Yoder IC, Pfister RC (1978) Radiology of colon loop diversion: anatomical and urodynamic studies of the conduit and ureters in children and adults. Radiology 127:85–92

Chapter 3

Percutaneous Litholapaxy and Extraction of Renal Calculi

Rolf W. Günther and P. Alken

Introduction

Operative treatment of urinary calculous disease has been the method of choice for many years, although the possibility of percutaneous manipulation was first demonstrated more than 40 years ago. On the path to modern endourology, Rupel and Brown (1941) set a milestone by endoscopic removal of a stone via the operative nephrostomy track. Only in the past 10 years, however, have technical innovations led to a breakthrough in the form of new nonoperative therapeutic modalities, including percutaneous stone manipulation and extracorporeal shock wave therapy.

Percutaneous stone manipulation is the logical consequence of percutaneous access to the upper urinary tract; this was recognized by Fernström and Johansson in 1976, who were able to extract stones nonoperatively. Apart from extraction, which is the simplest method of stone removal, fragmentation and chemolysis have become widely accepted [2, 13, 14, 22, 25].

On the basis of 6 years' experience [2], in this chapter we will deal with percutaneous stone manipulation via the nephrostomy tract, with special emphasis on litholapaxy and stone extraction from the pyelocalyceal system.

Renal Calculi

Classification of renal stones according to their radiopacity is still useful even in the era of extracorporeal shock wave therapy. Those stones that are radiopaque on conventional X-rays are mostly calcium oxalate, calcium phosphate, or struvite stones. Poor or lacking radiopacity is typical of uric acid, urate, xanthin, and matrix stones. Cystine calculi are usually faintly radiopaque. In vitro measurement of different renal stones by CT revealed the following maximal densities (K.J. Klose, Mainz, personal communication): cystine stones 150 HU, urate stones 650 HU, apatite stones more than 1000 HU, and whewellite stones more than 1000 HU. It is important to realize, however, that most stones are composed of several substances.

General Remarks on Litholapaxy

The terms litholapaxy and lithotripsy derive from the Greek and Latin (lithos = stone, lapaxy = triptos = to shear) and are used to denote stone fragmentation or disintegration. Kidney stones ranging from 8 to 10 mm in size may be extracted percutaneously from the collecting system following adequate dilatation of the nephrostomy track. Larger stones require fragmentation, which can be accomplished mechanically or using more elaborate techniques. The most important instruments used to break stones are:

1. Ultrasound lithotriptor
2. Electrohydraulic lithotriptor
3. Stone punch
4. Forceps

All these techniques are performed under direct endoscopic vision.

Simple mechanical fragmentation of small soft stones up to 2 cm in diameter is usually achieved using forceps. Only in a capacious collecting system may a stone punch be used. Ultrasound offers a safe and effective means of fragmenting larger stones [2, 3]. The lithotrite consists of a rigid metal probe which transmits ultrasonic waves (28 kHz, amplitude 20 µ) produced by a small generator (Fig. 3.5). The oscillating ultrasound probe is brought into direct contact with the stone and, similar to a drill, results in disintegration of the stone to sand at the site of contact. After early attempts at ultrasound destruction of calculi [10, 24], a lithotriptor was developed for fragmentation of vesical calculi [15, 29, 31, 34]. It was then applied in the upper urinary tract for removal of residual stones through a preexisting nephrostomy [21] and was modified and extended to the percutaneous approach by Alken and co-workers [2, 3]. Minimal damage in the form of mucosal edema may be caused by the ultrasound probe when it is directly applied to the tissue; by contrast electrohydraulic shock waves may cause more severe lesions (including perforation) when the probe is placed in direct contact with the tissue [35]. This can be prevented by maintaining a distance of 5–10 mm between the tip of the lithotrite and the tissue. Development of heat at the tip of the ultrasound lithotrite requires cooling and continuous flushing with saline. Liquid medium is also necessary for the transmission of the shock waves.

Similar to ultrasound disintegration, which is the most popular technique of stone fragmentation, electrohydraulic lithotripsy had been in use for crushing of bladder calculi for nearly a decade [29] before it was applied to renal stones [27].

The principle of the latter method is based on an electric spark discharge (DC, output 2.5 kV) between the two insulated electrodes at the tip of the probe.

Multiple short impulses of approx. 5 µs duration result in shock waves leading to stone disintegration. This technique seems to be quicker for large stones, but permits less controlled fragmentation than ultrasound. One advantage of the electrohydraulic lithotriptor is its small 5-F calibre and its flexibility (Fig. 3.6), whereas ultrasound is larger (10 F) and rigid.

Although many efforts have been made to break stones, including disintegration by laser [11, 26] or microexplosions [27], ultrasound litholapaxy seems to be the most practical and safest method for cracking large calculi.

Technique

Percutaneous stone manipulation was initially carried out under local anesthesia. However, since the procedure may be lengthy and cause discomfort to the patient, peridural anesthesia proved to be more convenient. General anesthesia is used only when a patient demands it. In the early part of our series, dilatation was performed successively in several sessions until the nephrostomy track was adequately dilated [2, 3]. Now puncture, dilatation, and stone removal are done in a single session without an increase in risk [5].

The equipment necessary for stone manipulation consists of: (a) a fluoroscope, (b) an ultrasound probe, (c) an endoscope, (d) a lithotrite, (e) a stone punch, and (f) forceps, basket, and balloon catheter.

The technical procedure comprises:

1. Puncture
2. Dilatation of the track
3. Endoscopy
4. Stone disintegration
5. Extraction

Puncture

The following instruments are required:

1. 5-F Longdwell needle (length 20 cm, Becton-Dickinson)
2. 1.0-mm J-tipped guide wire (length 100 cm)
   a) with torque control
   b) with movable core
   c) Lunderquist guide wire
3. 9-F introducer (total length 25 cm, outer sheath 15 cm, Vygon, Aachen)
4. Fine needle (ø 0.7 mm, length 20 cm) (W. Cook)

With the patient prone, the puncture is performed from posterolaterally, a hand's breadth plus 2 or 3 cm lateral from the midline between the 12th rib and the pelvic crest [16, 17]. A 5-F Teflon-sheathed needle (Longdwell) is now used for puncture. Some authors prefer a prone position with the affected side raised about

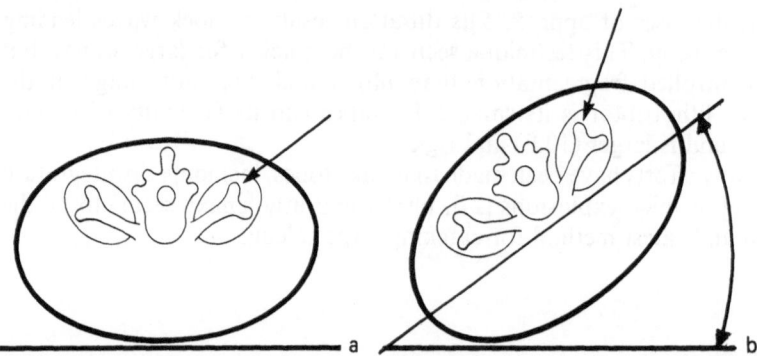

Fig. 3.1a,b. Positioning for percutaneous puncture of the renal collecting system. **a** prone position; **b** supine oblique position.

30°, so that the needle can be passed almost vertically into the collecting system (Fig. 3.1).

Correct puncture of the collecting system is one of the most important steps. In order to facilitate stone manipulation later on, the puncture channel should lead straight to the stone and without angulation to the renal pelvis.

The combination of real-time ultrasound monitoring and fluoroscopy at the same place is optimal for localization of the kidney and the stone and for insertion of the needle (Table 3.1). In our experience, a sector scanner is very useful. Intravenous contrast medium is injected for opacification of the renal collecting system. Puncture of a dilated system poses no major problems. Absence of obstruction, however, may render the procedure more difficult. Under these circumstances, intravenous contrast medium and fine needle puncture [18] are essential, particularly if real-time ultrasound is not available. Occasionally, a double needle technique may help to manage difficult cases. The renal collecting system is punctured directly from posteriorly with an 0.7-mm fine needle and constantly perfused with dilute contrast medium, while the definitive puncture for nephrostomy is done from posterolaterally. Another alternative is retrograde catheterization and contrast dye injection via the ureteral catheter.

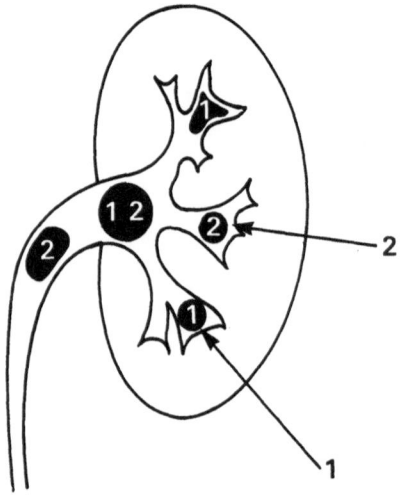

Fig. 3.2. Percutaneous access to kidney stones: stone in position *1* is reached by route *1*; stone in position *2* by route *2*.

In view of the distribution of the arterial vasculature as described by Kaye and Goldberg [19], a peripheral puncture aiming at the papilla or the fornix is advocated in order to avoid injury to major blood vessels. The posterior lower or middle calyx has proven to provide the best access to the renal collecting system (Fig. 3.2).

Ultrasound makes possible three-dimensional orientation and identification of the calyces, the stone, and the direction of the needle. Following localization of the lower posterior calyx using real-time ultrasound, the needle is advanced obliquely through the renal parenchyma. Injection of contrast medium verifies the position of the needle either within the calyx or malposition within a vein or renal parenchyma. Following correct placement, the needle is removed through the Teflon sheath, and exchanged for a J-tipped guide wire with torque control. Occasionally, a guide with a movable core may help to find the way out of the calyx through the infundibulum. Subsequently, the sheath is exchanged for a 9-F introducer which permits insertion of the coaxial rod of the telescopic bougie and a spare guide wire or ureteral catheter (Fig. 3.8).

Fig. 3.3. Teflon dilator set (Amplatz) (Cook, Europe). Metal telescopic bougies with guide rod shown in Fig. 3.5a.

Dilatation of the Track

Except for stone dissolution, manipulation of renal calculi requires dilatation of the nephrostomy track, usually to 26 F. Some authors even dilate up to 34 F [33]. Dilatation of the track can be accomplished using the following instruments:

1. Fascial dilators (Teflon of increasing calibre, maximum 26–34 F) (Cook, Europe)
2. Fascial dilators combined with introducer sheath (maximum 24–30 F) (Amplatz) (Cook, Europe) (Fig. 3.3)
3. Metal telescopic bougies (maximum 26 F) (Storz, Wolf, Olympus) (Fig. 3.5a)
4. Balloon catheters (maximum 26–30 F) (Grüntzig-type, Olbert-type) (Medi-Tech, W. Cook, Surgimed)

Teflon dilators are semiflexible and easily controlled, but may prove difficult in scar tissue. The advantage of the Amplatz set is that the nephroscope or nephrostomy tube can be placed through the introducer sheath, which is adjusted to the Teflon dilators. The Amplatz set requires dilatation greater than the size of the nephroscope. Balloon catheters are least traumatic and do not require serial passages, but may be difficult for dilatation of scar tissue. Balloon catheters are more expensive in the long run, since they cannot be reused very often.

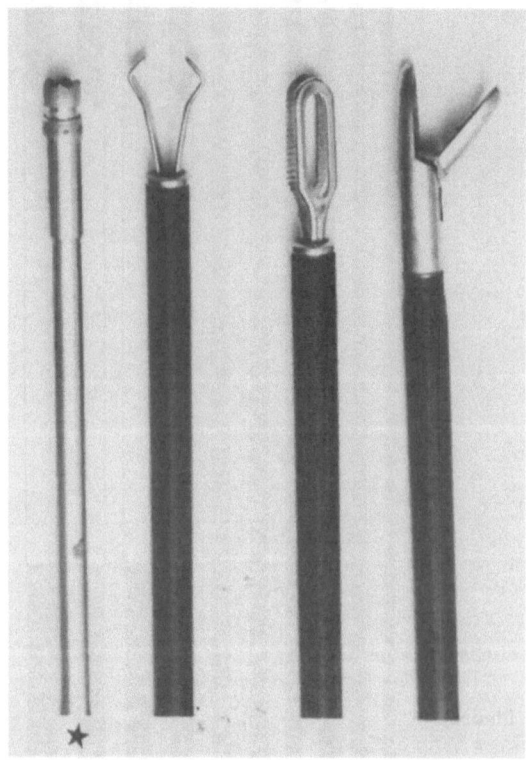

Fig. 3.4. Sonotrode (10 F) for stone crushing and various forceps for stone extraction.

We prefer the Alken metal telescopic bougies [1] (Fig. 3.5a), which are reusable and can be autoclaved. They are introduced over an axial rod or over a stiff Lunderquist guide wire which is provided with a flexible J-tip. The track is successively dilated up to a calibre of 18, 21, or 26 F depending on the diameter of the endoscope which is introduced through the last metal sheath. During dilatation, the rigid rod must be carefully observed fluoroscopically to avoid perforation. It should be noted that for the beginner a reserve guide wire or an antegrade ureteral catheter placed through the introducer sheath is advisable to ensure that the track can be reentered if it is lost during manipulation.

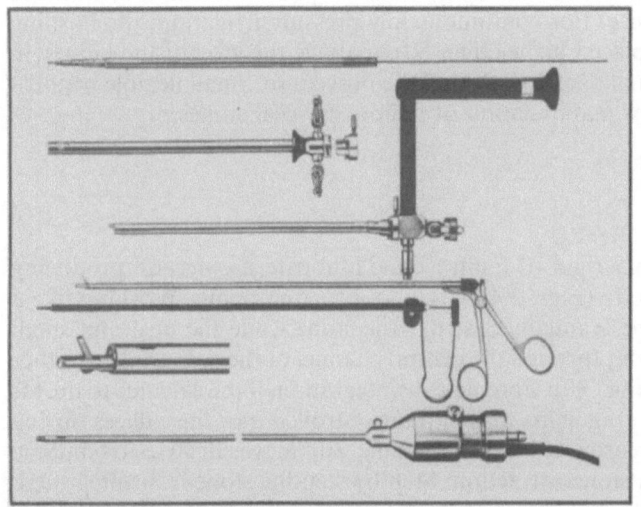

a

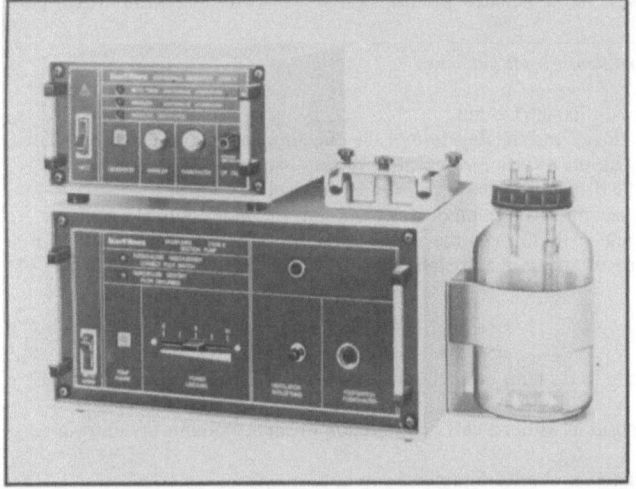

b

Fig. 3.5a,b. Assembly of instruments for percutaneous stone removal. **a** *Top to bottom*: telescopic dilators, sheath, rigid nephroscope, forceps, and ultrasound probe. **b** Ultrasound generator and suction pump. (By courtesy of Karl Storz AG)

Dilatation is usually done in one stage to 26 or even 34 F. Some authors, however, prefer a two-stage procedure: (1) the radiological insertion of a 14-F tube (Rüsch, W. Germany) and (2) urological stone removal 24 h later. A problem of the two-stage procedure may be dislocation of the nephrostomy tube.

Endoscopy

Both rigid (Storz, Wolf, Olympus) (Fig. 3.5) and flexible (Olympus, ACMI, Wolf) (Fig. 3.9c) endoscopes are available.

A rigid endoscope passed through the final metal sheath is needed for ultrasound litholapaxy since the lithotrite is not flexible. The endoscope consists of an optical system and a 5-mm instrumentation channel provided with a continuous flushing and suction device. For continuous low pressure irrigation, the flushing reservoir should not be placed higher than 80 cm above the level of the kidney in order to prevent pyelorenal backflow during the procedure. Small flexible nephroscopes (16 F) are used for manipulation of remote calyceal stones.

Stone Disintegration

The equipment consists of a rigid 10-F ultrasound lithotrite, a generator producing ultrasound of about 28 kHz (Figs. 3.4, 3.5), and a suction pump. Working like a drill, the oscillating probe gradually destroys the stone while the dust and small fragments are suctioned out through the central channel of the sonotrode together with the irrigation fluid (Fig. 3.9). Complete disintegration of the calculus to dust is not desirable since small fragments may slip uncontrolled into the calyces during the procedure. For this reason, it has proved safer and more effective to combine stone disintegration with stone extraction. Step by step the stone is disintegrated.

Table 3.1. Puncture techniques in the nondilated pyelocaliceal system (with and without real-time ultrasound guidance)

I. Combination of ultrasound und fluoroscopic guidance:
1. Obtain an IV urogram
2. Localize the kidney with real-time ultrasound
3. Check the position of the kidney and the direction of the puncture needle under fluoroscopic guidance and correlate it with the direction revealed by ultrasound
4. Advance the catheter needle (Longdwell needle 5 F) under ultrasound control
5. Check the correct needle position by injection of small amounts of dilute contrast medium
6. Insert a 1.0-mm J-tipped guide wire through the Teflon sleeve into the renal collecting system
7. Perform nephrostomy or percutaneous manipulations

II. Fluoroscopic guidance:

1. Obtain an IV urogram
2. Perform fine needle puncture (ø 0.7 mm) under fluoroscopic guidance (set as described in ref. 17)
3. Check the correct needle position within a calyx by injection of small amounts of contrast medium
4. Secure the needle tip by insertion of a 0.5-mm guide wire
5. Advance the outer cannula or Teflon sleeve (1.4 mm) into the collecting system
6. Remove the needle and insert a 1.0-mm J-tipped guide wire
7. Perform nephrostomy or percutaneous manipulations

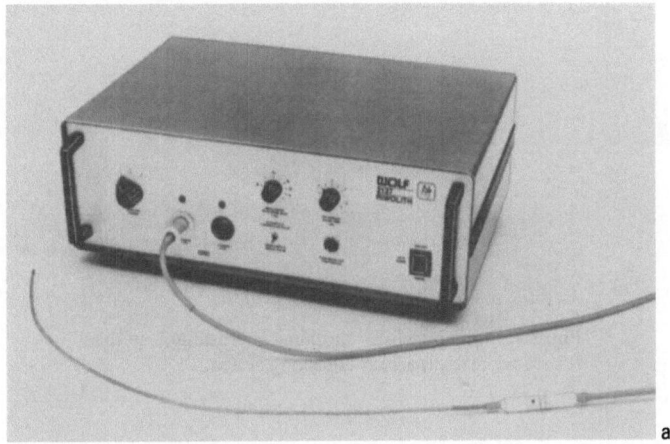

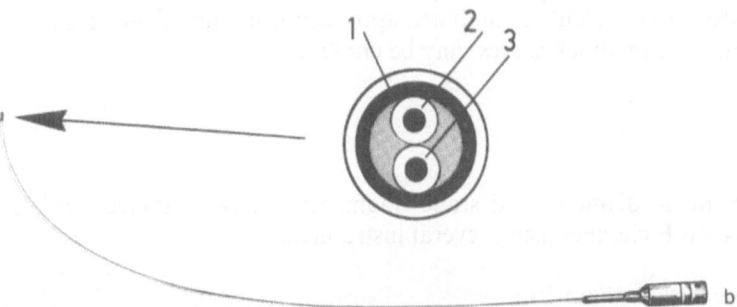

Fig. 3.6. Electrohydraulic lithotriptor comprising **a** a generator unit and **b** a flexible 5-F lithotrite probe. Cross section of the probe: *1* = insulation, *2,3* = electrodes for the electric discharge. (By courtesy of Richard Wolf GMBH)

As soon as a larger fragment breaks up, ultrasound litholapaxy is discontinued and the fragments are extracted by forceps through the shaft of the endoscope. This technique is more rapid and helps to avoid the problem of residual fragments. If no further stones are visible as verified by fluoroscopy and a plain radiograph, the nephroscope is exchanged for the telescopic dilators and a nephrostomy tube is inserted.

Electrohydraulic Litholapaxy

The equipment comprises a flexible 5-F probe and a portable generator (Wolff, Storz, Northgate-ACMI) (Fig. 3.6). At the tip of the insulated probe, which consists of two electrodes, an electric discharge produces shock waves. These are sufficiently strong to crack stones provided there is a surrounding liquid medium. Since the force of the shock wave decreases with the square of the distance, the electrode must be touching the stone.

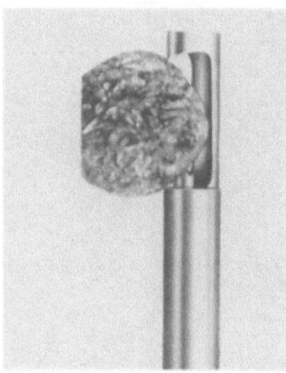

Fig. 3.7. Stone punch for mechanical crushing, suitable for stones in a capacious collecting system.

Stone Punch

Smith et al. [33] recently advocated the use of a stone punch for cracking renal calculi ranging from 1.5 to 2 cm in size (Fig. 3.7). This instrument is helpful in rare situations for stones in a large renal pelvis which offers enough space for manipulation. For larger calculi a combined approach using initial stone disintegration by ultrasound or shock waves may be chosen.

Extraction

Stones up to 8 mm in diameter and stone fragments can be extracted percutaneously via a 24–26 F channel using several instruments:

1. Dormia stone basket (4–6 wire)
2. Forceps (Randall's forceps, alligator-jaw forceps, or three-arm forceps) (Figs. 3.4, 3.8)
3. Snare

Stones in unfavorable positions in a calyx are first eased into the renal pelvis using a flexible scope, a 7-F angiographic catheter (Cordis, Cook), or a steerable catheter (Medi-Tech) aided by saline injection and then extracted. Stone dislocation may also be performed with the aid of a balloon catheter. As a final resort, Fernström and Johansson recommend percutaneous stone harpooning by a fine needle (ø 0.7 mm) in order to push the calculus into the renal pelvis [14]. Calyceal stones which are readily accessible in the lower posterior calyx or middle calyx are approached via the same calyx by direct puncture and are removed directly.

Selection of Patients

As in every therapeutic modality of stone treatment, the aims of percutaneous stone manipulation are the complete clearance of stones and a minimum of complications. There are two different aspects in patient selection: (1) the degree of

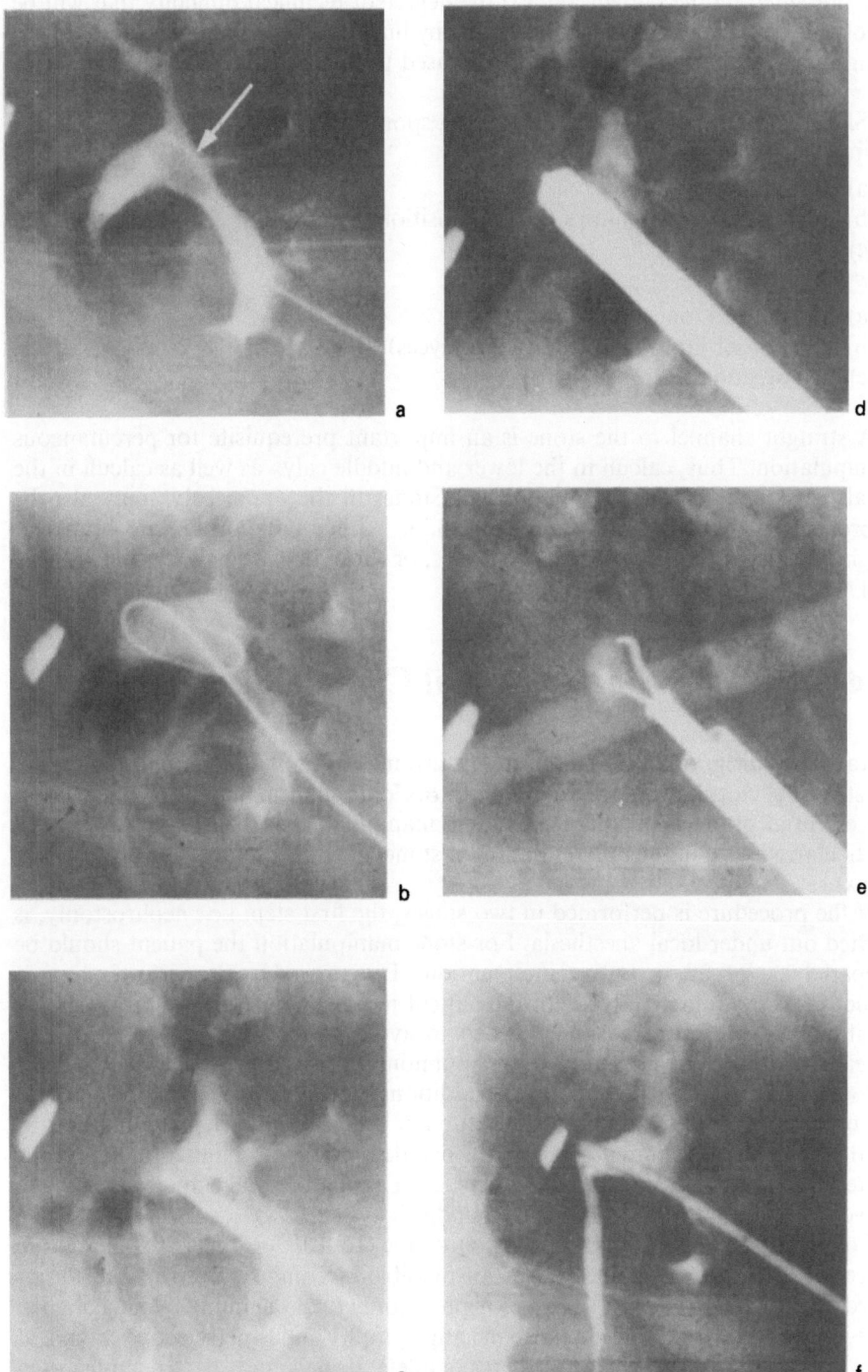

Fig. 3.8a–f. Percutaneous stone extraction. **a** puncture of the renal collecting system; **b** insertion of a J-tipped guide wire; **c** needle sheath exchanged for an introducer sheath (7 F) which permits insertion of the guide rod; **d** dilatation using telescopic bougies; **e** extraction of the stone; **f** nephrostogram following successful removal.

risk presented by the patient and (2) the degree of technical difficulty that will be involved. Problematic cases are presented by uncooperative patients or those with a high operative risk. The causes of increased technical difficulties may be:

1. Skeletal abnormalities (e.g., ankylosing spondylitis or gibbus)
2. The renal anatomy
   a) absence of dilatation
   b) congenital abnormalities (fusion, position, rotation)
   c) cysts
3. Calculi
   a) number of stones
   b) position of multiple stones (e.g., calyces)
   c) size of stones

A straight channel to the stone is an important prerequisite for percutaneous manipulation. Thus, calculi in the lower and middle calyx as well as calculi in the renal pelvis are best suited for removal. Stones in the upper calyx may also be approached via the inferior calyx (Fig. 3.2). Rather unfavorable are branched staghorn calculi, multiple peripheral stones, or those in extremely mobile kidneys [22].

Preparation and Postprocedural Care

Intravenous urogram and tomogram, ultrasound (CT only in complicated cases), chest X-ray, clotting screen, usual laboratory data, and matching of blood units are essential prior to percutaneous stone manipulation. Ultrasound has proved particularly useful in the differentiation of stone localization (anterior or posterior calyx).

If the procedure is performed in two stages, the first step, i.e., nephrostomy, is carried out under local anesthesia. For stone manipulation the patient should be prepared as for an operative intervention. The procedure is performed on a standard uroradiologic table with the patient in a prone or slightly raised supine position. A waterproof cover is needed to avoid cooling of the patient due to repeated flushing. In patients without pulmonary disease or renal insufficiency, 20% mannitol (1–2 ml per min) and additional intravenous fluids are given to increase urine production and prevent tubular reflux during the manipulation. A urethral catheter is required to empty the bladder of irrigation fluid drained via the ureter. Some authors prefer retrograde placement of a ureteral catheter in order to prevent stone fragments from being dislodged.

Following the procedure a nephrostomy tube (14–18 F) is reinserted and left in place for 2–4 days to enable control of possible bleeding or obstruction. Major bleeding may be managed by a larger nephrostomy tube or simply by plugging the tube. If gross persistent bleeding occurs, angiography and superselective embolization is the method of choice. When complete stone removal is demonstrated radiographically and free urinary flow is seen on the nephrostogram, the tube can be removed. In the immediate postprocedural period spasmolytics may be administered if necessary. Trimethoprim-sulfonamide is given for 2 weeks and the urine kept at a specific weight of 1010.

Contraindications

Patients with bleeding disorders and poorly controlled hypertension should be excluded from percutaneous nephrostomy and stone manipulation. Urinary infection is not considered a contraindication when adequate antibiotic treatment is administered. In stone obstruction complicated by infection, the kidney is decompressed by nephrostomy and antibacterial treatment is started prior to dilatation and stone disintegration.

Indications

Kidney Stones

The procedure is especially helpful for high risk patients and for those with multiple previous stone operations, as originally advocated by Alken et al. [2, 3]. Postoperative scar tissue does not prevent percutaneous manipulation. Apart from these indications, shortening of this method into a one-stage procedure without an increase in morbidity [38] has rendered it an attractive alternative to open surgery for a number of other patients who have had no previous operations or do not constitute a high risk. Thus, candidates considered for percutaneous stone manipulation are those with stones in an ideal position for extraction and litholapaxy independent of the patient's general condition. This obviates the need for operation to a considerable extent. Surgery is restricted to difficult stones such as branched staghorn calculi moulding the collecting system or multiple calyceal stones.

The decision as to whether a kidney stone should be dissolved, extracted, or fragmented depends on its size and composition. Our policy is: small stones are extracted (Fig. 3.8); for large stones a combined approach of ultrasound disintegration and extraction of the larger fragments is chosen (Fig. 3.9).

In principle, dissolution by direct irrigation is applicable for cystine or struvite calculi, or for obstructing urate stones. However, since dissolution may take as long as 10–30 days, disintegration and/or extraction are more advantageous.

Ureteral Stones

A definitive and generally accepted concept in the percutaneous management of ureteral stones has not yet been found. Ureteral stones are accessible via the retrograde transurethral or transrenal approach. Distal ureteral stones are still the domain of retrograde management if they do not pass spontaneously. Treatment of proximal ureteral stones may be attempted percutaneously, although this does not seem as effective as with kidney stones [8].

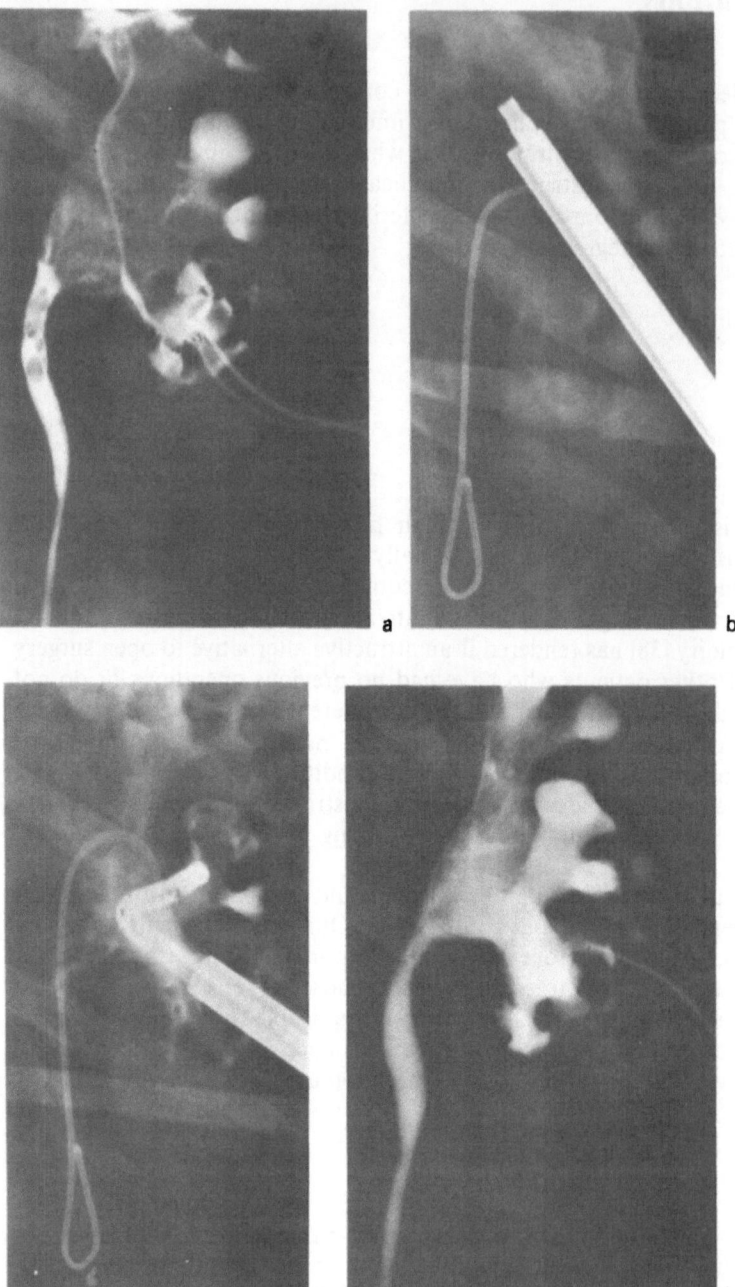

Fig. 3.9a–d. Ultrasound litholapaxy in a radiolucent staghorn calculus and ureteral stones (anuric patient due to bilateral stones). **a** emergency nephrostomy; **b** nephroscope sheath and tip of the ultrasound probe; loop introduced for removal of ureteral stones; **c** flexible nephroscope for removal of residual stones in a calyx following litholapaxy; **d** nephrostogram following successful stone manipulation completed in three sessions.

Results

Percutaneous stone manipulation is still in its infancy but has gained increasing popularity within the past few years [8, 12, 14, 20, 22, 23, 32, 38]. From 1977 to 1983 (Fig. 3.10) 200 kidneys were treated at the Urological Department of Mainz University; ultrasound disintegration was used in 112, electrohydraulic lithotripsy in 5, chemolysis in 20, and stone extraction in 53 alone or in combination. In the 200 kidneys, there were only 19 preexisting nephrostomies.

Percutaneous nephrostomy was feasible in 98%, although the majority of patients had a nondilated pyelocaliceal system. Stone removal was incomplete in 13 of 181 with percutaneous nephrostomy and in 9 of 19 with preexisting operative nephrostomy. In two instances surgical intervention was required because of residual stones. The better results in the percutaneous group may be attributed to the free choice of routes of access to the collecting system.

Similar results of percutaneous litholapaxy were obtained by other authors reporting on successful stone removal rates ranging from 71% to 89% [8, 12, 22, 32, 38]. The failure rate is subject to patient selection and technique; in particular, inappropriate course of the nephrostomy track, unfavorable stone position, or large stones not allowing insertion of the tube may be the reasons for failure. There has been no mortality in our series nor in the literature, and no kidney has been lost due to the procedure.

The average time required for the procedure, as measured in 105 patients in whom a one-stage procedure was attempted, was 75 min for extraction and 111 min for ultrasound disintegration. The hospital stay averaged 7–12 days depending on the necessary number of sessions for complete removal.

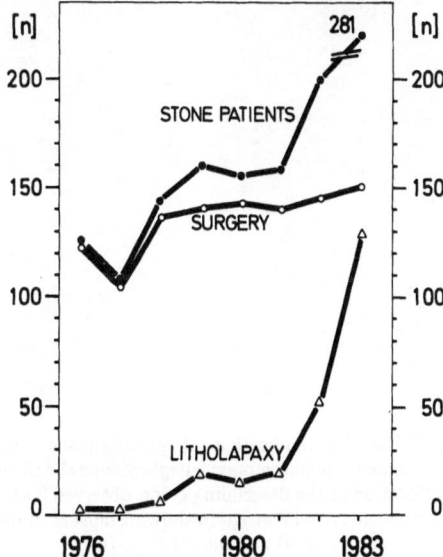

Fig. 3.10. Frequency of operative stone removal and percutaneous litholapaxy at the Department of Urology of Mainz University from 1976 to 1983.

Complications

Potential complications are bleeding, extravasation, and lesions of adjacent organs. In our series minor side-effects were encountered in nine patients: bleeding in six, catheter breakage and extravasation in one each, and an acute bout of pyelonephritis in one. Three major complications occurred: (1) perforation of the descending colon which became evident 2 days after the procedure and which was managed percutaneously by additional drainage of the colon (Fig. 3.11), (2) major persistent arterial bleeding which was eventually treated by selective transcatheter embolization, and (3) development of a uteropelvic junction stenosis following inadvertent dilatation of the proximal ureter up to 26 F. This complication had to

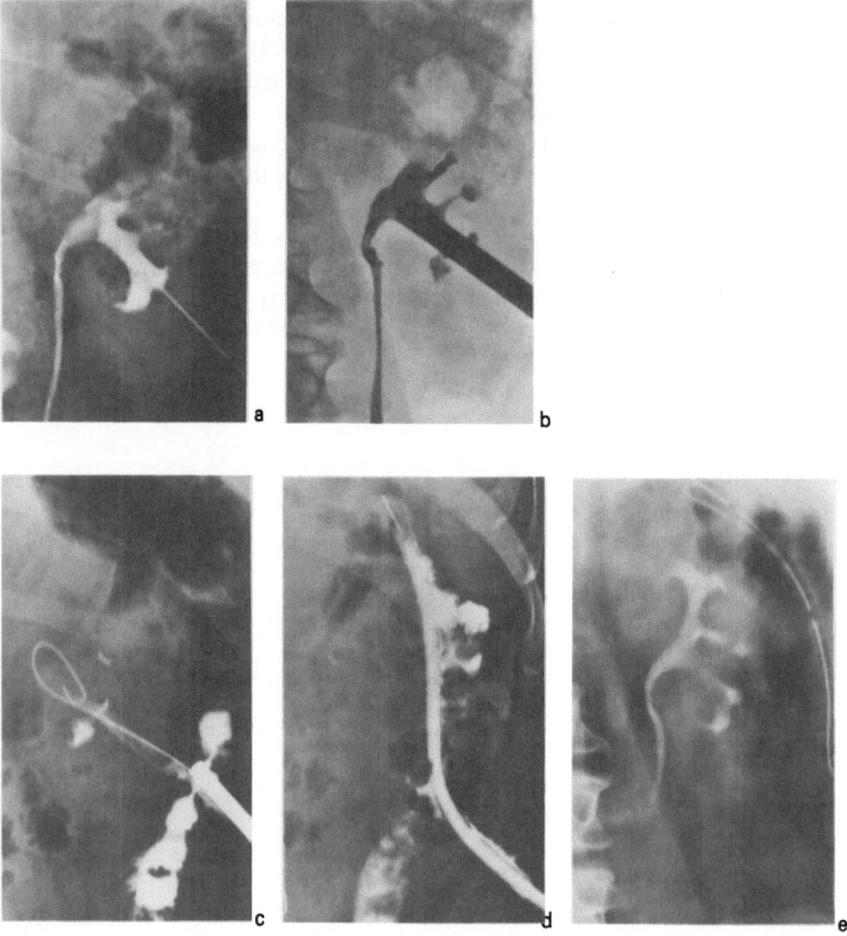

Fig. 3.11a–e. Complication of percutaneous stone extraction and percutaneous management. **a** percutaneous nephrostomy; **b** nephroscope sheath and guide wire following successful stone removal; **c** perforation of the descending colon observed 2 days after the procedure; **d** percutaneous colostomy for management; **e** IV urogram showing closure of the nephrostomy track; subsequently the colostomy catheter was removed and the fistula closed.

be corrected operatively later on. No deaths occurred. Minimal complications requiring no operative interventions have been reported by others [22, 38].

Percutaneous Stone Manipulation Versus Extracorporeal Shock Wave Lithotripsy (ESWL)

Very soon after the first clinical series of percutaneous stone manipulation, modern technology has made possible the extracorporeal treatment of stones by focused electrohydraulic shock waves [6]. This procedure is performed under peridural or general anesthesia with the patient positioned in a waterbath. Kidney stones can be fragmented provided they are radiopaque and there is no infection. Outflow obstruction hindering the stone particles from passing spontaneously must be ruled out.

This method will certainly reduce the indications for open surgery and percutaneous stone manipulation in a great number of patients. The major drawback of extracorporeal shock wave therapy is the expense of the equipment, which will limit it to large centers. More than 800 patients have been treated so far [7]. The high success rate is partially due to the fact that these patients were highly selected, e.g., complete staghorn calculi have not yet been treated. Nevertheless, it may well be that a combined percutaneous and extracorporeal procedure will lead to an exclusively nonoperative approach to renal calculi. On the other hand, if stone surgery should be necessary, ESWL may be a useful adjunct to the treatment of residual calculi.

Percutaneous litholapaxy prior to ESWL may be helpful in complicated stones, e.g., staghorn calculi, where the large mass of the stone is removed percutaneously and the remainder is disintegrated by ESWL (Fig. 3.12).

Conclusion

Percutaneous extraction and fragmentation of kidney stones performed as a single-stage or two-stage procedure is an effective and attractive alternative to open surgery. Its advantage is a significantly lower morbidity, a shorter hospital stay, and a short period of convalescence. Thus, surgery will be restricted to complicated stones. With the advent of extracorporeal shock wave therapy, the percutaneous approach has partly lost its attraction for those centers which can afford this equipment. Nevertheless, there are still some indications for the percutaneous approach, which is the method of second choice as compared with extracorporeal therapy.

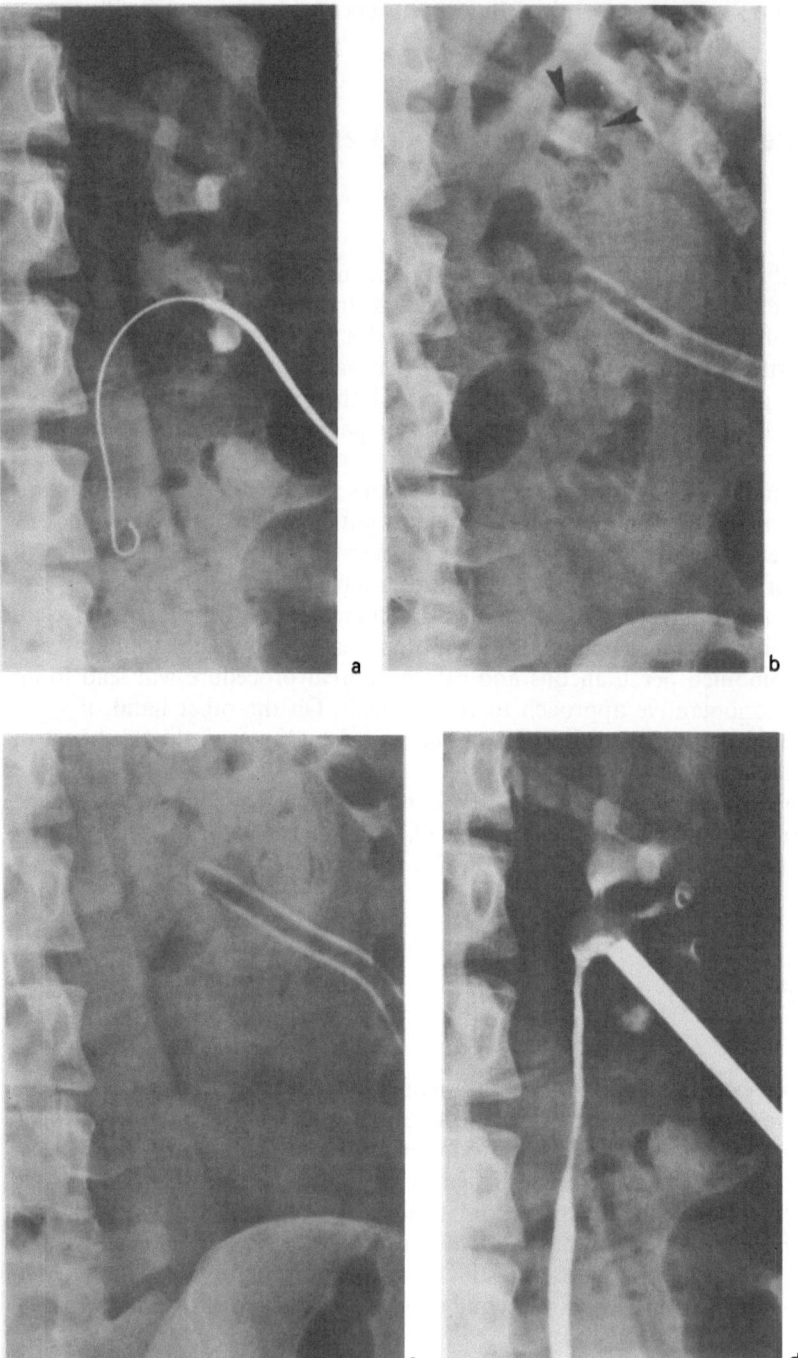

Fig. 3.12a–d. Combination of percutaneous lithotripsy and extracorporeal shockwave lithotripsy (ESWL). **a** Percutaneous nephrostomy showing radiopaque stone. **b, c** Percutaneous stone manipulation and removal of the pelvic stone. Primary ESWL was not indicated because of obstruction. **d** Following removal of the obstructing pelvic stone the calyceal stone was disintegrated by ESWL.

References

1. Alken P (1981) Teleskopbougierset zur perkutanen Nephrostomie. Akt Urol 12:216–219
2. Alken P, Altwein JE (1980) Die perkutane Nephrolitholapaxie. Verh Dtsch Ges Urol 31:109–112
3. Alken P, Hutschenreiter G, Günther R, Marberger M (1981) Percutaneous stone manipulation. J Urol 125:463–466
4. Alken P, Hutschenreiter G, Günther R (1982) Percutaneous kidney stone removal. Eur Urol 8:304–311
5. Alken P, Günther R, Thüroff J (1983) Percutaneous nephrolithotomy—A routine procedure? Br J Urol (Suppl): 1–5
6. Chaussy C, Schmiedt E, Jochan D, Brendel W, Forssmann B, Walther V (1982) First clinical experience with extracorporeally induced destruction of kidney stones by shock waves. J Urol 127:417–420
7. Chaussy C, Schmiedt E, Jochan D, Schüller J, Brendel H (1984) Extrakorporale Stoßwellen Lithotripsie—Beginn einer Umstrukturierung in der Behandlung des Harnsteinleidens. Urologe [Ausg A] 23:25–29
8. Clayman RV, Miller RP, Surya V, Castaneda-Zuniga WR, Smith AD, Amplatz K, Lange PH (1983) Nephrostolithotomy: Percutaneous removal of renal and ureteric calculi. Br J Urol (Suppl) 6–10
9. Coleman CC, Castaneda-Zuniga W, Miller R (1984) Logical approach to renal stone removal. Am J. Roentgenol 143:609–614
10. Coats EC (1956) The application of ultrasonic energy to urinary and biliary calculi. J Urol 75:865–870
11. Fair DF (1978) In vivo destruction of urinary calculi by laser induced stress waves. Med Instrum 12: 100–106
12. Fernström I (1983) Percutaneous extraction of renal calculi: Technique and results. Br J Urol (Suppl): 25–36
13. Fernström I, Johansson B (1976) Percutaneous pyelolithotomy. A new extraction technique. Scand J Urol Nephrol 10:257–259
14. Fernström I, Johansson B (1982) Percutaneous extraction of renal calculi. Front Eur Radiol 1:1–24
15. Gasteyer KH (1971) Eine neue Methode der Blasensteinzertrümmerung: Die Ultraschall-Lithotripsie. Urologe [Ausg A] 10:30–32
16. Goodwin WE, Casey WC, Woolf W (1955) Percutaneous trocar (needle) nephrostomy in hydronephrosis. JAMA 157:891–894
17. Günther R, Alken P, Altwein JE (1978) Perkutane Nephropyelostomy—Anwendungsmöglichkeiten und Ergebnisse. RöFo 128:720–726
18. Günther R, Alken P, Altwein JE (1979) Percutaneous nephropyelostomy using a fine-needle puncture set. Radiology 132:228–230
19. Kaye KW, Goldberg ME (1982) Applied anatomy of the kidney and ureter. Urol Clin Am 9:3–13
20. Korth K (1983) A new percutaneous pyeloscope with permanent irrigation. Br J Urol (Suppl): 31–33
21. Kurth KH, Hohenfellner R, Altwein JE (1977) Ultrasound litholapaxy of a staghorn calculus. J Urol 117:242–243
22. Marberger M (1983) Ultrasonic lithotripsy of renal calculi: A 3-year experience. Br J Urol (Suppl): 41–50
23. Miller RA, Wickham JEA, Kellett MJ (1983) Percutaneous destruction of renal calculi: Clinical and laboratory experience. Br J Urol (Suppl): 51–54
24. Mulvaney WD (1953) Attempted disintegration of calculi by ultrasonic vibrations. J Urol 70:704–706
25. Newhouse JR, Pfister RC (1981) Therapy for renal calculi via percutaneous nephrostomy: dissolution and extraction. Urol Radiol 2:157–164
26. Pensel J, Frank F, Rothenberger K, Hofstetter A, Unsöld E (1981) Destruction of urinary calculi by Neodym-Yag laser irradiation. Proc 4th Intern Soc Laser Surg, p 10, Tokyo
27. Raney AM, Handler J (1975) Electrohydraulic nephrolithotomy. Urology 6:439–446
28. Rathert P, Stumpff U, Pohlmann R, Lutzeyer W (1977) Ultraschall-Lithotripsie von Ureter- und Nierensteinen: experimentelle und erste klinische Untersuchungen. Verh Dtsch Ges Urol 28:365–369
29. Reuter HJ (1970) Electronic lithotripsy. Transurethral treatment of bladder stones in 50 cases. J.Urol 104:834–838

30. Rupel E, Brown R (1941) Nephroscopy with removal of stone following nephrostomy for obstructive calculous anuria J Urol 45:177–182
31. Sachse H (1970) Erfahrungen mit der Elektrolithotripsie. Verh Dtsch Ges Urol 23:171–173
32. Segura JW, Patterson DE, Le Roy AJ, McGough PF, Barrett DM (1982) Percutaneous removal of kidney stones. Preliminary report. Mayo Clin Proc 57:615–619
33. Smith AD, Clayman RV, Castaneda-Zuniga WR (1982) Use of Mauermeyer stone punch via percutaneous nephrostomy. J Urol 128:1285–1286
34. Terhorst B, Lutzeyer W, Cichos M, Pohlmann R (1972) Die Zerstörung von Harnsteinen durch Ultraschall. II. Ultraschall-Lithotripsie von Blasensteinen. Urol Int 27:458–467
35. Terhorst B, Cichos M, Versin F, Buss H (1975) Der Einfluss von elektrohydraulischer Schlagwelle und Ultraschall auf das Uroepithel. Urologe [Ausg A] 14:41–45
36. Walz PH, Riedmiller H. Alken P, Hutschenreiter G (1981) Technik und Fehlermöglichkeiten der perkutanen Nephrostomie unter sonographischer Kontrolle. Akt Urol 12:232–237
37. Watanabe H, Watanabe K, Shiino K, Oinuma S (1983) Micro-explosion cystolithotripsy. J Urol 129:23–28
38. Wickham JEA, Kellett MJ, Miller RA (1981) Elective percutaneous nephrolithotomy in 50 patients: an analysis of the technique, results and complications. Br J Urol 53: 297–299

Chapter 4

Percutaneous Approach to Urinary Tract Calculi

N. Reed Dunnick

Introduction

Urinary tract calculi are a major cause of morbidity and mortality, as they are responsible for over 7 out of every 1000 general hospital admissions. In certain areas of the United States, particularly the southeast, this rate of hospital admission for stone disease more than doubles [11]. Stones predispose to urinary tract infection by causing obstruction and stasis, and by providing a nidus which may harbor bacteria. In addition, infection of the urinary tract by urea splitting bacteria induces struvite stone formation by making the urine more alkaline, which results in the precipitation of magnesium ammonium phosphate and calcium apatite. Stones are also associated with an increased incidence of squamous cell carcinomas of the urinary tract.

Although many small stones may be passed spontaneously with the help of hydration and analgesia, the definitive therapy for renal stones has been surgical. However, surgery usually requires 1–2 weeks of hospitalization followed by a convalescence ranging from 4 to 8 weeks. Furthermore, not all patients with symptomatic renal stones are appropriate surgical candidates. Thus, the development of percutaneous techniques for removal of urinary tract calculi has been greeted with enthusiasm by internists, urologists, and radiologists. These techniques have proven to be effective methods of therapy as in most cases the entire renal stone can be removed through the nephrostomy tract. Many of the problems of surgery are avoided and the patient may return to normal activities within 7–10 days of the procedure. This chapter reviews the percutaneous approach to urinary tract stone disease, including perioperative assessment of the patient, technical details of stone manipulation, and an assessment of the results.

Patient Assessment

The percutaneous approach is one method of removing urinary tract calculi. Patients referred for this procedure should be those patients in whom surgery would otherwise be considered. For the most part, such patients will be symptomatic with pain, hematuria, or recurrent urinary tract infections. With percutaneous techniques, the patient does not necessarily have to undergo general anesthesia, nor must the patient be an adequate surgical candidate; however, complications of the procedure may arise in which surgery is necessary, and this must be considered before embarking upon the procedure.

Since the percutaneous nephrostomy is an invasive procedure, and blood vessels as well as fascial planes will be traversed, the patient must have normal bleeding parameters. We routinely obtain a complete blood count as well as measure the prothrombin and partial thromboplastin times as screening laboratory studies for a bleeding diathesis. If these parameters are abnormal or if there is a history of unusual bleeding or a tendency to hemorrhage, a hematology consultation should be obtained. A careful history of contrast and drug allergy or intolerance must also be obtained. Approximately 5% of patients will exhibit an adverse reaction to intravenous contrast material [18], and a variety of medication and analgesics may be required before, during, or after the procedure. Evidence of urinary tract infection should be sought by urinalysis and culture, if indicated. We prefer to treat patients with active infections with appropriate antibiotics to clear the infection before performing a percutaneous nephrostomy. In patients with urinary tract sepsis and an obstructing stone, nevertheless, a percutaneous nephrostomy may be indicated to drain an infected collecting system. In all patients, however, the infection must be controlled before further manipulations are attempted.

A good quality urogram with oblique projections or tomograms of the collecting system is essential to assess the presence, location, and route of access for stone removal. Stones in the renal pelvis can almost always be successfully removed regardless of the access route. Stones in an infundibulum or calyx, however, must be approached either directly with the nephrostomy placed through the calyx which contains the stone, or through an infundibulum which will allow manipulation of the catheter, stone basket, or forceps into the calyx containing the stone. Stones in upper pole calyces or kidneys which are relatively cephalad in location are the most difficult, as the rib cage, pleural sulcus, liver, and spleen restrict the location of the percutaneous nephrostomy tract. The position of the liver and spleen should also be noted, and if there is any question about their location from the abdominal radiographs, additional studies such as computed tomography (CT) can be obtained.

Previous surgery makes the approach to these patients more difficult. There may be extensive scarring around the kidney which makes passage of the needle, fascial dilators, and catheters more difficult. Furthermore, these adhesions may restrict motion of the kidney such that manipulation with rigid instruments is more hazardous. However, the operative approach to these patients is also significantly compromised and it is this group of patients who may be best served by the percutaneous approach. Prior abdominal operations may also have resulted in alterations in normal anatomy such as an incisional hernia in which bowel may be interposed along the nephrostomy tract.

Finally, a thorough discussion with the patient of the procedure and its goals is essential. Since only the final nephrostomy tract dilatation and stone removal are routinely performed under general anesthesia, patient cooperation is mandatory. Despite large amounts of parenteral analgesia, many portions of the percutaneous nephrostomy as well as subsequent tube checks and catheter manipulations may be painful, and it is important for the patient to understand the necessity for these procedures and the part each plays in the overall process [20]. A discussion of the position of the nephrostomy catheters and the difficulty in placing them if their position is lost will ensure optimal patient cooperation in caring for the tubes. These percutaneous procedures are physician intensive, for both the radiologist and the urologist, and they require a high degree of patient understanding and cooperation. Nevertheless, the success rate has been high [8, 13, 17], and those patients who have undergone both an open surgical procedure for stone removal as well as a percutaneous stone manipulation have uniformly preferred the percutaneous procedure [20].

Placement of the Percutaneous Nephrostomy

After careful examination of the intravenous pyelogram, the number and location of the urinary calculi are assessed. Occasionally, additional studies such as computed tomography may be required for better appreciation of the renal or perirenal anatomy. The percutaneous nephrostomy must be placed through a track which will allow access to the stone and avoids adjacent organs including bowel, liver, spleen, and pleura. It is preferable to enter below the 12th rib, but in some patients an entry site between the 11th and 12th ribs may be required, particularly when access to the upper pole collecting system is necessary [14]. This, however, will restrict the mobility of the manipulating tools, particularly if rigid instruments are used.

Once the proposed route has been determined, the collecting system must be opacified to provide a target for the percutaneous needle puncture. Several methods are available to provide opacification including: (1) intravenous contrast injection with normal renal excretion; (2) retrograde injection into a ureteral stent catheter placed by a urologist; and (3) an antegrade pyelogram. Each of these methods has obvious advantages and disadvantages and the choice will vary with individual patients and anatomic problems. In general, we prefer to perform an antegrade pyelogram with a 22-gauge thin needle. This frequently can be done using the radiopaque stone as a landmark and entering the renal pelvis adjacent to the stone. In such cases the patient is placed in a prone position and the 22-gauge fine needle passed percutaneously from a posterior position directly into the renal pelvis. This usually requires a depth of 10–12 cm at which time the needle tip can be seen to move with the renal stone. If biplane fluoroscopy is available, the relationship of the stone and needle tip can be determined in two planes, which is a further aid in precise needle placement. The stylet of the needle is removed and gentle suction applied via venotubing.

If there is no return of urine, the needle is slowly withdrawn until urine flow is identified. It is best to withdraw only a small amount of urine through this needle to prevent collapse of the collecting system which may oppose the opposite wall of the pelvis or infundibulum against the needle, making passage of the guide wire

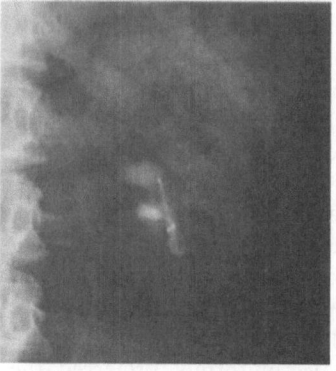 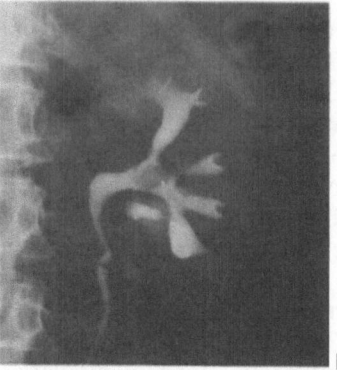

a   b

Fig. 4.1. a Intravenous injection of 50 cc of contrast material only faintly opacifies the collecting system. **b** Injection of contrast through the 3-F dilator densely opacifies and mildly distends the collecting system.

more likely to perforate into the perirenal space. Although this same needle may be used to inject contrast material and opacify the collecting system, we prefer to pass a 0.018-in. guide wire into the collecting system, remove the needle, and then follow the guide wire with a 3-F multi side hole dilator. After removal of the guide wire, this dilator can be taped to the skin and used for repeated injections of contrast material to opacify the collecting system for placement of the nephrostomy catheter (Fig. 4.1). The dilator enables movement of the patient without the danger of laceration of the collecting system or dislodgement of the needle [3].

Placement of a ureteral stent by a member of the urology team accomplishes a similar goal, as contrast can be injected into the stent catheter to opacify the collecting system and provide a dense target for the permanent nephrostomy catheter placement (Fig. 4.2). An additional advantage of this procedure is that there is no bleeding into the collecting system and this precludes possible confusion in predicting the location of the needle or catheter when fluid is withdrawn. This does, however, require cystoscopy, and in most cases we have not found this necessary.

The simplest method for providing opacification of the collecting system is intravenous injection of contrast material. This relies on normal renal function for contrast excretion. The disadvantages of this method are the less than optimal opacification of the collecting system and the absence of the augmented dilatation which can be accomplished by the direct injection techniques. Occasionally, the technique of antegrade pyelography may be combined with intravenous contrast injection.

Once the target is well opacified and the route of the percutaneous nephrostomy has been determined, the patient is positioned to optimize the nephrostomy placement. This is usually a prone oblique position with elevation of the kidney to be manipulated. A supine oblique position which allows entry from a lateral access can also be used. This improves the ability of the operator to manipulate needle, guide wire, and catheter under direct fluoroscopic vision while maintaining his/her hands out of the fluoroscopic field. However, the direction of the fine needle is usually more difficult to control with this horizontal approach than with a perpendicular approach.

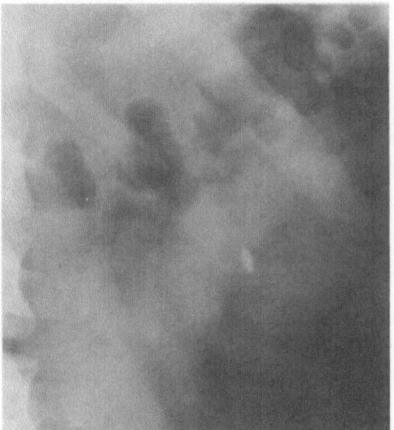
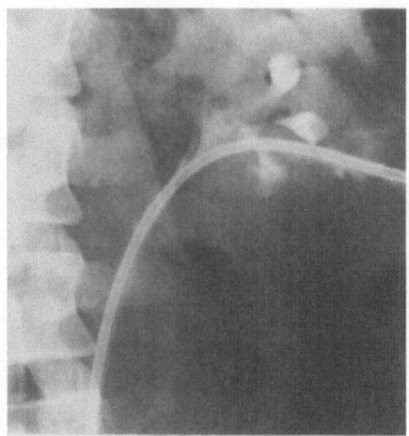
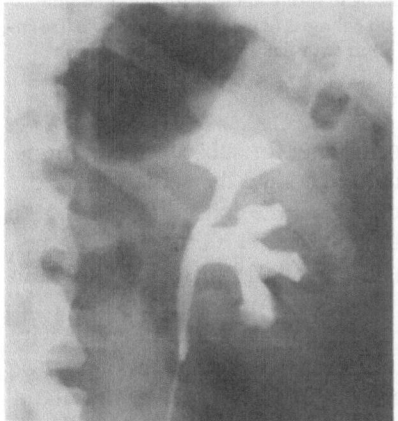

Fig. 4.2. a A 9-mm stone is present in the left lower pole infundibulum. b A ureteral stent, passed cystoscopically, provides a route for direct opacification and mild distension of the collecting system which aids in performing the percutaneous nephrostomy. c The nephrostomy track has been dilated to accommodate a 10-F catheter which enters the collecting system adjacent to the stone and passes down the ureter.

Local anesthesia is used liberally. After infiltrating the skin and subcutaneous tissues with 0.5% bupivacaine, a 3.5-in. needle is used to infiltrate fascial planes toward the kidney. A small incision is made in the skin which will allow manipulation of dilators up to 11 F without constriction by the skin or subcutaneous fascia. The initial puncture of the collecting system along the nephrostomy catheter tract may be made with a variety of needles. We generally prefer to use the smaller 21- or 22-gauge needles as this allows several passes with only minimal renal damage or bleeding. Larger needles are easier to direct and allow passage of a larger guide wire which will result in fewer dilator and catheter manipulations. In some instances this may be the least traumatic method of accomplishing the percutaneous nephrostomy.

The fine needle is passed into the appropriate calyx or infundibulum under fluoroscopic guidance, and once the tip of the needle is seen to be within the collecting system, the stylet is withdrawn and venotubing attached for gentle aspiration. This is the same technique used in performing the initial antegrade pyelogram. When urine is seen in the venotubing, a 0.018-in. guide wire is passed through the needle into the collecting system. If this wire can be maneuvered down

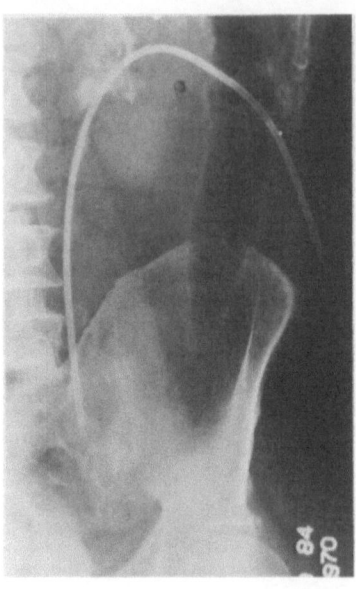

Fig. 4.3. A straight 10-F catheter with multiple side holes and a tip enlarged to accommodate two 0.038-in. guide wires is left with the tip of the catheter in the mid ureter.

the ureter, it will provide much more secure positioning for subsequent dilations. However, it will not always pass down the ureter and coiling the guide wire in the renal pelvis may suffice. With the 0.018-in. guide wire in the collecting system, the 6.3-F Cope system (Cope Catheter Introduction System, #70653A, Cook Inc., Bloomington, IN 47402) may be used to convert this 0.018-in. guide wire to a 0.038-in. guide wire. This system requires that the 6.3-F Cope catheter follow the 0.018-in. guide wire without dislodging the wire, and that the 0.038-in. guide wire pass out the larger side hole. Despite recommendations of the manufacturer, we have not always found this to be the case. We have thus developed a 4/6 dilator system which can be used if this problem ensues [4]. This consists of a 6-F dilator mounted on a longer 4-F dilator (JCD4.0-25-25 SET SYSTEM, VSVSS-4.0-21 SET SYSTEM, Cook Inc., Bloomington, IN 47402). This pair is passed in tandom over the 0.018-in. guide wire and once the collecting system is reached by the 6-F dilator, both the guide wire and the 4-F dilator are removed. The 6-F dilator allows passage of the 0.038-in. guide wire, which can then be used to secure passage of larger dilators. It is still preferable to have the dilator passed down the ureter for more secure positioning, and the use of a steerable angiographic catheter (such as a Cobra configuration) may be useful in this situation.

Once a secure position has been attained, preferably with a 0.038-in. heavy duty or "coathanger" guide wire down the ureter, a series of dilators may be used to enlarge the track to accommodate a 10-F catheter. We routinely enlarge the track using 7-, 9-, and 11-F fascial dilators. At this point, a modified 10-F straight 40-cm catheter with multiple side holes is passed over the guide wire and approximately half-way down the ureter (Fig. 4.3). This catheter has been modified such that the tip of the catheter is tapered to accommodate two 0.038-in. guide wires, and is available commercially (VA10.0-68-40-P-305-FORD-051783, Cook Inc., Bloomington, Indiana 47402). This is extremely important as it will allow the immediate passage of a safety guide wire before subsequent intraoperative dilations and catheter manipulations are performed.

Stone Manipulation

The nephrostomy track must be dilated to a size large enough to remove the stone or allow passage of the nephroscope which will accommodate the ultrasonic lithotrite. In view of the painful nature of the track dilatation as well as the subsequent manipulations for stone removal, we routinely perform this portion of the procedure in the operating room with the patient under general anesthesia. The patient may be brought to the operating room immediately after placement of the percutaneous nephrostomy, later the same day, or on the day after the placement of the nephrostomy tract. If the stones to be removed are relatively small or if the patient has tolerated the initial placement well, this procedure can be performed with only local anesthesia supplemented with analgesia. Although polyethylene tapered-tip fascial dilators [15] and the use of a balloon catheter [9] have been recommended for tract dilatation, we prefer to use the concentric stainless steel dilators with fluoroscopic guidance, particularly on those patients who have had previous renal surgery.

The initial step in this procedure is to pass two angiographic guide wires down the 10-F ureteral catheter and into the bladder. One of these guide wires is then fixed to the patient's skin, placed under a surgical drape, and kept in reserve as a safety wire to be used only if the working wire is dislodged. With a series of concentric stainless steel dilators passed over the working wire, the track is dilated to 24 F, which will then accommodate the nephroscope (Fig. 4.4). The ultrasonic lithotrite is passed through the nephroscope and the irrigating solution tubing attached to the nephroscope to remove blood and stone fragments. After irrigation removes the blood and blood clot, the safety wire can be identified through the nephroscope, and the renal pelvis and ureteropelvic junction located for orientation. If there is a large amount of bleeding, vision may be impaired; however, the continuous irrigation through the nephroscope should soon clear the blood and enable adequate vision to identify the stone. The lithotrite is then brought into contact with the stone and the dissolution process begun. The length of this process will depend upon the size and hardness of the stone, but usually can be

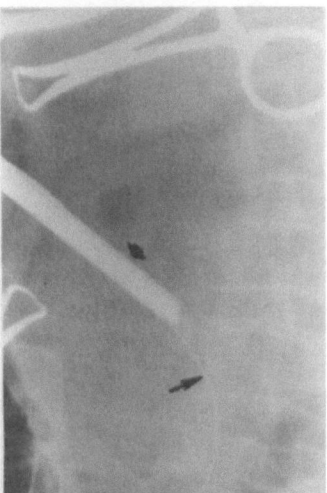

Fig. 4.4. The nephrostomy track has been dilated with concentric stainless steel dilators up to 24 F, which will accommodate the nephroscope (*arrowhead*). The safety wire remains in position (*arrow*) through the nephrostomy track and down the ureter.

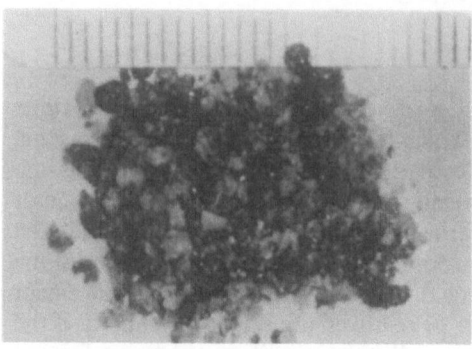

Fig. 4.5. Tiny stone fragments are removed with the constant irrigation during ultrasonic lithotripsy. These are captured in the suction trap and may be sent for analysis.

accomplished in 15–45 min. The lithotrite may be used to dissolve the stone completely, with the tiny stone fragments (sand) being removed by constant irrigation. These fragments are captured in the irrigant suction catch bottle and may be used for stone analysis (Fig. 4.5). However, not all of these small fragments flow out with the irrigating solution and some may be lost down the ureter or into other calyces. For this reason, we prefer to break the stone into larger fragments and remove them with forceps. When the stone has been completely removed, all portions of the collecting system which are accessible through the nephroscope are examined for any remaining fragments. If none are seen either through the nephroscope or on fluoroscopy, an abdominal radiograph is obtained (Fig. 4.6). Attempts are made to remove any remaining fragments which are accessible with the nephroscope. If none are present, this procedure is terminated. A 5-F Gensini catheter is passed over the safety wire and down into the bladder. The outer tip of the Gensini catheter is then occluded, as its purpose is to stent the region of the

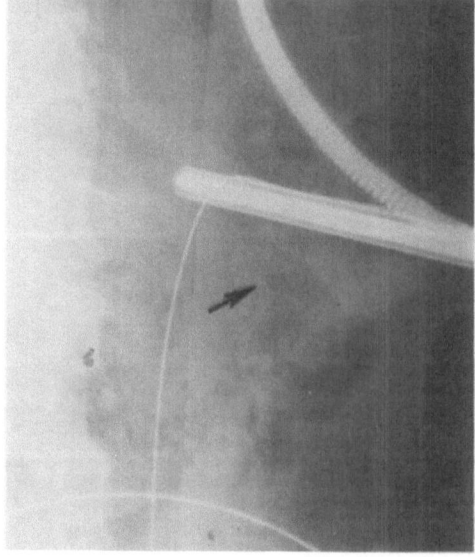

Fig. 4.6. Retained stone fragments are a common problem. A radiograph obtained at the end of the ultrasonic lithotripsy procedure may identify small fragments (*arrow*) which cannot be seen with fluoroscopy.

ureteropelvic junction, which may have received significant trauma during the procedure, and to provide a safety access in case of dislodgement of the percutaneous nephrostomy catheter. A 10-F self-retaining Cope catheter is then passed over the working wire and coiled in the renal pelvis. When proper position of the loop of the catheter is ascertained, the holding thread is tied in position. These two catheters are then fixed to the skin using a Molnar disc (Molnar Retention Disc #61119, Cook Inc., Bloomington, IN 47402), and the percutaneous nephrostomy catheter is connected to external tubing and a urine bag for external drainage.

Postprocedure Care

The patient is allowed to recuperate for 48 h after the stone manipulation with the percutaneous nephrostomy catheter left to external drainage. This period of time is usually sufficient to allow healing of any trauma to the collecting system, clearing of blood from the collecting system, and resolution of edema. On the second postoperative day, 48 h after stone removal, the patient is brought to the radiology department for a tube check. Careful plain films are obtained to look for any residual stone fragments. If any are identified, additional manipulations with the stone basket or forceps may be performed in an attempt to remove residual fragments. If no stone fragments are seen, contrast is injected through the percutaneous nephrostomy catheter and the collecting system examined for patency and extravasation. If there is no significant contrast extravasation, the 5-F Gensini catheter may be removed. If contrast readily reaches the bladder, the percutaneous nephrostomy catheter may be occluded to force internal drainage. If contrast does not reach the bladder, this is most likely due to residual edema in the ureter or ureteropelvic junction and removal of the Gensini catheter may hasten its resolution. The percutaneous nephrostomy catheter, however, must be left to external drainage until this edema subsides and allows passage of urine into the bladder. If there is significant extravasation, particularly at the region of the ureteropelvic junction, it is best to leave the Gensini catheter in position to stent this region and encourage proper healing.

Once the nephrostomy catheter has been turned to internal drainage and the patient tolerates this for a period of 24 h, it may be removed without further radiographic evaluation. Intolerance to internal drainage may result from either ureteral edema or a small stone fragment causing obstruction of the ureter. Small stone fragments frequently pass spontaneously, but if there is persistence, basket removal may be successful. Ureteral edema will subside spontaneously although in some cases it may take as long as 2 weeks for this to do so and allow internal drainage of urine.

These are frequently difficult times for the patient who is feeling well but continues to need the percutaneous nephrostomy for external urine drainage. These patients may be discharged to return at convenient intervals of 2–7 days for an additional tube check, trial of internal drainage, and subsequent catheter removal. However, a collection bag may be attached to the percutaneous nephrostomy catheter which allows many of these patients to return to work and resume nearly normal activities.

Results

The many cases of percutaneous stone removal that have been reported attest to the enthusiasm with which these percutaneous procedures have been received by both physicians and patients. Several groups have reported large numbers of patients, and although there are variations in technique, the results have been similar [1, 2, 8, 13, 17, 21].

Successful removal of renal pelvic stones is accomplished in almost every patient. Calyceal stones can also be removed, particularly if their location allows placement of the percutaneous nephrostomy directly into the calyx containing the stone. Even in those patients with upper pole calyceal stones in whom the entry for the percutaneous nephrostomy must be in a middle or lower pole calyx, the stones can be removed directly or maneuvered into the renal pelvis where they are amenable to dissolution by the ultrasonic lithotripter. This high success rate has led some to recommend a percutaneous approach to virtually any patient. Although this can be accomplished, the difficulty of certain stone positions and anatomic configurations means that the procedure will be prolonged and possibly require multiple attempts before successful stone removal can be attained. These patients may be better served with conventional stone surgery.

The success rate in removal of ureteral stones via percutaneous techniques has been disappointing. Using the conventional four wire basket we have successfully removed less than 50% of ureteral stones [13]. The reasons for this are several, and include failure to pass the guide wire beyond the ureteral stone, failure to capture the stone within the basket, and a stone which cannot be removed because it is adherent to the ureteral mucosa. We have recently adapted an older urologic stone basket which is similar to the four wire basket, but whose wire strutts are larger in caliber and stiffer. Use of this basket has enabled us to remove successfully more ureteral stones, possibly by distending the ureteral mucosa and more successful engagement of the stone within the basket [6].

In addition to the disintegration of stones with ultrasonic lithotripsy, there are a variety of grasping instruments which may be used to extract stones directly. This direct stone extraction is best applied to smaller stones as the track required for their removal will be proportional to the axis of the stone. This technique has the advantage that since the stone is not broken, stone fragments cannot be lost.

We will try to remove any stone 10 mm or smaller with a four wire basket (Fig. 4.7) [12]. If the stone can be engaged in the basket, the second wire can be used to

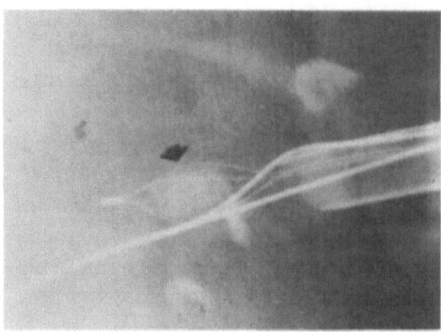

Fig. 4.7. The four-wire basket has been passed through an Amplatz dilator and has engaged the stone (*arrow*), which can easily be removed through the dilator.

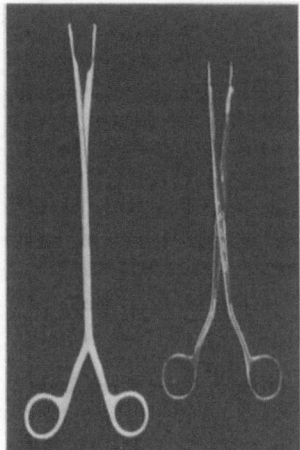

Fig. 4.8. The scissors action of the Randall forceps (*right*) limits the degree to which they may be opened through a nephrostomy track or dilator. The Mazzariello-Caprini forceps (*left*) have a rotating connection which allows a larger opening through restricting tracts.

dilate the nephrostomy track and the stone removed. If the stone lies in a calyx the basket often cannot be manipulated beyond the stone and the stone will not be engaged. In this situation forceps can be used to grasp and extract the stone.

Two types of forceps available for this purpose are the Randall forceps and the Mazzariello-Caprini forceps. The Randall forceps open with a scissoring action which does not allow a large opening to grasp the stone. Thus, it has limited usefulness through a sheath or narrow track. The Mazzariello-Caprini forceps, on the other hand, open with a rotational motion (Fig. 4.8). This mechanism allows the jaws to be fully spread with little change in the shaft diameter (Fig. 4.9). When a groove is made in the jaws to accommodate an angiographic guide wire, either of these forceps may be introduced over the wire, precluding the need for a sheath [10].

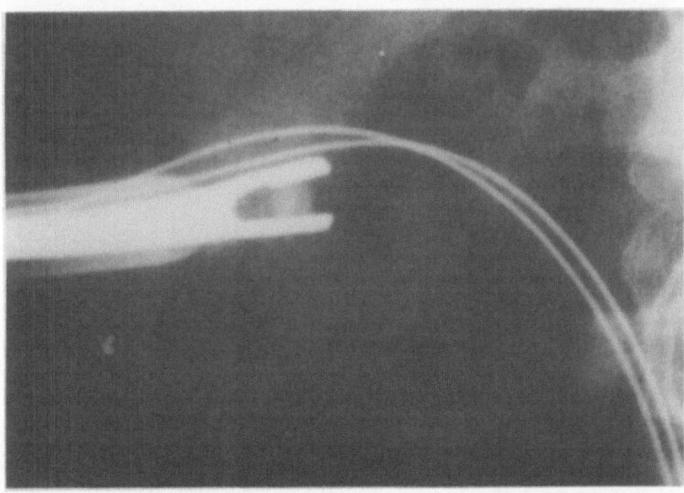

Fig. 4.9. Mazzariello-Caprini forceps are used to capture a stone and withdraw it through the dilator. The safety and working wires are also seen.

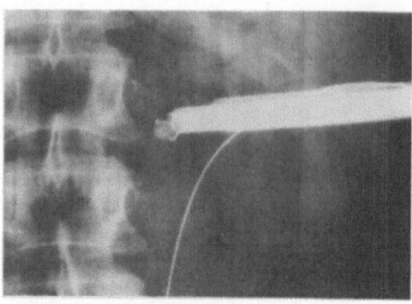

Fig. 4.10. After identifying the stone through the nephroscopy, the four-prong forceps can be used to extract the stone.

An additional instrument that may be used is the four-pronged grasping forceps (Fig. 4.10). If used blindly, however, a portion of the normal kidney may be grasped; therefore, these forceps are usually reserved for use under direct vision through the nephroscope.

Complications

A variety of complications have been reported resulting from these percutaneous procedures for stone removal. Bleeding into the collecting system (Fig. 4.11) and extravasation of urine and contrast material outside the collecting system (Fig. 4.12) are to be expected and not considered complications [5]. Hemorrhage to the extent that blood transfusion is required has occurred in only 3% of our patients [13]. Extravasation from the renal collecting system may result in urinoma formation. As long as adequate drainage of the collecting system is maintained, however, these fluid collections should be readily resorbed.

With multiple renal punctures an arterial venous fistula may be created [8]. If these do not close spontaneously, angiographic demonstration and vascular occlusion could be performed [7, 19].

The most serious complication we have experienced is the development of tense

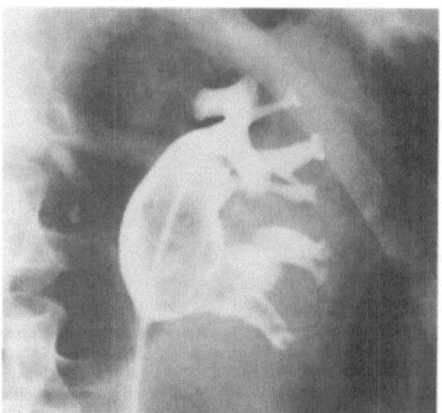

Fig. 4.11. Bleeding into the collecting system is expected during the percutaneous nephrostomy placement. The blood clot is a filling defect which conforms to the collecting system.

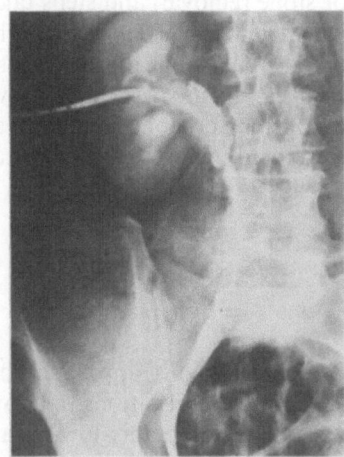

Fig. 4.12. Extravasation of contrast is most frequently at the renal pelvis. These small performations heal quickly and do not retard the procedure. Blood clot can also be seen in the ureter.

ascites with the irrigating solution used for the ultrasonic lithotripsy [13]. The route of contrast extravasation into the peritoneum is unclear but could result from perforation of the renal pelvis into the peritoneal cavity or from a peritoneal reflection which is more lateral and posterior than one normally encounters and is traversed by the percutaneous nephrostomy. We have encountered this complication in 3% of our first 100 procedures. The ascitic fluid in the peritoneal cavity readily exchanges electrolytes with the serum, and since we have been using a glycine irrigant this quickly results in an electrolyte imbalance, most noticeably hyponatremia. Fortunately, each of these were recognized immediately after the procedure when the patient was returned to the supine position, and percutaneous aspiration of the ascites quickly alleviated the problem. The use of an irrigant solution which more closely resembles the serum electrolyte concentration than the glycine solution would also diminish the hazard of this procedure [16].

Residual stone fragments, however, remain a problem. Fragments were left in 30% of our patients [13]. Although some of these could be removed percutaneously under radiographic control, and others were passed spontaneously, 20% of our patients still left the hospital with residual stone fragments within the renal collecting system. It is still not clear whether these small fragments will be subsequently passed or whether they will remain and form the nidus for future stone formation. This relatively high rate of residual fragments has led us to attempt initial basket or forceps removal whenever possible. We also tend to use the ultrasonic lithotriptor to break large stone fragments into pieces which can then be removed with the forceps rather than rely on complete disintegration of the stones with the lithotriptor.

Patient Monitoring

After the immediate problem has been handled and the renal stone has been removed, the patients must be evaluated for the etiology of nephrolithiasis. This should be done soon (and in some cases can even be done during hospitalization for stone removal) and steps taken to prevent stone recurrence. We have had one patient whose workup revealed hyperparathyroidism and who developed a symptomatic renal stone on the opposite side before the parathyroid adenoma could be removed. In most patients, however, dietary and/or genetic factors are largely responsible for stone formation and these patients can be controlled by alterations in diet and increases in fluid intake.

Discussion

The percutaneous approach to urinary tract calculi has been developed and undergone modifications to allow removal of symptomatic stones. The complication rate is acceptably low in large series from several different institutions, and follow-up studies in occasional patients show no apparent renal damage.

Since much of the procedure, and sometimes all of it, is performed with local anesthesia and parenteral analgesia, the hazards of general anesthesia are minimized or avoided. Some portions of the procedure are uncomfortable and not all patients are suitable candidates for percutaneous stone extraction. However, we have removed stones from many patients who have also had conventional urologic surgery for stone disease, and they uniformly prefer the percutaneous approach.

The single greatest advantage of the percutaneous techniques over conventional surgery for urinary tract calculi is the shorter convalescent time before patients may return to normal activities. The duration of hospitalization has also been shorter with the percutaneous procedures as compared with conventional surgery; however, this has not been a dramatic difference. Patients undergoing percutaneous stone manipulation average 10 days of hospitalization. Those patients who are able to undergo direct removal of the stone by basket or forceps average only 8 days of hospitalization as opposed to almost 11 days for those patients undergoing ultrasonic lithotripsy. In many of these patients, however, the additional hospitalization days are due to evaluation of other medical problems or merely due to persistent edema preventing contrast from reaching the bladder and necessitating external drainage. These patients could easily be managed on an outpatient basis and many of them could return to work and nearly normal activity.

References

1. Alken P, Hutschenreiter G, Gunther R, Marbarger M (1981) Percutaneous stone manipulation. J Urol 125:463–466
2. Banner MP, Pollack HM (1982) Percutaneous extraction of renal and ureteral calculi. Radiology 144:753–758
3. Braun SD, Moore AV Jr, Miller GA, Ford KK, Dunnick NR (to be published) A technique to facilitate percutaneous nephrostomy in nonobstructed kidneys. Cardiovasc Intervent Radiol
4. Braun SD, Moore AV Jr, Miller GA, Ford KK, Dunnick NR (1984) A technique for conversion from small (0.018″) to large (0.038″) guidewires for drainage procedures. Urol Radiol 6:227
5. Carson CC, Moore AV, Weinerth JL, Ford KK, Dunnick NR (1984) Percutaneous dissolution of renal calculi using ultrasonic litholapaxy. South Med J 77:196–199

6. Carson CC, Braun SD, Weinerth JL, Dunnick NR (1984) Modified Johnson basket for antegrade stone extraction. Urology 24:359
7. Castaneda-Zuniga WR, Tadavarthy SM, Murphy W, Beranei KI, Amplatz K (1976) Nonsurgical closure of a large arteriovenous fistula. JAMA 236:2649
8. Castaneda-Zuniga WR, Clayman R, Smith A, Rusnak B, Herrera M, Amplatz K (1982) Nephrostolithotomy: percutaneous techniques for urinary calculus removal. AJR 139:721–726
9. Clayman RV, Castaneda-Zuniga WR, Hunter DW, Miller RP, Lange PH, Amplatz K (1983) Rapid balloon dilatation of the nephrostomy track for nephrostolithotomy. Radiology 147:884–885
10. Clayman RV, Surya V, Castaneda-Zuniga WR, Miller RP, Lange PH (1983) Percutaneous nephrolithotomy with Mazzariello-Caprini forceps. J Urol 129:1213–1215
11. Drach GW (1978) Urinary lithiasis. In: Campbell's urology, 4th edn. W.B. Saunders, Philadelphia, pp 784–790
12. Dunnick NR, Braun SB (1985) Imaging and access to the urinary tract. In: Dunnick NR, Carson CC (eds) Endourology. Churchill Livingstone, New York
13. Dunnick NR, Carson CC, Moore AV Jr, Ford K, Miller GA, Braun SD, Newman GE, Weinerth JL (1985) Percutaneous approach to nephrolithiasis. AJR 144:451
14. Ford K, Weinerth JL (1985) Renal anatomy. In: Carson CC, Dunnick NR (eds) Endourology. Churchill Livingstone, New York
15. LeRoy AJ, May GR, Segura JW, Patterson DE, McGough PF (1984) Rapid dilatation of percutaneous nephrostomy tracks. AJR 142:355–357
16. Schultz RE, Hanno PM, Wein AJ, Levin RM, Pollack HM, Van Arsdalen KN (1983) Percutaneous ultrasonic lithotripsy: choice of irrigant. J Urol 130:858–860
17. Segura JW, Patterson DE, LeRoy AJ, May GR, Smith LH (1983) Percutaneous lithotripsy. J Urol 130:1051–1054
18. Shehadi WH, Toniolo G (1980) Adverse reactions to contrast media. Radiology 137:299–302
19. Wallace S, Schwarten DE, Smith DC, Gerson LP, Davis LJ (1978) Intrarenal arteriovenous fistulas: transcatheter steel coil occlusion. J Urol 120:282–286
20. Weinerth JL, Dunnick NR (1985) Perioperative management. In: Carson CC, Dunnick NR (eds) Endourology. Churchill Livingstone, New York
21. Wickham JEA, Kellett MJ, Miller RA (1983) Elective percutaneous nephrolithotomy in 50 patients: an analysis of the technique, results, and complications. J Urol 129:904–906

Chapter 5

Antegrade and Retrograde Ureteral Stenting

Peggy J. Fritzsche

Introduction

Ureteral stents have been used for many years to provide both short- and long-term drainage of the urinary tract. Early stents were primarily placed in conjunction with ureteral surgery. The efficacy of polyethylene in ureteral catheters was described in 1951 [11]. Retrograde placement of indwelling silicone rubber ureteral tubing was reported in 1967 for use in patients with ureteral obstruction [62].

The major problem with the early stents was migration of the catheter. Modifications of the catheter material and methods of insertion ensued [36, 41, 48]. In 1976, Gibbons et al. introduced an indwelling silicone stent with side wings and a distal flange which resisted upward migration and expulsion [18], but this stent proved to be technically difficult for many others to position properly. In 1978, Hepperlen et al. adapted angiographic materials and techniques to the urinary tract [24]. A pigtail catheter in the renal pelvis was cystoscopically placed using the Seldinger technique. A distal flange in the urinary bladder allowed the catheter to be indwelling. A pigtail curve was later added to the distal portion of the catheter to stabilize catheter position and to reduce irritation caused by the flange [12, 34]. The same year, Finney described a double J catheter made of flexible silicone which was designed to prevent migration and remain indwelling [15].

The first percutaneous nephrostomy for temporary urinary tract drainage was reported in 1955 by Goodwin [20]. More than 20 years later, the percutaneous approach was revived for access to urinary tract calculi and to place ureteral stents when the retrograde approach had failed [19, 60]. Percutaneous nephrostomy became a conduit to the urinary tract for stent placement and a variety of interventional procedures [13, 22, 26, 28, 30, 31, 39, 43, 53, 55, 57, 59]. The percutaneous approach gained popularity because of the widespread use of angiographic techniques which could be applied to the urinary tract and because of the convenience of accomplishing the procedure outside the surgical suite without general anesthesia [12].

This chapter reviews the status of ureteral stenting from the literature and discusses the technical details of both the antegrade and the retrograde approach.

Clinical Considerations

Indwelling ureteral stents are particularly attractive because the patient is able to void naturally and is not bothered with an external appliance. However, cystoscopy is required for adjustment, exchange, or removal of the stent. It is, therefore, advisable to allow the catheter to extend from the flank when the antegrade approach has been used and adjustments are anticipated (Fig. 5.1). It is unacceptable for the distal portion of the stent to extend beyond the urethra except for very short-term use during hospitalization.

The choice between antegrade and retrograde placement varies in each case based on the course of the ureter in relation to the fistulous tract [19, 30, 32]. Torque control of the catheter must also be considered, especially in a redundant ureter.

retrograde placement is the logical choice if cystoscopy is necessary for other reasons. It is not uncommon for one approach to be impossible, and, subsequently, for the other method to proceed smoothly. The antegrade approach is preferred in obstruction because the proximal dilatation enhances catheter and guide wire manipulations. In cases of fistula, one approach is often favored over the other, based on the course of the ureter in relation to the fistulous tract [19,30, 32]. Torque control of the catheter must also be considered, especially in a redundant ureter.

It is sometimes possible to predict the most suitable approach, but usually the best approach is the first one that succeeds. If cystoscopy is not necessary for other reasons, the antegrade approach is desirable because it avoids operating room expenses and anesthesia. Furthermore, fluoroscopy and ultrasound are superior in quality and more readily available outside the surgical suite in most hospitals.

In the event of ureteral damage from trauma or surgery, stricture formation is prone to occur. Therefore, ureteral stents are commonly placed during surgical procedures involving the ureters. Intraoperative stent placement is used in antici-

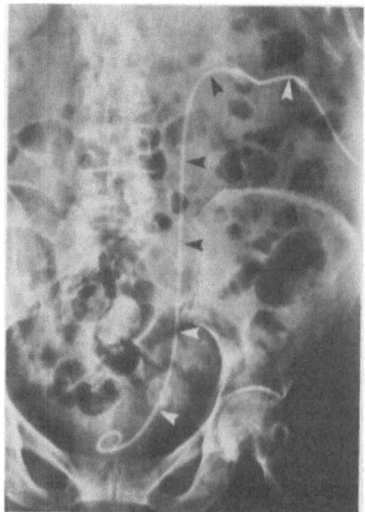

Fig. 5.1. Ureteral catheter extending through the flank for future access. An angiographic pigtail catheter (*arrows*) has been introduced percutaneously into the urinary tract, past staghorn calculus in the renal pelvis. The catheter extends from the flank for future manipulations.

pation of problems and rarely as primary treatment of existing problems. The established success of the antegrade and retrograde approach to stent placement has replaced the operative approach except in unusual circumstances.

A combined approach using the nephrostomy tract for access and retrieval of the guide wire and/or catheter via the bladder or ileostomy permits dual access to the ureteral problem. This approach has been used to position stents and to retrieve calculi [5, 6, 7, 16, 46, 51, 52].

Regardless of the selected approach to the urinary tract, it is important that infection be under control prior to urothelial trauma which occurs during catheter and guide wire manipulation. In cases of infected obstruction, a percutaneous nephrostomy should be followed by irrigation and antibiotics before any attempt is made to insert a stent. Another consideration before placing a stent is whether there is distal outlet obstruction at either the bladder or the intestinal conduit. A functioning indwelling stent would be rendered useless if outlet obstruction existed. If a percutaneous nephrostomy must be placed for access, bleeding disorders are a relative contraindication.

Dilute, uninfected, acidic urine resists encrustations of the catheter. However, encrustations are a persistent problem in some patients. It is controversial whether silicone or polyethylene is less prone to encrustations [15, 24]. Mardis et al. reported no difference in reactivity or efficiency of drainage with either silicone or polyethylene catheters [34]. Regardless of the catheter material, encrustations are almost certain to occur when infection is present [9]. Stents should be changed periodically to avoid obliteration of the catheter lumen, and patency should be checked every 4–6 weeks in newly placed stents to establish the necessary exchange interval. Stents can sometimes be effective for 6 months before exchange is necessary, but it would be unwise to assume this long interval to be appropriate without evaluation in each individual case.

Patency of the lumen can be verified by reflux demonstrated on a static cystogram. Intravesical pressure may require increase in volume of as much as 100 cm of water to produce reflux. Intravenous methylene blue will also indicate patency if seen effluxing from a stent. If there is a solitary kidney or only one kidney is functioning with a stent, then patency can be followed with serum creatinine levels.

Description of Materials

Silicone has been used in the urinary tract for many years without problem, primarily because it is soft and essentially inert. However, silicone stents are most often used with intraoperative placement. The soft, flexible silicone material is poorly suited to placement over guide wires unless there is dual access to the ureter so that the stent can be pulled into position rather than pushed. Historically, the internal diameter of silicone double J stents was considerably smaller than polyethylene double pigtail stents with resultant lower flow rates [35]. Recently, the internal diameter of the double J stents has been increased, but there are no data on flow comparisons of the new material.

Polyethylene became very popular as stent material when nonoperative stent placement became more common. Angiographers were well acquainted with the torque control of polyethylene catheters. However, it was found that polyethylene became brittle if left in the urinary tract for extended periods. The manufacturers of the polyethylene catheter stents converted to polyurethane material, which has received enthusiastic support in the past 1–2 years. Polyurethane is softer and has better memory characteristics than polyethylene. The preliminary unpublished reports from Cook Urological, Inc. indicate decrease in polyurethane stent breakage, particularly in patients receiving chemotherapy.

External Ureteral Stent

Long ureteral stents measuring 90 cm in length can be used in the urinary tract. One end of the stent has a Luer lock connector and remains external for access to the urinary tract. The universal stent is an 8-F tube of silicone rubber popularized by Smith [50] (Heyer-Schulte, Goleta, California). Long pigtail, polyethylene catheters (Cook, Inc. Bloomington, Indiana) can be used in a similar fashion. Because of the external exposure, these catheters are best suited to short-term use.

Indwelling Ureteral Stent

Double pigtail polyurethane ureteral stents are available in diameters of 5 F, 6 F, 7 F, and 8 F and lengths of 8–30 cm (Cook Urological, Inc. Spencer, Indiana). The stent set includes a 0.038-in. flexible tip guide wire, an open-end ureteral catheter with pigtail curves at each end, and a pusher.

Double-J silicone ureteral stents are available in a stent kit which contains an 8.5-F ureteral catheter either 26 or 28 cm in length and a push catheter plus a 10-ml vial of sterile mineral oil. The lubricant is included to overcome the friction which exists between the guide wire and the silicone catheter. A positioning thread retractor is attached to the proximal end of the J (Medical Engineering Corp., Racine, Wisconsin).

Technique of Stent Placement

Antegrade Approach

Successful antegrade stenting of the ureter depends on a well placed nephrostomy. When establishing a new nephrostomy tract, it is important to select a mid or upper pole calyx because it provides a more favorable angle to the ureter than the lower pole calyx (Fig. 5.2). Respiration will assist in selecting the calyx most suitable for puncture. When converting a nephrostomy previously placed in a lower pole calyx, it is worthwhile to repuncture an appropriate calyx. The unfavorable angle of the lower pole calyx will cause unnecessary distress. Even when one is successful in directing the guide wire and catheter down the ureter from a lower pole calyx, the torque control necessary to negotiate the ureter will have been lost.

Torque control is so important for antegrade placement that polyethylene or

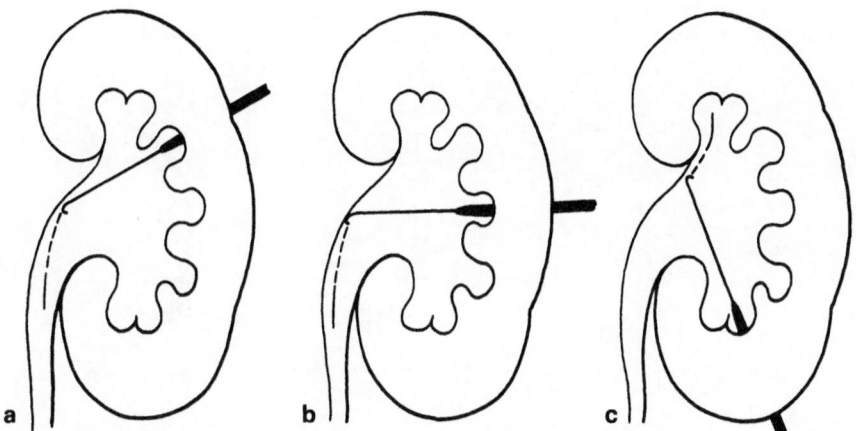

Fig. 5.2a–c. Calyx selection for percutaneous entry. The upper and mid calyceal groups (**a,b**) provide better guide wire access to the ureter than the lower pole calyx (**c**).

polyurethane catheters are usually selected. The soft, silicone catheters are usually reserved for intraoperative or uncomplicated retrograde placement. Silicone catheters can theoretically be placed in an antegrade manner in mature tracts or with the aid of a vascular introducer. However, the reports of antegrade placement of silicone catheters in the literature describe dual control with pulling the stent into position [5, 51, 52].

Contrast opacification of the ureter outlines the course to follow and suggests the most appropriate catheter and guide wire combination. The contrast should be diluted so that the guide wire and catheter are not obscured.

A straight, flexible, or J-shaped guide wire is inserted and ideally passes directly into the ureter. Sometimes the guide wire will coil in the pelvis, requiring manipulation under fluoroscopy. It is safe to remove the needle sheath or previous nephrostomy catheter when the guide wire is coiled in the pelvis and to insert a slightly curved tip, torque control catheter. After the catheter tip is well into the pelvis, the guide wire is retracted until it can be directed toward the ureteropelvic junction. The wire is advanced carefully under fluoroscopic control as the catheter is rotated, probing for the ureter. Sometimes the guide wire will pass into the ureter and continue down to the bladder easily. The guide wire should precede the catheter in the ureter to prevent perforation.

Detailed suggestions for advancing guide wires and catheters past obstacles have been described [8, 16, 17, 23, 30, 38, 47]. If resistance is encountered because of angulations, a catheter should be advanced to the level of the obstacle and dilute contrast injected to outline the ureteral path. A slightly curved tip catheter can be used in combination with a variety of guide wires in order to pass the obstacle (Fig. 5.3). A J-shaped guide wire, particularly one with a tapered, movable core, or a floppy tip Bentson guide wire (Cook, Inc. Bloomington, Indiana) is useful in angulated ureters because the guide wire will often hit the back wall of the ureteral curve and buckle toward the new direction (Fig. 5.4). The advancing catheter will follow in the new direction. Change in patient respiratory effort will sometimes alter the degree of angulation sufficiently for successful catheterization (Fig. 5.5). If one is unsuccessful in bypassing the redundant ureteral curves after a reasonable length of time, such as 15–20 min, a nephrostomy catheter should be left in the

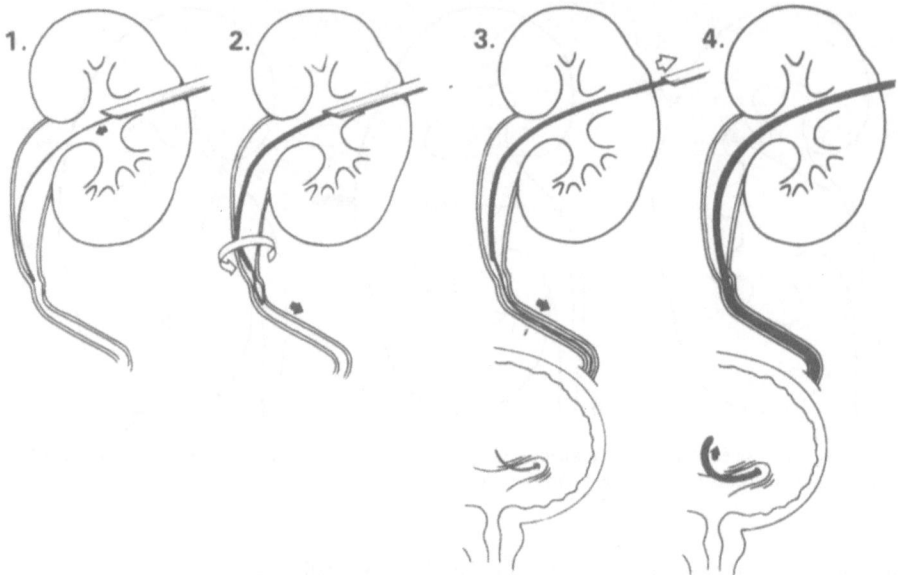

Fig. 5.3. *Transrenal approach*
1. Introduce guide wire through the nephrostomy tract.
2. Probe with floppy tip guide wire and rotate the end hole, slightly curved tip torque catheter.
3. Advance guide wire past obstacle into the urinary bladder.
4. Advance catheter over guide wire into the urinary bladder. Removal of guide wire under fluoroscopic control.

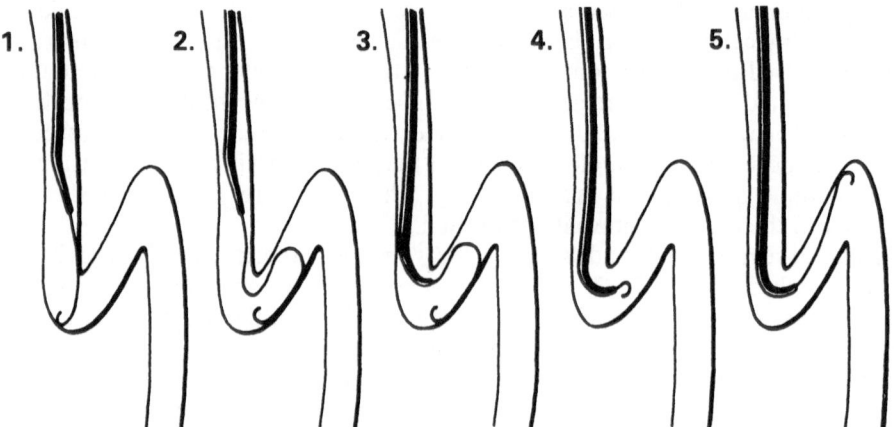

Fig. 5.4. *Technique of bypassing angulated ureter*
1. A slightly curved tip, end hole catheter is placed near the obstacle and the J guide wire advanced until it strikes the opposite wall.
2. The guide wire will buckle toward new direction with continued advancement.
3. Advance catheter to take advantage of new guide wire direction.
4. Retract guide wire close to tip of catheter.
5. Advance guide wire in new direction and repeat procedure.

INSPIRATION   EXPIRATION

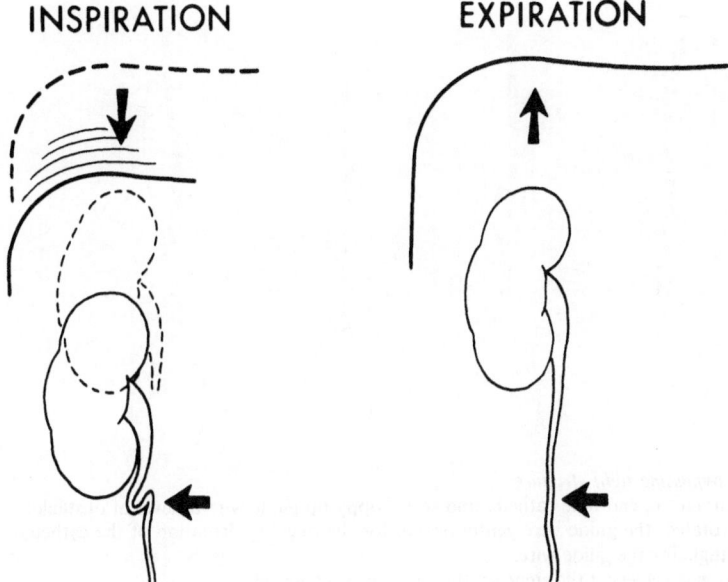

Fig. 5.5. Change in respiration to alter ureteral course. *Inspiration*: Redundancy of the ureter. *Expiration*: Ureter straightened to aid in guide wire and catheter manipulations.

renal pelvis. A delay of 5–14 days sometimes solves the problem because the edema subsides and the ureter becomes less redundant after decompression.

Resistance secondary to stricture or fistulas requires a few extra steps (Figs. 5.6, 5.7). A catheter is introduced to the level of the obstacle and dilute contrast injected to map the ureteral course. The slightly curved tip catheter is positioned about 1 cm above the obstacle and a floppy tip Bentson guide wire is inserted. Rotation of the catheter while gently probing allows the guide wire to approach the stenoses at a multiplicity of angles until the opening is located. It is even possible to use this technique successfully in ureters which are not opacified beyond the obstruction. Ring has described probing a stenosis with the Lunderquist-Ring torque control guide wire after adding a right angle bend 1.5 cm from the tip [47]. The opening to a stenotic lesion is often eccentric and not necessarily at the tip of the contrast column. After the guide wire enters the stenotic area, the catheter is advanced to secure the position. Additional contrast can be injected at this point to distend the stenosis and review the ureteral path. The floppy tip guide wire is reinserted and probing is resumed until both the catheter and the guide wire reach the bladder. If difficulties are encountered in reaching the bladder with the initial single end hole catheter, it is wise to leave this access catheter in place for 5–10 days to mature the tract before attempting to insert the double pigtail catheter (Fig. 5.8).

The stent catheter length needed can be estimated from the radiographs, allowing for magnification. The 25–26 cm length stent catheter is usually acceptable for most average adults. Exact length can be measured by marking the distance between the bladder and the renal pelvis on the guide wire (Fig. 5.9). Both the guide wire and the catheter must reach the bladder for measurement purposes. The distal pigtail should be at least 1 cm beyond the ureter. Therefore, the guide wire should be bent at the catheter hub when it is approximately 1 cm beyond the ureterovesical junction or across the midline in the expected region of the catheter

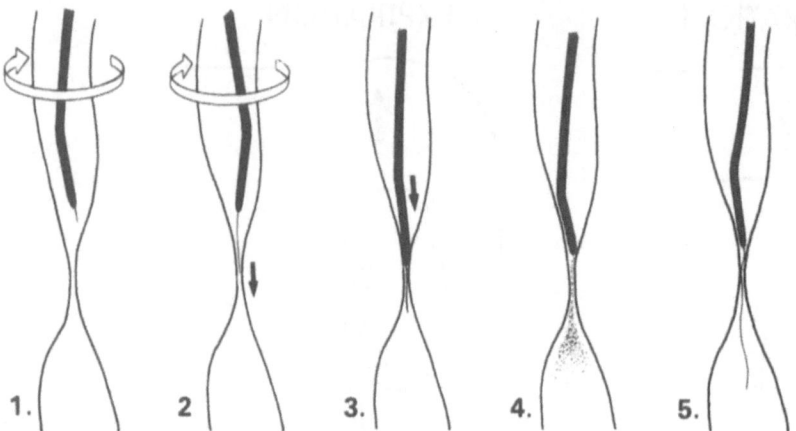

Fig. 5.6. *Technique of bypassing tight stricture*
1. Advance slightly curved tip, end hole catheter and soft, floppy tip guide wire to level of obstacle.
2. As the catheter is rotated, the guide wire gently probes for the opening. Rotation of the catheter changes the entry angle for the guide wire.
3. After the guide wire has traversed the stenosis, the catheter is advanced.
4. If the catheter and guide wire will not advance further, remove guide wire and inject contrast to outline ureteral course.
5. Continue rotation of catheter and gentle probing with soft, floppy tip guide wire. Repeat procedure as needed until both the guide wire and catheter extend beyond the stricture.

curve. The guide wire is then withdrawn until it is located in the desired region of the proximal catheter curve, at least 1 cm above the ureteropelvic junction, where a second guide wire bend is made. The guide wire is then removed to be used as the measure for the final catheter length. The access catheter is left in place.

An exchange guide wire can now be inserted through the access catheter. Selection of a stiff guide wire allows the double pigtail catheter to follow more easily and prevents buckling in the soft tissues and/or renal pelvis. The rigid guide wire popularized by Lunderquist is commonly used. This Lunderquist exchange guide wire, known as the "coat hanger" guide wire, is made of stainless steel cannula material with a short flexible tip. The exchange guide wire of Lunderquist should not be confused with the Lunderquist-Ring torque control guide wire, which is a coiled stainless steel wire with multiple distal solder joints (Cook, Inc., Bloomington, Indiana).

Insertion of the double pigtail catheter should be done while holding the guide wire steady and straight to reduce the possibility of buckling. Fluoroscopy is required for safe insertion. Inexperienced trainees frequently use too much backward tension on the guide wire, which quickly destroys position, or too little backward tension, which allows the guide wire to be carried forward as the catheter is advanced and may result in damage to the urothelium. If the pigtail catheter will not pass a stenotic segment, the slightly curved tip catheter should be reinserted and left in place for several days to increase the caliber of the stricture. Alternatively, the stenosis could be dilated with an angioplasty balloon or the endoscopist could retrieve the guide wire in the bladder. Control both proximally and distally allows one to attach an appropriate stent catheter which can then be pulled into position past the stricture.

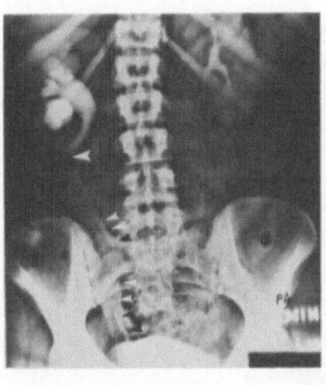

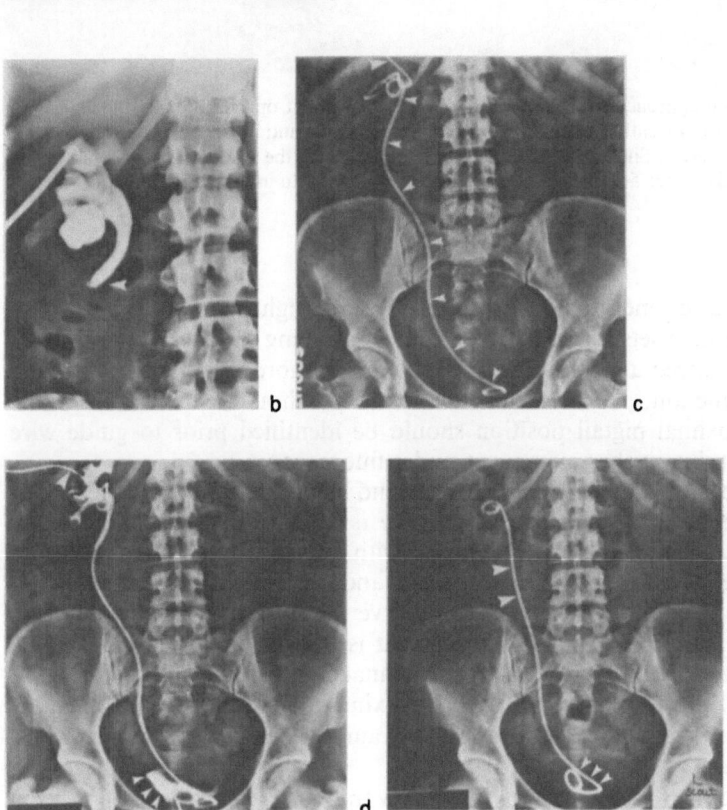

Fig. 5.7a–e. Ureteral stent after ureteral lithotomy. **a** Postoperative urogram showing partial obstruction of the proximal ureter at the site of previous surgery (*large arrow*); note contrast in distal ureter (*small arrows*). **b** Introduction of contrast via percutaneous nephrostomy demonstrates displacement and obstruction of the proximal ureter at the site of previous surgery (*arrow*). **c** A double pigtail ureteral stent catheter (*small arrows*) has been placed percutaneously and traverses the obstruction. The nephrostomy pigtail (*large arrow*) catheter remains in place for 24–48 h, until function of the ureteral stent is confirmed. **d** Introduction of contrast via nephrostomy catheter (*large arrow*) demonstrates good drainage into the bladder (*small arrows*). **e** The nephrostomy catheter has been removed and this plain abdominal film taken 2 weeks later shows straightening of the ureter (*large arrows*) and migration of excess stent into the bladder (*small arrows*). Prior to removal of the stent catheter, a guide wire is cystoscopically inserted and a single end hole catheter is placed in the renal pelvis. Patency is confirmed before removal of the catheter.

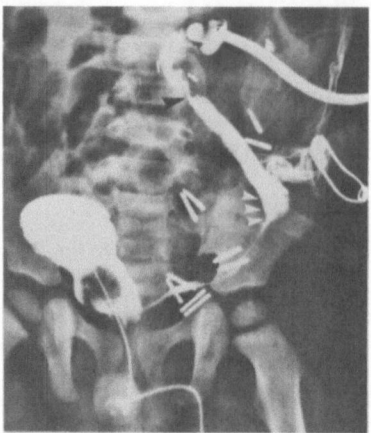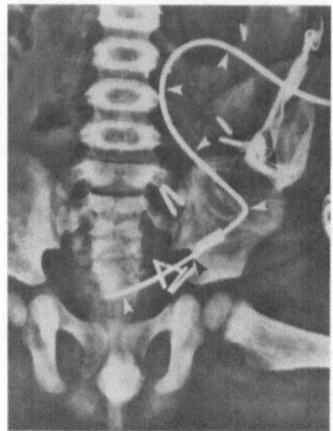

a   b

Fig. 5.8a,b. Transrenal approach to postoperative ureter. **a** Contrast opacification of the collecting system via the nephrostomy catheter shows narrowing (*large arrow*) and angulation (*small arrows*) of the ureter postoperatively. **b** Single end hole catheter advanced into the bladder (*arrows*) and left in place as an access catheter for 5–7 days to mature the pathway prior to insertion of a pigtail catheter.

The catheter positioner or pusher is a short straight nontapered catheter supplied with the stent sets necessary to push the indwelling catheters into position. The pusher is advanced until the distal pigtail reaches more than 1 cm beyond the ureterovesical junction, which means the catheter should extend across the midline. The proximal pigtail position should be identified prior to guide wire removal by observing pusher movement under fluoroscopy.

The guide wire should be long enough to extend beyond the combined length of the stent catheter and pusher. The guide wire is always removed prior to the pusher. The stent position must be maintained with forward pressure on the pusher as the guide wire is removed. Fluoroscopy is mandatory to ensure that the distal position remains near the midline and to observe the distal and proximal curves forming in the expected positions. If placement is too distal, corrections can be made via the safety thread attached to the proximal end and side holes of the stent catheter (Fig. 5.10). If placement is too proximal, cystoscopic adjustment is necessary because a catheter cannot be left to drain into renal parenchyma or into the perirenal space.

The pusher provides final access to the urinary tract for confirmation of position and function of the stent with contrast instillation. Occasionally, a nephrostomy is left in place to confirm desired function of the stent or to instill medications for stone dissolution.

Retrograde Approach

Whenever cystoscopy is planned for diagnostic reasons, it is advantageous to try the retrograde approach for stent placement. The patient is spared the anxiety of another procedure. The transvesical approach to the ureter is familiar to the practice of everyday urology and successful in the majority of patients.

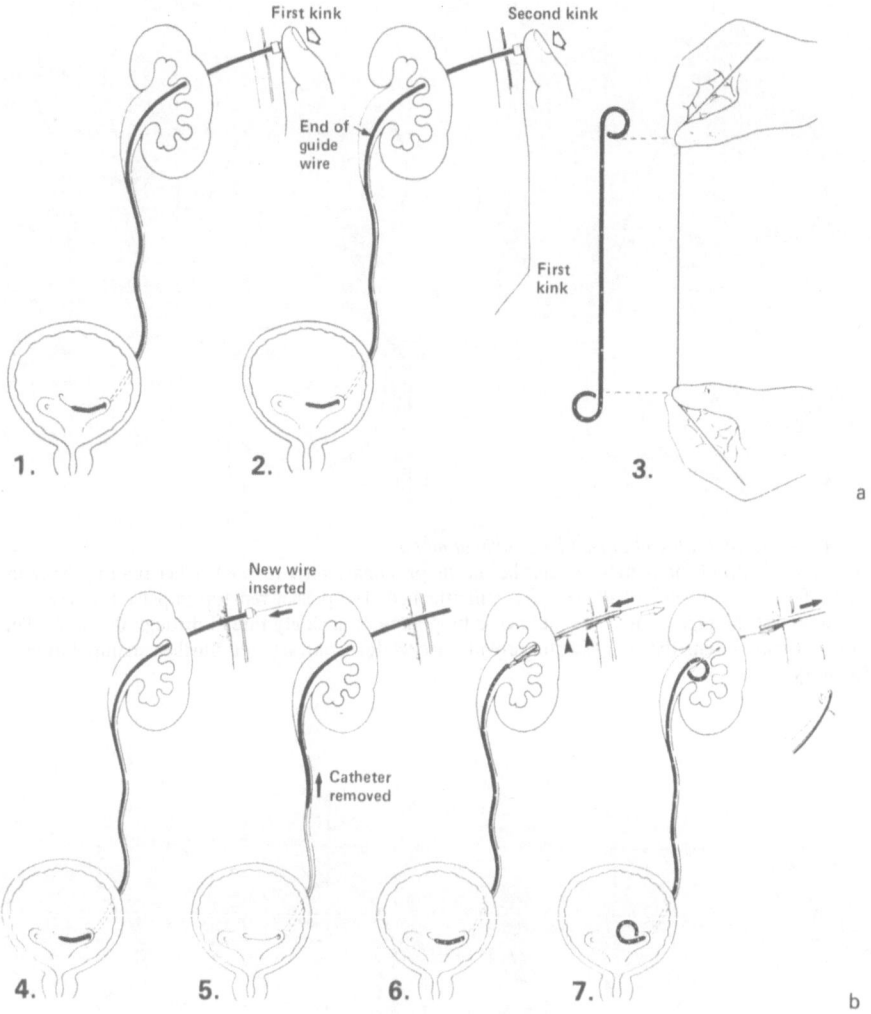

Fig. 5.9a,b. *Measuring the ureter to determine stent catheter length*

1. The guide wire and catheter extend past the ureterovesical junction. When the guide wire is across the midline, the guide wire extending from the flank is bent at the catheter hub.
2. The guide wire is retracted until the tip is located in the renal pelvis approximately 1 cm above the ureteral pelvic junction, and a second bend is made in the guide wire at the catheter hub.
3. The distance between the two bends in the guide wire will determine the length of catheter between the pigtail curves.
4. Insert a new guide wire such as a Lunderquist exchange guide wire.
5. Remove catheter under fluoroscopic control. Advance the guide wire as the catheter is removed to ensure bladder position of guide wire.
6. Introduce double pigtail catheter over guide wire. Note the safety suture attached to the proximal portion of the catheter (*vertical arrows*). The pusher is advanced until the distal pigtail reaches across the midline of the bony pelvis. Observe pusher movement in the renal pelvis to ensure that the proximal tip of the catheter is within the renal pelvis. Remove guide wire under fluoroscopic control to ensure distal position in the bladder and reforming of pigtail shape.
7. Remove pusher last, after confirming both the distal and proximal curves to be within the urinary tract.

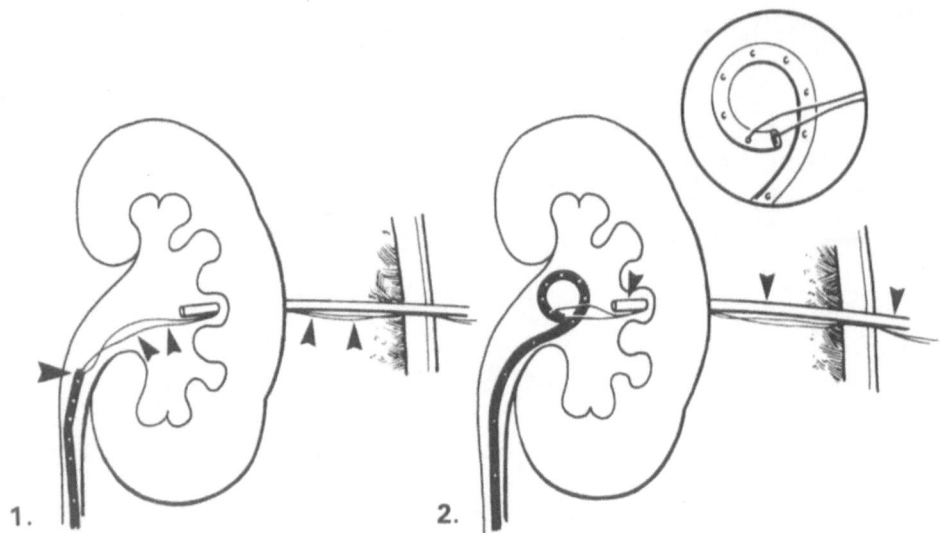

Fig. 5.10. *Use of safety thread to position proximal pigtail*
1. The proximal tip of the pigtail catheter lies in the proximal ureter (*arrow*) rather than in the renal pelvis. The safety thread (*small arrows*) is still attached. The pusher remains in place for access.
2. Retraction of the pigtail into the renal pelvis by pulling on a safety thread through the flank. The pusher (*arrows*) remains in place to provide access for contrast and further manipulation if necessary.

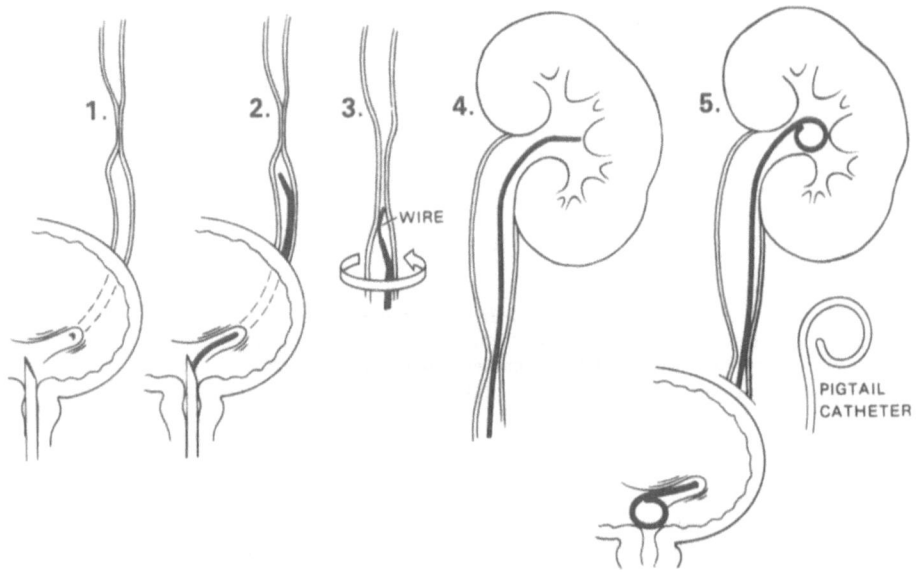

Fig. 5.11. *Transvesical approach*
1. The cystoscope is introduced into the bladder and the ureterovesical junction identified.
2. A single end hole, slightly curved tip torque catheter is inserted.
3. A soft, floppy tip guide wire probes for entry as the catheter is simultaneously rotated.
4. The catheter is advanced beyond the obstacle into the renal pelvis.
5. Catheter exchange over stiff guide wire for double pigtail catheter.

The initial catheter is inserted past the ureterovesical junction and the guide wire advanced until it reaches the renal pelvis. Resistance to guide wire advancement is handled as described and illustrated under the previous section on antegrade placement (Fig. 5.11). Measurements for stent length can be made by bending the guide wire in the expected positions of the stent curves as described in the previous section. The access catheter should be left in place until the exchange guide wire has been inserted.

The pigtail catheter is advanced while holding the exchange guide wire in a steady position. Fluoroscopy should be used to ensure that the catheter is not advancing the guide wire unnecessarily, because the guide wire can easily extend beyond the collecting system. Fluoroscopy is sometimes less than optimal in the operating room. It is tempting to try blind stent insertion to save time, but renal damage is often the result and additional time is required to correct the mistake after films confirm the proximal curve to be outside the collecting system.

After the proximal stent curve is documented to be in the renal pelvis, the guide wire is removed while applying forward pressure on the stent catheter with the pusher. Fluoroscopy is vital to proper positioning of the stent curves. Minor adjustments can be made via the cystoscopic access.

Modified Approach for Ureterointestinal Conduits

Ureterointestinal diversions require a modified approach. If the anastomosis is easily identified with an endoscope in the conduit, access can be obtained in a retrograde manner (Fig. 5.12). A sharply angled, end hole catheter is placed at the anastomosis and a guide wire is inserted into the ureter as far as possible for stability. If there is an obstacle to negotiate, replace the sharply angled catheter with a slightly curved tip, torque catheter and probe with various guide wires. A J-

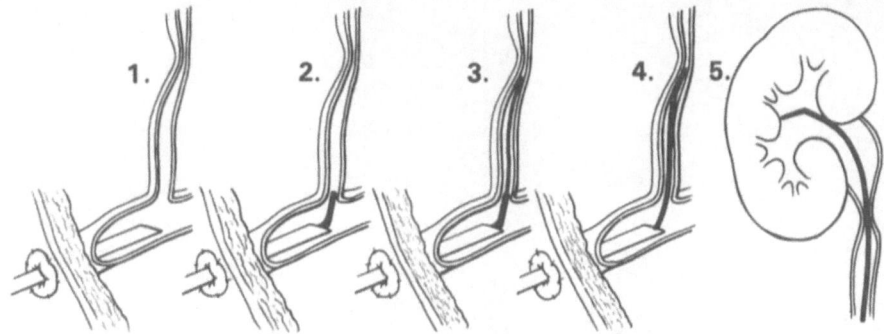

Fig. 5.12. *Transconduit approach*
1. The cystoscope is placed into the intestinal loop and the ureterointestinal anastomosis identified.
2. An angled tip catheter is placed at the ureteral orifice.
3. The guide wire is advanced to the level of the obstacle.
4. Angle tip catheter exchange for single end hole slightly curved tip catheter. The guide wire and catheter are advanced beyond the obstacle.
5. The catheter is advanced into the renal pelvis and the guide wire removed. If a pigtail catheter is desired in the renal pelvis, a stiff guide wire should be introduced into the renal pelvis for the exchange.

shaped guide wire will usually be successful. Other guide wires such as a floppy tip Bentson wire or a torque control, Lunderquist-Ring guide wire may be necessary. After the guide wire reaches the renal pelvis, the appropriate stent catheter can be advanced over the guide wire. The more difficult the placement of the initial guide wire and catheter into the renal pelvis, the greater the need for leaving an access catheter in place for several days before attempting to advance a stent catheter past the obstacle.

The antegrade approach for stent placement after ureterointestinal diversion is usually required because the anastomosis is frequently difficult to locate for retrograde placement (Fig. 5.13). The advantage to the antegrade approach is that dual access naturally occurs when the guide wire reaches the intestinal conduit. The guide wire is usually easily found by sweeping the finger in a circular motion in the conduit. Rarely is endoscopy required to retrieve the guide wire. The stent catheter can be attached and pulled into proper position once dual access to the urinary tract is established.

Double pigtail catheters are usually chosen when placing an antegrade stent. It does not matter whether the stent is a single or double pigtail catheter when using the retrograde approach because the distal tip will be accessible in the intestinal conduit. A distal tip which extends too far beyond the stoma is susceptible to accidental withdrawal.

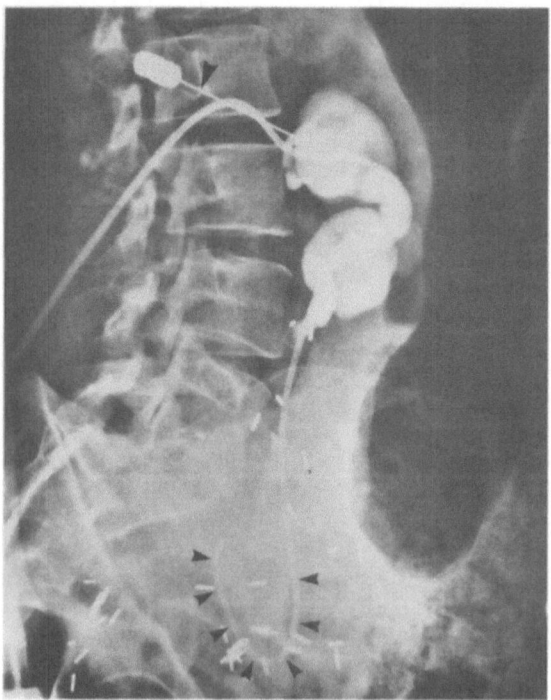

Fig. 5.13. *Antegrade approach in ureterointestinal diversion.* A slightly curved tip catheter has been introduced percutaneously into the urinary tract and the tip reaches the intestinal loop (*small arrows*). The tip of the catheter can be retrieved manually via the intestinal stoma. Note that the localizing needle (*large arrow*) is still in place to provide contrast for localization and distension.

Applications and Results

Postoperative

Ureteral stents have been used for many years at the time of ureteral surgery to keep the ureter open during the healing process. In the past there was often controversy because the results were poor whether or not a stent was used. Because the stents drained externally, patients were eager to have them removed, resulting in premature extraction before healing was complete. Infection was a problem because the stents were rarely indwelling. The early stents were small and probably did not provide adequate urine drainage. With the advent of larger indwelling stents, these problems were corrected and ureteral stenting is now routinely used successfully in the postoperative period (Figs. 5.14–5.16).

Postsurgical ureteral leaks are unwelcome, but not uncommon, particularly after radical surgery (Figs. 5.17–5.19) [58, 61]. Ureteral stents have proven to be extremely desirable in the postoperative period when additional surgery is inappropriate (Fig. 5.20) [5, 14, 30].

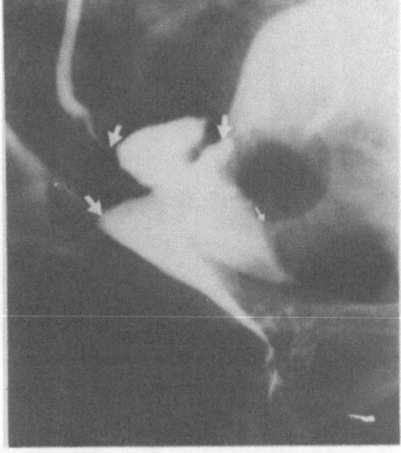

Fig. 5.14. Following a vaginal hysterectomy this patient developed a urine leak. Cystograms failed to show a vesicovaginal fistula. This antegrade pyelogram, however, demonstrates a right-sided ureterovaginal fistula with the ureter ending in the cuff of the vagina. (From Lang [30], with permission)

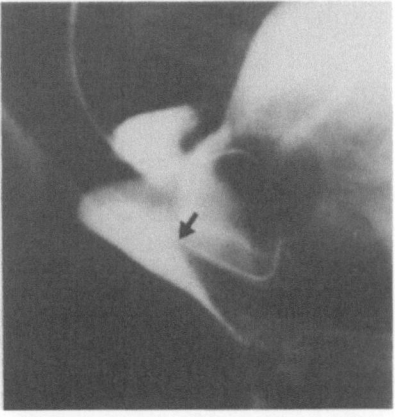

Fig. 5.15. Initial attempts to regain entry into the bladder failed and the guide wire (*arrow*), passed from an antegrade approach, repeatedly coiled in the vaginal fornix. (From Lang [30], with permission)

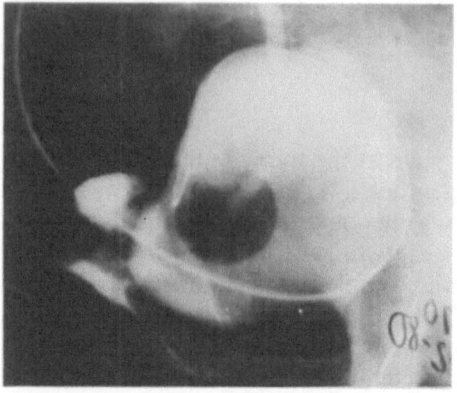

Fig. 5.16. Reentry into the bladder was accomplished with the use of a perforating guide wire. An antegrade stent catheter was then advanced over this guide wire into the bladder. This catheter is equipped with side holes located at the level of the renal pelvis and thus draining the renal unit either downward into the bladder or to an outside receptacle. Satisfactory healing without stricture occurred after retaining the stent catheter in position for 7 weeks. (From Lang [30], with permission)

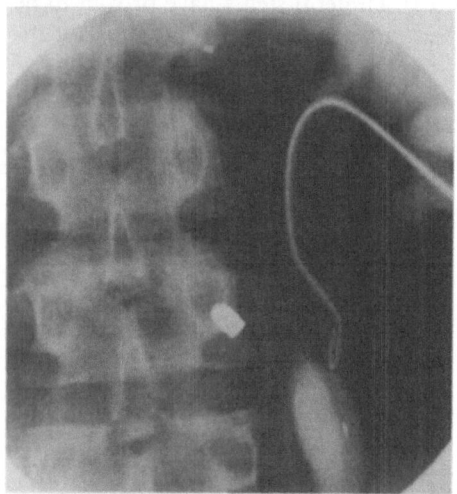

Fig. 5.17. An attempt to pass a guide wire along existing tissue bridges across a partial dehiscence of the ureter fails. (By courtesy of Lang EK)

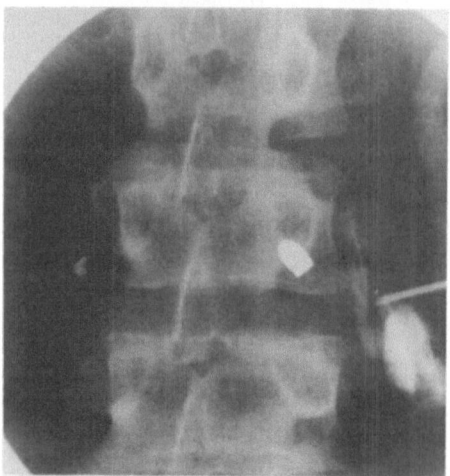

5.18. The urinoma responsible for increased separation of the dehiscent ureteral ends is aspirated under fluoroscopic guidance. This results in a closer approximation of the ureteral ends and should facilitate passage of a guide wire. (By courtesy of Lang EK)

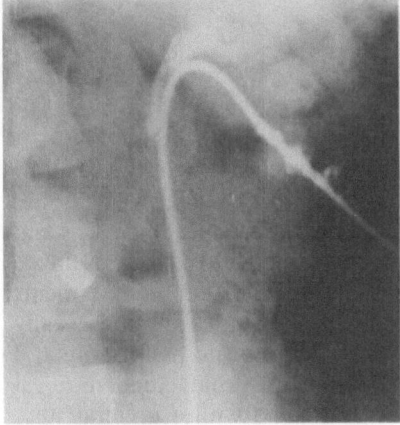

Fig. 5.19. Following the aspiration procedure of the urinoma, a guide wire is successfully passed across this partial dehiscence and a stent catheter introduced via this antegrade approach. Prior attempts to place a stent catheter via a retrograde cystoscopic approach had failed. The combination of aspiration of the urinoma and attendant reduction of dehiscence of the partially severed ureteral ends and the better alignment of the ureteral ends retained in position by tissue bridges is credited with the success of the procedure. (By courtesy of Lang EK)

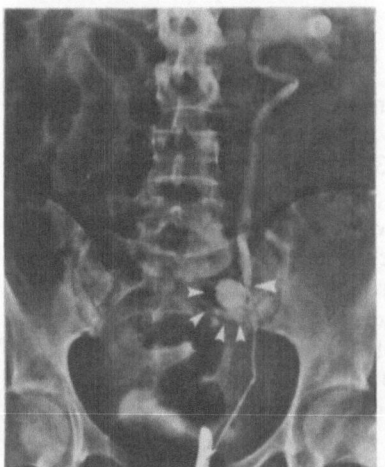
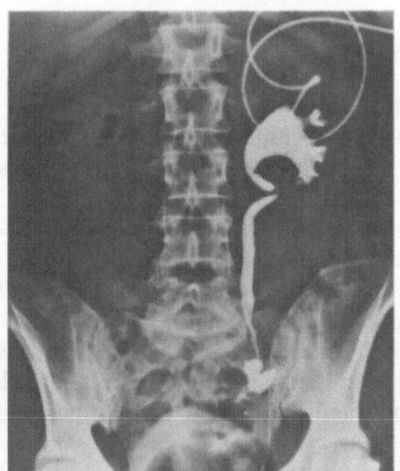

Fig. 5.20a,b. Ureteral stenosis and fistula after hysterectomy, **a** Retrograde visualization of the urinary tract shows caliber change (*large arrow*) and medial extension of contrast outside the ureter (*small arrows*). Retrograde attempts to pass a ureteral stent were unsuccessful. **b** Percutaneous nephrostomy in place prior to passing antegrade ureteral stent.

Obstruction

Another popular use of the ureteral stent is with ureteral obstruction, whether it be secondary to intraluminal blockage, edema, periureteral fibrosis, or malignant encasement [10, 25, 29, 42, 49]. Patients with malignancy may present with ureteral obstruction prior to treatment and should not be denied the benefit of renal salvage during the treatment period. Even in patients with poor treatment response, the physician is often obliged to preserve the patient's life for as long as possible in the hope that the tumor will respond to other modalities. Indwelling ureteral stents are a substitute to a nephrostomy, which burdens the patient with an external drainage bag. Open nephrostomy carries a 3%–6% mortality in patients with cancer [21,

27]. The indwelling ureteral stent often allows the cancer patient to enjoy family support and arrange personal business.

Stone Management

The management of urinary tract calculi has changed dramatically in the past few years via dissolution, retrieval, and lithotripsy [1, 13, 43]. Ureteral stents are coupled with these procedures to maintain drainage during chemical infusions and following manipulation (Fig. 5.21). It is imperative that adequate urinary drainage be established prior to many stone dissolution methods [13, 33, 40, 54]. Patients with ileal conduits are particularly prone to form struvite stones and are usually poorly suited to additional surgery. Placement of a ureteral stent assures ureteral drainage during the infusion of hemiacridin. Lithotripsy and stone retrieval techniques damage the urothelium, which is wisely treated with a ureteral stent until the edema subsides and small fragments have passed.

Dilatations

Ureteral dilatations are undergoing a revival since the widespread acceptance of balloon catheter techniques for dilating stenotic blood vessels. Barbaric et al. first dilated artificially created obstructions in dogs [3]. Several authors have described successful dilatation of ureteral strictures [2, 33, 44, 56]. The results suggest that recent postoperative strictures are amenable to dilatation, whereas older, densely fibrotic strictures and strictures secondary to ischemia are not responsive. Therefore, strictures that present years after ureteroneocystostomy are unlikely to respond to dilatation. Ureteral strictures that develop after radical hysterectomy are also not amenable to dilatation, probably because of ureteral ischemia secondary to ureteral stripping. Fistulas are also common following radical pelvic surgery and the urine leakage compounds the problem with ureteral and periureteral fibrosis.

Long-term stents show crystalloid deposits which are accelerated in patients with urinary tract infections and those receiving cancer chemotherapy. It is

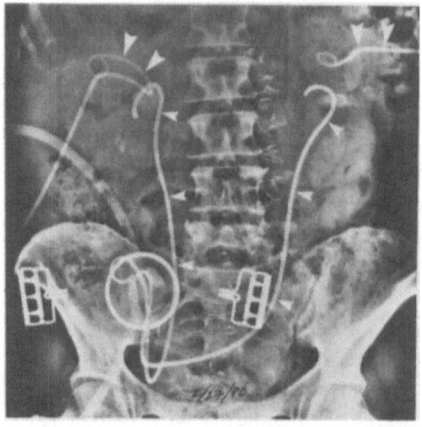

Fig. 5.21. Bilateral ureteral stents and pigtail nephrostomies prior to infusion of hemiacridin. Plain abdominal film of patient with urinary diversion. Uretera; stent catheters are in place to ensure adequate drainage during infusion of hemiacridrin through the pigtail nephrostomy catheters (*arrows*).

advisable to reduce these encrustations by controlling infection, acidifying the urine, and encouraging high fluid intake. If the catheter stent lumen becomes plugged so that a guide wire will not pass, it is possible to maintain access to the urinary tract by placing a large introducer sheath, such as a Desilets-Hoffman sheath, over the smaller stent catheter. This exchange method has been reported for changing flank and ileostomy stent catheters [4, 45].

Summary

The use of ureteral stents has evolved dramatically in the past few years, largely because of the widespread acceptance of the percutaneous approach to the kidney and the application of angiographic techniques and materials to the urinary tract.

Endourologic placement of ureteral stents was originally indicated in patients who were poor surgical risks and now represents an often preferred approach in the management of complex ureteral problems. Ureteral stents are probably most commonly used now as an accompaniment to the varied endoscopic ureteral manipulations involving calculi.

References

1. Banner MP, Pollack HM (1982) Percutaneous extraction of renal and ureteral calculi. Radiology 144:753–758
2. Banner MP, Pollack HM, Ring EJ, Wein AJ (1983) Catheter dilatation of benign ureteral strictures. Radiology 147:427–433
3. Barbaric ZL, Gothlin JH, Davies RS (1977) Transluminal dilatation and stent placement in obstructed ureters in dogs through the use of percutaneous nephropyelostomy. Invest Radiol 12:534–536
4. Baron RL, McClennan BL (1981) Replacing the occluded percutaneous nephrostomy catheter. Radiology 141:824
5. Bettmann MA, Murray PD, Perlmutt LM, Whitmore WF III, Richie JP (1983) Ureteroileal anastomotic leaks: percutaneous treatment. Radiology 148:95–100
6. Bigongiari LR, Lee KR, Mebust WK, Foret J, Weigel J (1978) Transurethral conversion of a percutaneous ureteral stent to an indwelling stent. Am J Roentgenol 131:1098–1099
7. Bigongiari LR, Lee KR, Moffat RE, Mebust WK, Foret J, Weigel J (1979) Percutaneous ureteral stent placement for stricture management and internal urinary drainage. Am J Roentgenol 133:865–868
8. Bigongiari LR, Lee KR, Moffat RE, Mebust WK, Foret J, Weigel J (1980) Conversion of percutaneous ureteral stent to indwelling pigtail stent over guidewire. Urology 15:461–465
9. Blum J, Skemp C, Reiser M (1963) Silicone rubber ureteral prosthesis. J Urol 90:276–280
10. Brin EN, Schiff M Jr, Weiss RM (1975) Palliative urinary diversion for pelvic malignancy. J Urol 113:619–622
11. Brown HP, Harrison JH (1951) The efficacy of plastic ureteral and urethral catheters for constant drainage. J Urol 66:85–93
12. Camacho MF, Pereiras R, Carrion H, Bondhus M, Politano VA (1979) Double-ended pigtail ureteral stent: useful modification to single end ureteral stent. Urology 13:516–520
13. Dretler SP, Pfister RC, Newhouse JH (1979) Renal-stone dissolution via percutaneous nephrostomy. N Engl J Med 300:341–343
14. Druy EM, Gharib M, Finder CA (1983) Percutaneous nephroureteral drainage and stenting for postsurgical ureteral leaks. Am J Roentgenol 141:389–394

15. Finney RP (1978) Experience with new double J ureteral catheter stent. J Urol 120:678–681
16. Fritzsche P, Moorhead JD, Axford PD, Torrey RR (1981) Urologic applications of angiographic guide wire and catheter techniques. J Urol 125:774–779
17. Fritzsche P. Senac M, Moorhead JD (1981) Guide wire probe technique of the urinary tract. Radiographics 1:38–48
18. Gibbons RP, Correa RJ Jr, Cummings KB, Tate Mason J (1976) Experience with indwelling ureteral stent catheters. J Urol 115:22–26
19. Goldin AR (1977) Percutaneous ureteral splinting. Urology 10:165–168
20. Goodwin WE, Casey WC, Woolf W (1955) Percutaneous trocar (needle) nephrostomy in hydronephrosis. JAMA 157:891–894
21. Grabstald H, McPhee M (1973) Nephrostomy and the cancer patient. South Med J 66:217–219
22. Gunther R, Alken P, Altwein JE (1978) Ureterobstruktion: perkutane transrenale Uretersplintung. Aktuelle Urol 4:195–199
23. Gunther R, Altwein JE, Alken P (1980) Internal urinary diversion by a percutaneous ureteric splint. Br J Urol 52:165
24. Hepperlen TW, Mardis HK, Kammandel H (1978) Self-retained internal ureteral stents: a new approach. J Urol 119:731–734
25. Hepperlen TW, Mardis HK, Kammandel H (1979) The pigtail ureteral stent in the cancer patient. J Urol 121:17–18
26. Ho PC, Talner LB, Parsons CL, Schmidt JD (1980) Percutaneous nephrostomy: experience in 107 kidneys. Urology 16:532–535
27. Holden S, McPhee M, Grabstald H (1979) The rationale of urinary diversion in cancer patients. J Urol 121:19–21
28. Jaffe RB, Middleton AW Jr (1980) Whitaker test: differentiation of obstructive from nonobstructive uropathy. AJR 134:9–15
29. Kearney GP, Mahoney EM, Brown HP (1979) Useful technique for long-term urinary drainage by inlying ureteral stent. Urology 14:126–134
30. Lang EK (1981) Diagnosis and management of ureteral fistulas by percutaneous nephrostomy and antegrade stent catheter. Radiology 138:311–317
31. Lang EK, Alexander R, Barnett T, Palomar J, Hamway S (1978) Brush biopsy of pyelocalyceal lesions via a percutaneous translumbar approach. Radiology 129:623–627
32. Lang EK, Lanasa JA, Garrett J, Stripling J, Palomar J (1979) The management of urinary fistulas and strictures with percutaneous ureteral stent catheters. J Urol 122:736–740
33. Lang EK, Price ET (1983) Redefinitions of indications for percutaneous nephrostomy. Radiology 147:419–426
34. Mardis HK, Hepperlen TW, Kammandel H (1979) Double pigtail ureteral stent. Urology 14:23–26
35. Mardis HK, Kroeger RM, Hepperlen TW, Mazer MJ, Kammandel H (1982) Polyethylene double-pigtail ureteral stents. Urol Clin North Am 9:95–101
36. Marmar JL (1970) The management of ureteral obstruction with silicone rubber splint catheters. J Urol 104:386–389
37. Mazer MJ, LeVeen RF, Call JE, Wolf G, Baltaxe HA (1979) Permanent percutaneous antegrade ureteral stent placement without trans-urethral assistance. Urology 14:413–419
38. Miller RP, Reinke DB, Clayman RV, Lange PH (1982) Percutaneous approach to the ureter. Urol Clin North Am 9:31–40
39. Mitty HA, Gribetz ME (1982) The status of interventional uroradiology. J Urol 127:2–9
40. Mulvaney WP (1960) The clinical use of Renacidin in urinary calcifications. J Urol 84:206–212
41. Orikasa S, Tsuji I, Siba T, Ohashi N (1973) A new technique for transurethral insertion of a silicone rubber tree into an obstructed ureter. J Urol 110:184–187
42. Pais VM, Spellman RM, Stiles RE, Mahoney SA (1975) Internal ureteral splints. Urology 4:32–36
43. Pfister RC, Yoder IC, Newhouse JH (1981) Percutaneous uroradiologic procedures. Semin Roentgenol 16:135–151
44. Pingoud EG, Bagley DH, Zeman, RD, Glancy KE, Pais OS (1980) Percutaneous antegrade bilateral ureteral dilatation and stent placement for internal drainage. Radiology 134:780
45. Pollack HM, Banner MP (1982) Replacing blocked or dislodged percutaneous nephrostomy and ureteral stent catheters. Radiology 145:203–205
46. Rosen RJ, McLean GK, Freiman DB, Oleaga JA, Wein AJ, Ring EJ (1980) Obstructed ureteroileal conduits: antegrade catheter drainage. Am J Roentgenol 135:1201–1204
47. Ring EJ, McLean GK (1981) Interventional radiology: principles and techniques. Little, Brown and Company, Boston, p 379–410
48. Rutner AB, Fucilla IS (1976) Flexible tip ureteral catheters in clinical practice. J Urol 115:18–21
49. Singh B, Kim H, Was SH (1979) Stent versus nephrostomy: Is there a choice? J Urol 121:268–270

50. Smith AD (1982) The universal ureteral stent. Urol Clin North Am 9:103–107
51. Smith AD, Lange PH, Miller RP, Reinke DB (1978) Introduction of the Gibbons ureteral stent facilitated by antecedent percutaneous nephrostomy. J Urol 120:543–544
52. Smith AD, Lange PH, Reinke DB, Miller RP (1978) Extraction of ureteral calculi from patients with ileal loops: a new technique. J Urol 120:623–625
53. Smith AD, Lange PH, Miller RP, Reinke DB (1979) Percutaneous dilatation of ureteroileal strictures and insertion of Gibbons ureteral stents. Urology 13:24–26
54. Smith AD, Lange PH, Miller RP, Reinke DB (1979) Dissolution of cystine calculi by irrigation with acetylcysteine through percutaneous nephrostomy. Urology 13:422–423
55. Smith AD, Lange PH, Miller RP, Reinke DB (1979) Controlled ureteral meatotomy. J Urol 121:587–589
56. Smith AD, Miller RP, Reinke DB, Lange PH, Fraley EE (1979) Insertion of Gibbons ureteral stents using endourologic techniques. Urology 14:330–336
57. Smith AD, Reinke DB, Miller RP, Lange PH (1979) Percutaneous nephrostomy in the management of ureteral and renal calculi. Radiology 133:49–54
58. Sullivan JW, Grabstald H, Whitmore WF Jr (1980) Complications of ureteroileal conduit with radical cystectomy: review of 336 cases. J Urol 124:797–801
59. Whitaker RH (1973) Methods of assessing obstruction in dilated ureters. Br J Urol 45:15–22
60. Wiess EQ, Leyva A, Hernandez A (1976) Treatment of lithiasis by the forced injection of liquid and ureteral catheterization by the translumbar route. Int Surg 61:419–422
61. Wrigley JV, Prem KA, Fraley EE (1976) Pelvic exenteration: complications of urinary diversion. J Urol 116:428–430
62. Zimskind PD, Fetter TR, Wilkerson JL (1967) Clinical use of long-term indwelling silicone rubber ureteral splints inserted cystoscopically. J Urol 97:840–844

Chapter 6

Transluminal Dilatation of Ureteral Strictures

Lawrence R. Bigongiari

Dilatation of ureteral strictures was first performed in the 1890s shortly after the introduction of the cystoscope [9]. The procedure fell into disrepute and disuse as modern anesthesia and surgical techniques were developed. With the advent of percutaneous nephrostomy and the techniques of endourology, catheters can be easily placed in the ureter from above as well as from below. Any minimally invasive nonsurgical therapy which replaces an invasive surgical procedure will minimize hospital stay. Cost containment warrants a review of the efficiency of catheter dilatation of ureteral strictures.

Ureteral strictures can be dilated by the passage of a catheter of larger caliber or by a balloon catheter inflated in the stricture. A catheter traversing the narrowed area or a balloon distending it enlarges the lumen by stretching the process in the ureteral wall which is narrowing the lumen. Progressively larger dilating catheters or a catheter with a long taper may also be used. The principal advantage of a dilating balloon is the ability to stretch the wall to a size much larger than the caliber of the catheter itself, without multiple manipulations (Fig. 6.1). A stent catheter may then be left in the ureter to ensure drainage of the collecting system and to serve as a mold for the desired residual lumen. This stent may be left in place until the inflammatory process has run its course. The hydrostatic pressure of flowing urine will then maintain patency.

Modern descriptions of this approach to ureteral strictures are scant and scattered, with even the largest series consisting of only 80 cases. We found reports of 124 cases since 1977. Acknowledging the difficulty of comparing data reported from diverse sources, we will try to summarize recent experience categorized by type of lesion. We have excluded cases in which information was not adequate for our categorization. Success of the procedure was determined by varying periods of subsequent adequate drainage.

We found 43 cases involving strictures occurring after various operative procedures. These cases are divided into those occurring within 2 months of surgery (Table 6.1) and those occurring after 2 months (Table 6.2).

Even with the total number of cases in the literature being small and the variation in techniques, some patterns seem to be emerging.

Ureteral strictures occurring shortly after surgical procedures for benign conditions seem to respond favorably to dilatation. In three of three cases after ureterolithotomy and in three of three cases after gynecologic surgery, dilatation was successful. This finding should be expected from theoretical considerations. The lumen is remolded to the desired caliber and stented until the postoperative healing process is completed. Ureteropelvic junction obstruction may be an exception, with two of three cases failing. This finding may be due more to the nature of the underlying abnormality than to the nature of either the surgery or the dilatation. Multiple long-term dilatations up to 16 h per day for 4 days were used in the one successful case. The possibility of ischemic necrosis of the mucosa must be considered. The overall success rate in this group was 77.8% (7/9).

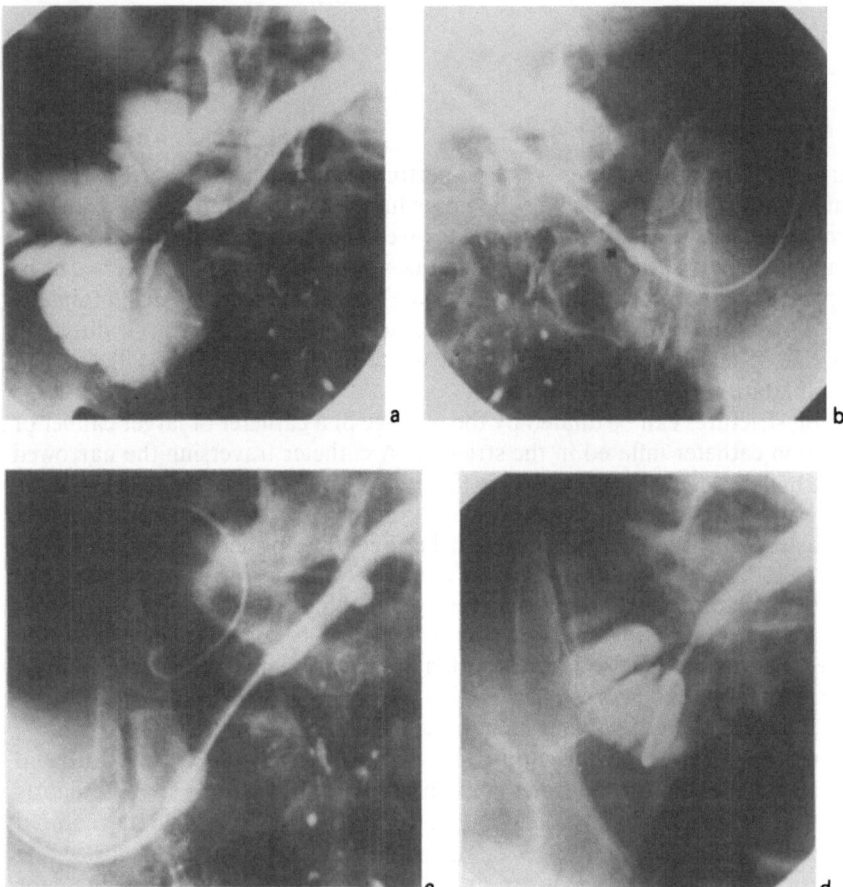

Fig. 6.1. a A catheter introduced via the percutaneous nephrostomy approach has been advanced to the level of a stricture at the ureteroileostomy site. The injection phase clearly delineates the stricture. **b** The guide wire is passed through the stricture and after initial dilatation with a Bougie catheter, an 8-mm Gruntzig balloon catheter is placed across the stricture. Initially there is considerable deformity of the balloon when being inflated, indicating constraints by the stricture. **c** After several attempts the balloon dilates fully, indicating salutory stretching of the lesion. The caliber of the balloon chosen is slightly larger than that of the normal ureter. **d** Following the dilatation procedure a double J Cook stent catheter (8 F) is placed across the lesion to help retain the lumen during the phase of healing. (All four photographs by courtesy of E. K. Lang)

Table 6.1. Postoperative strictures occurring within 2 months

		Interval postop.	Success (+/−)	Stent	Comment
UPJ repair					
Banner et al. [1]	Case 26	6 wks	−	1 mo	One of these two cases
	Case 27	1 mo	−	1 wk	had urinemia and peripelvic abscess
Kadir et al. [4]		6 wks	+	4 days	Balloon inflated up to 16 h/day for 4 days
Ureterolithotomy					
Banner et al. [1]	Case 1	2 wks	+	3 mo	
	Case 2	1 mo	+	4 days	
	Case 3	2 wks	+	7 days	
Ureteroileostomy					
Banner et al. [1]	Case 6	3 wks	+	4 days	Left
Goldin [3]	Case 3	?	+	6 wks	Right complicated by transient infection
	Case 4	3 wks	+	3 wks	Right
	Case 5	1 wk	−	6 wks	Right
Kaufman and Ehrlich [6]	Case 1	2 wks	+	3 wks	Left
After radical hysterectomy					
Banner et al. [1]	Case 18	7 wks	−	3 wks	Ureteral strip
	Case 19	2 wks	−	4½ mo	Preop. radiation
	Case 20	5 wks	−	2½ mo	Ureteral strip
	Case 21	7 days	+	5 wks	
After gynecologic surgery for benign disease					
Reimer and Oswalt [12]		6 wks	+	—	Ligation at Marshall-Marchetti suspension
Kaplan et al. [5]		2 wks	+	1 wk	Emergency cesarean section
Witherington and Shelor [13]	Case 2	5 wks	+	None	Abdominal hysterectomy, 4 dilatations over 6 weeks
Ureteroneocystostomy					
Banner et al. [1]	Case 4	10 days	−	7 days	Ureteral stripping separate from radical hysterectomy
Lang et al. [7]	Case 4	"Several days"	+	10 wks	
Miscellaneous					
Banner et al. [1]	Case 25	2 wks	−	Indefinite	Ureterolysis for retroperitoneal fibrosis
Total success			14/21 66.7%		

Ureteral strictures occurring 3 months to 7½ years after gynecologic surgery for benign disease were successfully treated by the technique in four of five cases, but a stricture occurring at the site of a ureteral anastomosis 10 years after surgery did not respond. At this late stage, one would expect more fibrosis than edema. This 66.6% (4/6) success rate is still encouraging.

In strictured ureteroileal anastomoses, four of five recent and seven of eleven older strictures responded to the techniques. The success rate was 68.8% overall (11/16).

In ureteral strictures after radical hysterectomy, three of four recent cases failed and two of three older cases succeeded. All of these cases except the recent success

Table 6.2. Postoperative strictures occurring after more than 2 months

		Interval postop.	Success (+/−)	Stent	Comment
Ureteroileal anastomoses					
Banner et al. [1]	Case 7	17 mo	+	6 mo	Left
	Case 8	6 mo	+	7 days	Right
	Case 9	6 mo	−	7 days	Left
	Case 10	2 yrs	−	4 days	Right ureteral stripping
	Case 11	2 yr	−	4 days	Right
	Case 12	4½ yr	+	0	Left
	Case 13	2½ yr	−	7 days	Right
	Case 14	4 mo	+	2 wks	Left
	Case 15	4 mo	+	2 wks	Right
	Case 16	5 mo	+	2 wks	Left
Dixon et al. [2]		5½ mo	+	6 wks	Left multiple dilatations over 6 weeks
After radical hysterectomy					
Banner et al. [1]	Case 17	4 mo	−	10 days	Ureteral stripping
Lang et al. [7]	Case 2	5 mo	+	6 wks	Ureteral stripping
	Case 3	2½ yrs	+	4 wks	External radiation therapy, surgery, and radium implant
After gynecologic surgery for benign disease					
Banner et al. [1]	Case 22	3 mo	+	4 days	After tubal ligation
	Case 23	10 yr	−	5 days	Ureteral ligation surgically repaired with anastomosis
	Case 24	10 wks	−	1 day	Abdominal hysterectomy
Witherington and Shelor [13]	Case 1	3 mo	+	3 days	Abdominal hysterectomy and Marshall-Marchetti Then dilated ×4 over next month
	Case 3	3 mo	−	6 wks	Transabdominal hysterectomy
	Case 4	7 yrs	+	2 wks	Transabdominal hysterectomy and left oophorectomy. Indwelling catheter for 2 days postop. Seven years later severe symptoms
Ureteroneocystostomy					
Banner et al. [1]	Case 5	18 mo	−	4 days	Transplant
Renal allograft transplant stenosis					
Lieberman et al. [8]		16 yrs	+	3 wks	7 mo follow-up
Total success			14/22 63.6%		

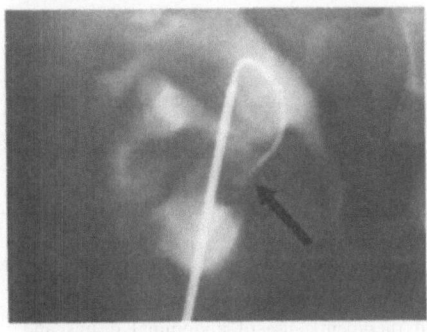

Fig. 6.2. A steerable Wilson Eskridge brush has been introduced via a coaxial sheath into the renal pelvis. The brush element is then negotiated under fluoroscopic control into the infundibulum of the inferior calyx and a brush biopsy obtained from the suspect lesion. The coaxial sheath protects against dissemination of tumor cells along the tract. [By courtesy of E. K. Lang and Radiology (1978) 129:623]

had preoperative radiation or ureteral stripping which could have impaired the blood supply to the ureter and impaired the healing process. We must assume the strictures were related to postoperative fibrosis, not malignant encasement.

In patients with a previous history of tumor, particularly if ureteroileal conduit was created for uroepithelial malignancy, cytologic studies should be obtained to differentiate between benign and malignant structure. Transabdominal skinny needle aspiration biopsy or brush biopsy via a ureteral catheter are alternatives. Any brush biopsy obtained should be via a coaxial sheathed catheter to prevent seeding to other mucosal sites or along a nephrostomy tract (Fig. 6.2).

Dilatation by itself seems to have little place in the palliation of malignant encasement. Ureteral stenting may maintain drainage in supravesical obstruction while radiation or chemotherapy is being applied. If treatment shrinks the obstructing tumor, the stent may even be removed for a period of time. The underlying pathologic process is not such that lasting patency can be expected.

Pingoud et al. [11] reported the use of balloon dilatation of a channel through a malignant ureteral obstruction to facilitate placement of an indwelling stent. Such dilatation risks intravascular dissemination of tumor cells.

Tuberculous ureteral strictures result from a chronic granulomatous fibrotic process. Murphy et al. [10] reported successful transurethral dilatation in 51 of 80 (64%) ureters with tubercular strictures. The technique was applied but failed in 29 ureters and could not be applied because of technical difficulties in 17 other ureters. All patients were on a regimen of triple antitubercular chemotherapy. Either a single 8-F or two 5-F ureteral catheters were passed through the stenotic area. The dilatation was repeated weekly or biweekly at first, then monthly or bimonthly until the upper tract stabilized. All patients in the series were followed for 5 years.

The 60% success reported in tuberculous strictures using multiple dilatations suggests that persistence may have ultimately led to success in some of the postoperative failures.

Banner et al. [1] reported failure of ureteral dilatation in a case of retroperitoneal fibrosis. Although dilatation to a caliber larger than that of the stent may facilitate placement, lasting ureteral patency should not be expected from dilatation alone in this relentless densely fibrotic process.

Catheter dilatation will find its place in the treatment of ureteral strictures, though at this early stage it is difficult to predict what that place will be. The minimal invasiveness of ureteral catheterization warrants further investigation. The financial, physical, and emotional cost of inpatient surgical procedures for these conditions must be weighed against the same costs of repeated outpatient procedures.

References

1. Banner MP, Pollack HM, Ring EJ, Wein AJ (1983) Catheter dilatation of benign ureteral strictures. Radiology 147: 427–433
2. Dixon GD, Moore JD, Stockton R (1982) Successful dilatation of ureteroileal anastomotic stenosis using Gruntzig catheter. Urology 19:555–558
3. Goldin AR (1977) Percutaneous ureteral splinting. Urology 10:165–168
4. Kadir S, White RI, Engel R (1982) Balloon dilatation of a ureteropelvic junction obstruction. Radiology 143:263–264
5. Kaplan JO, Winslow OP, Sneider SE, Pryor TH, Caplan LH, Messinger NH (1982) Dilatation of a surgically ligated ureter through a percutaneous nephrostomy. AJR 139:188–189
6. Kaufman JJ, Ehrlich RM (1982) Prophylactic and therapeutic use of abdominal drains and percutaneous nephrostomies and stents for treatment of precarious ureteroileal anastomosis. Urology 20:118–120
7. Lang EK, Lanasa JA, Garrett J, Stripling J, Palomar J (1979) The management of urinary fistulas and strictures with percutaneous ureteral stent catheters. J Urol 122:736–740
8. Lieberman SF, Keller FS, Barry JM, Rosch J (1982) Percutaneous antegrade transluminal ureteroplasty for renal allograft ureteral stenosis. J Urol 128:122–124
9. Murphy LJF (ed) (1972) In: The history of urology. CC Thomas, Springfield, Ill. 281–332
10. Murphy DM, Fallon B, Lane V, O'Flynn JD (1982) Tuberculous strictures of ureter. Urology 20:382–384
11. Pingoud EG, Bagley DH, Zemian RK, Glancy KE, Pais OS (1980) Percutaneous antegrade bilateral ureteral dilatation and stent placement for internal drainage. Radiology 134:780
12. Reimer DE, Oswalt GC (1981) Iatrogenic ureteral obstruction treated with balloon dilation. J Urol 126:689–690
13. Witherington R, Shelor WC (1980) Treatment of postoperative ureteral stricture by catheter dilation: A forgotten procedure. Urology 16:592–595

Chapter 7

Percutaneous Drainage of Abscesses, Urinomas, and Hematomas of the Genitourinary Tract and Retroperitoneum

Bruce R. Baumgartner and Michael E. Bernardino

Introduction

Considerable attention has been given to abdominal abscesses in the recent literature and to the importance of the role of the radiologist in their diagnosis and treatment. Untreated intra-abdominal abscesses continue to be associated with high mortality, especially in the subphrenic and upper abdominal regions [5]. Most of these cases are seen following intra-abdominal surgery, and the clinical presentation is often subtle with today's widespread use of antibiotics in the post-operative period. The etiology of retroperitoneal abscesses differs with the three various subdivisions of that region. Anterior pararenal abscesses tend to originate in the gastrointestinal tract secondary to pancreatitis, diverticulitis, or ulcer perforation [34]. An isolated abscess in the perinephric space, however, is most often the result of direct extension from a primary infectious process in the kidney [30]. With the decline of hematogenous staphylococcal renal abscesses, postoperative abscesses now account for an increasing proportion of lesions in this space. Postoperative and primary renal infections are also the source of the majority of the abscesses in the posterior pararenal space [8]. As with intraperitoneal abscesses, there is a need for prompt diagnosis and treatment of those in the retroperitoneal space. Thus, these abscesses are ideal lesions to respond to percutaneous aspiration and drainage combined with appropriate antibiotic therapy. This report will discuss the anatomy, diagnosis, accuracy, technique, and indications of interventional procedures in patients with abnormal renal or perirenal fluid collections.

Anatomy

The anatomy of the retroperitoneum has been well described in the literature [25]. The region is divided into three distinct spaces that are readily delineated by computed tomography (CT) [21]. The retroperitoneum is bounded anteriorly by the posterior parietal peritoneum and posteriorly by the transversalis fascia and extends from the diaphragm superiorly to the pelvic brim inferiorly. The anterior pararenal space lies between the posterior peritoneum and the anterior renal (Gerota's) fascia, contains the pancreas, duodenum, and retroperitoneal portions of the colon, and is continuous across the midline. The perinephric space lies between the anterior and posterior renal (Gerota's) fasciae and includes the kidneys, adrenals, and perinephric fat. Although the perinephric space has been considered to be interrupted at the midline, communication between the right and left perirenal spaces has been demonstrated by CT [33]. The posterior pararenal space lies between the posterior renal (Gerota's) fascia and the transversalis fascia, contains no organs, and does not communicate with the contralateral posterior pararenal space.

Retroperitoneal fluid collections, whether pus, blood, or urine, tend to observe fascial boundaries (Fig. 7.1), although with severe infection or hemorrhage there may be spread from one compartment to another. The retroperitoneum is a difficult area to evaluate clinically and, before the advent of cross-sectional imaging, was also hard to study radiographically. The diagnosis of retroperitoneal abscess or inflammation was overlooked in 20%–50% of patients [34]. Morbidity and mortality increase with delayed diagnosis of abscess, and mortality approaches 100% when there is failure to drain an abscess.

Most retroperitoneal inflammatory fluid collections occur in the anterior pararenal space related to the pancreas or the retroperitoneal intestine, with the former being a more frequent source [1]. Fluid collections confined to the posterior pararenal space are rare, as there are no organs in this space, but they may occur

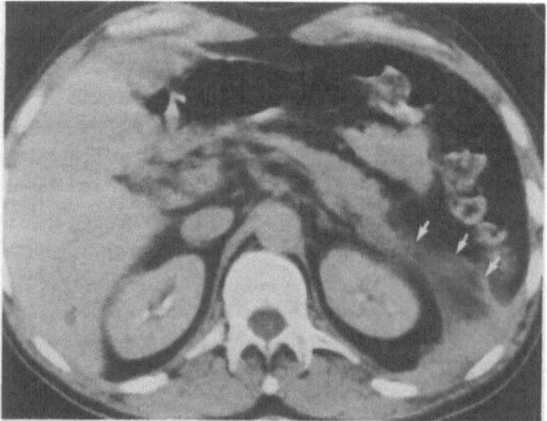

Fig. 7.1. CT scan several days following percutaneous nephrolithotomy reveals inhomogeneous density extending from the tail of the pancreas posterolaterally (*arrows*). Note thickening of Gerota's fascia anteriorly and preservation of perinephric fat planes with this hematoma involving the anterior and posterior pararenal spaces.

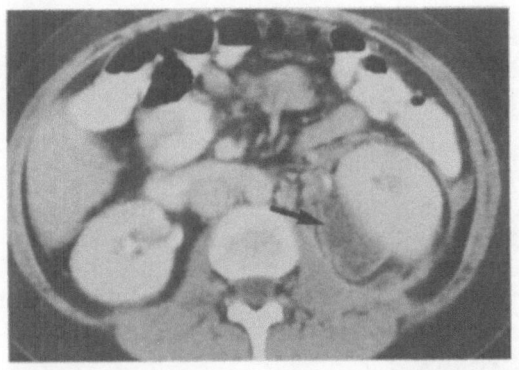

a

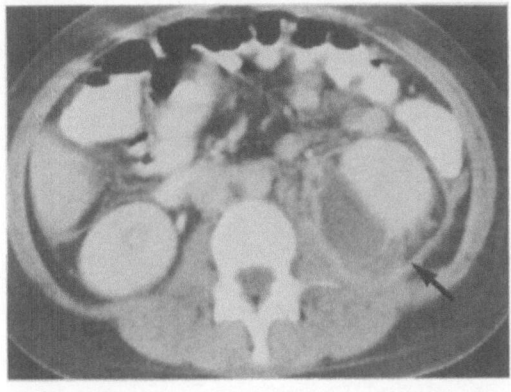

b

Fig. 7.2.a CT scan 1 week after left renal biopsy demonstrates a subcapsular fluid collection (*arrow*) displacing the kidney anteriorly. **b** More caudad CT section demonstrates extension of the hematoma into the perinephric and medial posterior pararenal spaces with thickening of Gerota's fascia (*arrow*).

secondary to severe infection or hemorrhage in another space (Fig. 7.2). Of intermediate frequency are those fluid collections or abscesses in the perirenal space. Over 80% occur as direct extension from the kidney [23].

Pathology of Renal Infections

Infectious involvement of the kidney may have no radiographic manifestations. The kidney may be swollen with diffuse pyelonephritis, although a more discrete mass effect may be seen with acute focal bacterial nephritis (AFBN) [20]. This latter entity has also been termed acute lobar nephronia [28]. The radiographic findings in this form of infection include a localized mass on excretory urography and a relatively sonolucent mass disrupting the corticomedullary junction on ultrasonography [20, 28]. AFBN may be seen on CT as a focal or generalized enlargement of the kidney, usually with patchy or wedge-shaped areas having variable degrees of diminished contrast enhancement [27, 36]. The fluid content

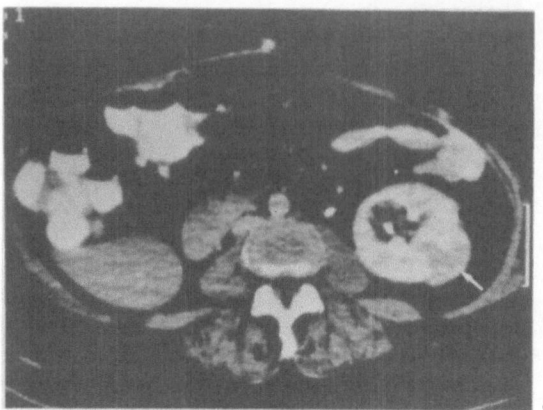

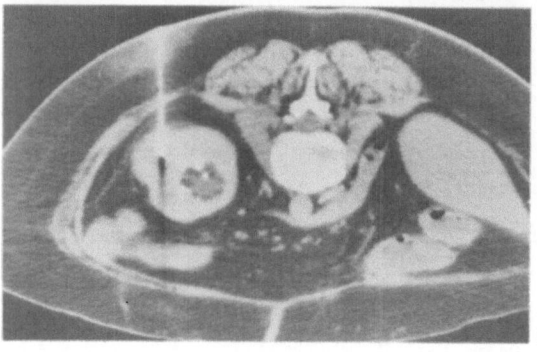

Fig. 7.3. a 69-year-old female with previous right nephrectomy developed fever, chills, and left flank pain following resection of gangrenous bowel. CT scan demonstrates a wedge-shaped irregular area of diminished attenuation posterolaterally (*arrow*). **b** Prone CT-directed needle aspiration yielded no pus or fluid, but tissue fragments were positive for infection. These findings are consistent with acute focal bacterial nephritis.

characteristic of abscess is usually not delineated (Fig. 7.3). AFBN generally resolves with antibiotic therapy, but may progress into an abscess cavity. Once an abscess has formed, drainage is usually required. The abscess may remain confined to the kidney, but, if untreated, may extend to involve the perinephric space (Fig. 7.4).

Hoddick et al. described 12 patients with urosepsis and severe renal or perinephric infection evaluated by CT and ultrasound [15]. Six patients had renal or perinephric abscesses larger than 2 cm, one patient had multiple abscesses smaller than 1 cm, and five patients had AFBN. All diagnoses were made correctly by CT, but there were several false-negatives with ultrasound. They concluded, "CT seems to be more sensitive than ultrasound in evaluating severe renal and perirenal infections." Infections involving the kidney and perinephric space may be thought of as a pathologic spectrum from a bacterial nephritis that usually responds to antibiotic treatment through frank perinephric abscess requiring drainage. A consistent CT feature among Hoddick et al.'s patients was the sharp delineation of abscesses from adjacent enhancing renal parenchyma as opposed to the poorly defined areas of AFBN, usually in a lobar distribution.

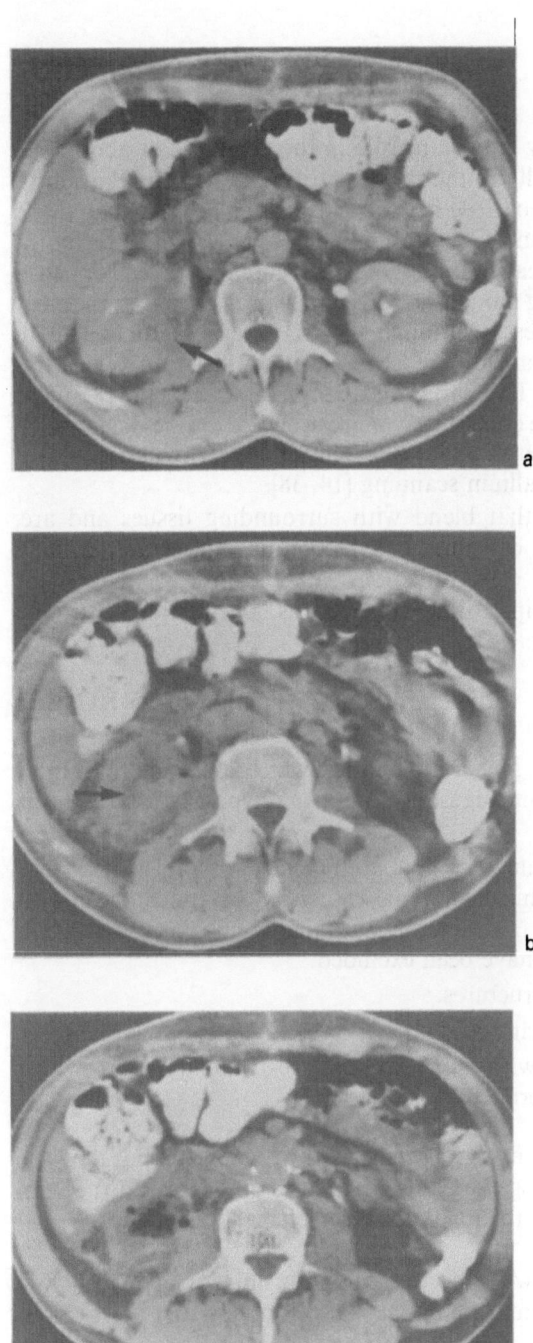

Fig. 7.4. a CT scan demonstrates a vague, irregular area of decreased attenuation in the medial right kidney (*arrow*) in a 50-year-old man with fever. **b** More caudad CT section shows a lobulated fluid density in the lower pole of the kidney (*arrow*) with one small gas pocket, as well as loss of the normal perinephric fat planes. **c** Additional gas collections are seen more inferiorly in the abscess, which extends into the perinephric space, causing thickening of Gerota's fascia.

Diagnosis

The radiologist plays an extremely important role in the diagnosis of abdominal abscess. The clinical signs, especially in the retroperitoneal space, may be subtle. Conventional radiographs may be of little help, as the fluid collections may blend with adjacent structures. The presence of extraluminal gas may be detected on the films, but may be confused with fecal debris or intestinal gas. The advent of newer isotope and cross-sectional imaging modalities has significantly enhanced the early diagnosis of retroperitoneal abscess. Although earlier reports were unable to demonstrate a statistically significant difference in accuracy between CT, ultrasound, and gallium-67 scanning in the search for abdominal abscess [6, 18], more recent studies have shown CT to be consistently more accurate for the diagnosis of abdominal abscess and for the determination of extent of disease, with significant advantages over ultrasound and gallium scanning [14, 38].

Abscesses are fluid collections that blend with surrounding tissues and are, therefore, usually not apparent on conventional radiographs unless they contain gas. Cross-sectional imaging will clearly demonstrate the abscess, as well as delineate its extent and relationships to adjacent organs. The characteristic CT signs of abscess are [7, 8, 11]:

1. Round or oval soft tissue mass with central low attenuation (0–25 HU) and smooth or irregular margins.

2. A surrounding region of slightly higher attenuation which often enhances after IV contrast to form the so-called rind sign, resulting from hypervascularity in the abscess wall (Fig. 7.5).

3. The presence of gas within the mass, seen as multiple small bubbles or a large solitary collection. This finding is unusual in renal abscess but not uncommon with abscesses in the perinephric space; it is virtually pathognomonic of abscess when fistulas and iatrogenic gas sources have been excluded.

4. Displacement of surrounding structures.

5. Edema of surrounding tissues with obliteration of contiguous tissue planes.

6. Thickening of Gerota's fascia with any retroperitoneal inflammation, which may also extend to involve the lateral conal fascia.

There are several sonographic signs that may be seen with abscess, but they are variable and depend upon the echogenicity of the lesion's contents and the scan technique. The ultrasound findings for renal abscess include [7, 8, 11]:

1. A round or oval echo-free mass with good through transmission. The wall may be smooth or irregular. At times it may be difficult to distinguish an abscess from simple renal cyst on ultrasound.

2. Occasional low-level internal echoes which may be seen to layer.

3. A highly echogenic mass caused by gas bubbles in the abscess [19]. A large anterior collection of gas within the abscess may prevent delineation of a more dependent fluid collection. This is more likely with perinephric than intrarenal abscesses. Internal septation is also more common with the former than the latter [7].

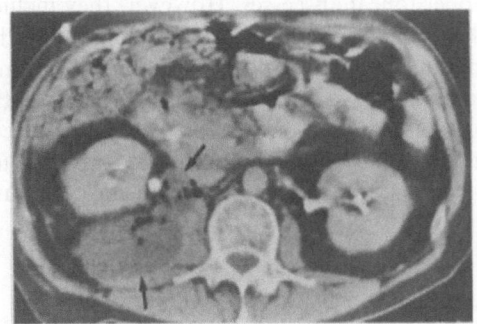

a

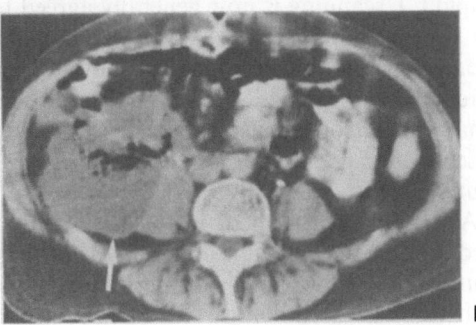

b

Fig. 7.5. a CT scan demonstrates a lobulated fluid collection (*arrows*) with gas involving the perinephric space in a 60-year-old man who developed sepsis following cholecystectomy. There is thickening of the psoas and quadratus lumborum muscles and anterior displacement of the kidney. **b** More caudad CT section reveals the considerable extent of the abscess. Note the enhanced rim (*arrow*) of the peripheral margin of the abscess ("rind sign").

These CT and ultrasound findings are nonspecific, and other fluid collections may mimic abscess. Gerzof has devised a mnemonic for the differential diagnosis in the postoperative period: *BLUSH*—which represents biloma, lymphocele, urinoma, seroma, and hematoma [11]. Pancreatic pseudocyst and other cysts, fluid-filled or distended bowel, dilated genitourinary structures, and primary and secondary neoplasms may have the same CT or ultrasound appearance as abscess. It must be emphasized that neither CT nor ultrasound can differentiate sterile from infected fluid collections. Interpretation of CT and ultrasound must be made in light of the clinical history. In the patient with clinical signs of sepsis, including fever, flank pain, and/or elevated WBC, the ultrasound or CT demonstration of a renal or perinephric mass or fluid collection should suggest guided needle aspiration as the most effective diagnostic modality.

Percutaneous Abscess Drainage

When the diagnosis of retroperitoneal abscess seems likely on the basis of the clinical picture as well as the CT and/or ultrasound findings, percutaneous drainage must be considered in the therapeutic approach. Indications for this procedure include [7–9, 11, 13]: (1) a well defined, unilocular abscess, (2) a safe percutaneous drainage route, and (3) surgical consultation and backup in the event of failure or a complication. Contraindications are unusual, especially in renal or retroperitoneal abscesses. However, they include absence of a safe drainage route and a bleeding diathesis or coagulopathy, although this latter condition may be overcome at least temporarily for the duration of the procedure. A multiseptated abscess is not a contraindication, because the vast majority may be drained successfully. Only one catheter may be needed in most situations, since the compartments of the multiseptated abscess usually communicate or the single catheter disrupts the septation, causing communication between the compartments [4].

Technique

Rapid CT scanning is now generally agreed to be the preferred imaging modality for suspected abdominal abscess, including renal and perinephric locations. It has been shown to be accurate for both diagnosis and route planning prior to percutaneous drainage. Ultrasound has also been considered adequate for imaging renal and retroperitoneal abscesses [9]. We prefer to use CT guidance for all abscess drainage, because it better delineates the extent of the abscess and access routes.

After the institution of intravenous antibiotics and appropriate preoperative medications, the patient is placed in the prone position in the CT gantry; the needle route should always be extraperitoneal with renal or perinephric abscesses. A catheter filled with contrast is taped to the patient's skin in the cephalocaudad direction along the anticipated needle entry site as determined by preliminary diagnostic CT scans. The patient may be rotated into an oblique position if this is necessary for drainage. The percutaneous catheter must be placed so that drainage will be dependent but in such a manner that it will cause as little discomfort to the patient as possible. A digital abdominal image is obtained, and sections through the abscess are made for reference. Measurements are made of the distance from the contrast-filled catheter to the appropriate entry site on the skin. This location is marked on the patient's skin utilizing the laser light of the CT gantry for reference. The angle of entry and the depth from the skin to the near wall of the abscess are measured from the appropriate CT scans. The skin is then prepared with Betadine solution, draped appropriately, and anesthetized with 2% lidocaine. A small dermotomy is made with a No. 11 scalpel blade and widened with a curved hemostat. The size of the catheter anticipated to be used determines the slit length, as well as the amount of skin dissection to be made by the hemostat. An 18-gauge Teflon sheathed needle is then marked with a Steristrip or sterile clamp at the maximum length to be inserted through the skin. The needle is then advanced half the distance between the skin and the abscess. Repeat CT scan is made and, if the trajectory appears correct, the needle is then advanced the full distance into the abscess. Another scan is obtained to confirm the needle location within the abscess and, after removal of the stylet, approximately 10 cc of fluid is aspirated through the sheath for Gram stain and culture for both aerobes and anaerobes (Fig. 7.6a, b). Only a small amount of fluid is removed, so that the remainder provides an adequate target for subsequent catheter insertion [8]. The antibiotics given before aspiration may be changed, pending the results of the Gram stain and bacterial sensitivity studies. If the aspirate is purulent, percutaneous drainage should proceed immediately without moving the patient, as that may alter the anatomic relationships shown on earlier scans and thereby change the drainage

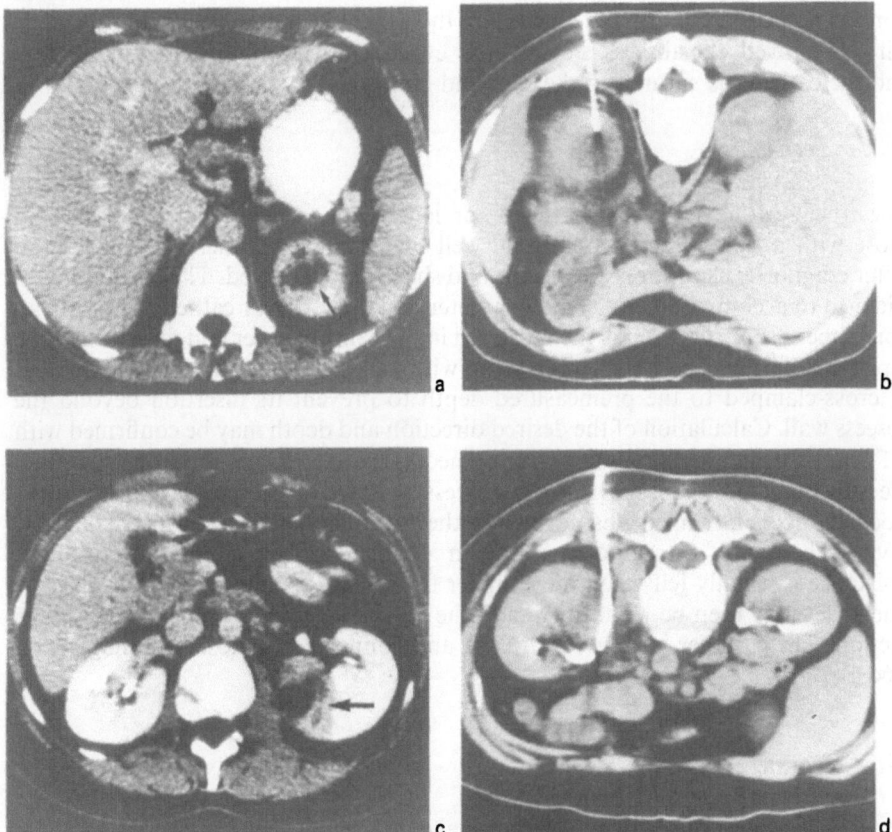

Fig. 7.6. a CT scan in a 30-year-old female with fever of unknown origin and bacteremia demonstrates an area of decreased attenuation and probable necrosis involving the upper pole of the left kidney (*arrow*). **b** With CT guidance in the prone position, an 18-gauge needle was placed into the abscess and purulent material aspirated. **c** An additional, larger abscess is located by CT scan in the medial left kidney (*arrow*). **d** With the patient in the prone position, an 8.3-F trocar catheter is placed into this abscess and, after aspiration of pus, the catheter is connected to closed drainage.

route [11]. If the fluid is clear and appears sterile, it may be aspirated and the sheath removed; if findings are indeterminate, one may await the results of Gram stain before evacuating the fluid or inserting a drainage catheter. This latter procedure may be accomplished by either of two methods: (1) modified Seldinger catheter technique, or (2) the trocar technique.

Modified Seldinger Technique

The 8.3-F pigtail catheter is used for smaller and deeper retroperitoneal abscesses and most renal parenchymal abscesses. An 0.038-in. angiographic guide wire is inserted through the Teflon sheath into the abscess cavity, and the sheath is removed. The tract is then dilated with angiographic dilators over the guide wire. An 8.3-F pigtail or nephrostomy catheter is then passed over the guide wire into the abscess. The catheter will assume its curved shape after passing beyond the end of the wire, which should prevent perforation of the abscess wall. CT scans may be done as needed to confirm the location of the wire and/or catheter. After the guide wire is removed, the abscess is completely evacuated with manual syringe suction, and the catheter is sutured to the skin and connected to closed drainage.

Trocar Technique

The trocar catheter is recommended for larger, more superficial abscesses and those with a safe percutaneous route well removed from other vital structures. After diagnostic aspiration, the needle and sheath are removed. The dermatomy is widened to accommodate the larger catheter. An 8.3-F trocar catheter to 14-F van Sonnenberg sump catheter is then inserted in the same manner and direction as the aspiration needle. The trocar has a stylet with a cutting edge and must be marked or cross-clamped to the premeasured depth to prevent its insertion beyond the abscess wall. Calculation of the desired direction and depth may be confirmed with CT scan. Considerable pressure may be necessary to advance the trocar through the subcutaneous tissues. Once the abscess is entered, the central stylet of the trocar is held in a fixed position while the outer catheter is advanced into the cavity. The end of the catheter will again assume a curved configuration. Slight resistance is usually felt when the catheter tip reaches the far wall of the abscess. The stylet may then be withdrawn, and the abscess is emptied by manual syringe suction. The catheter is sutured in place and connected to closed drainage (Fig. 7.6c,d).

After Drainage

Repeat CT scans are obtained after drainage, to exclude areas of residual abscess that have not been drained. Contrast may be injected into the cavity as a baseline for follow-up CT scans or sinograms. Once in position, the percutaneously placed catheters are managed in the same manner as surgical drains. It is important to position the catheter so that gravity will assist drainage, but also so that the patient has as little discomfort as possible. The catheter may be removed after drainage has stopped, if there is a good clinical response and if follow-up scans indicate complete resolution of the abscess. This usually happens within 10–14 days [7]. Antibiotic therapy is continued during this period. If symptoms do not improve in 2–3 days after the percutaneous drainage catheter has been placed, the patient should be rescanned to confirm catheter location and to exclude the presence of undrained material. Catheter irrigation under pressure is generally contraindicated in the immediate postdrainage period, as it may precipitate bacteremia [7]. Although these techniques of abscess drainage have been described for renal and perirenal locations, the principles are the same for other retroperitoneal abscesses, retroperitoneal hematomas, and urinomas.

Urinoma and Hematoma

The urinoma or "perinephric uriniferous pseudocyst" [24], caused by extravasation of urine into the retroperitoneum, is most often secondary to trauma, either extraneous or iatrogenic. It has also been reported with urinary tract obstruction

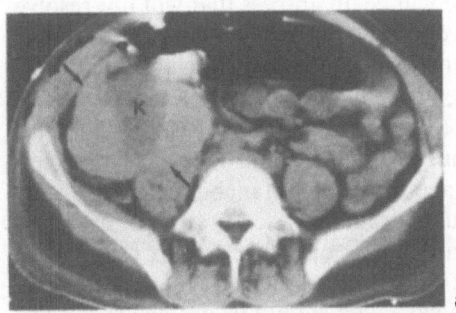

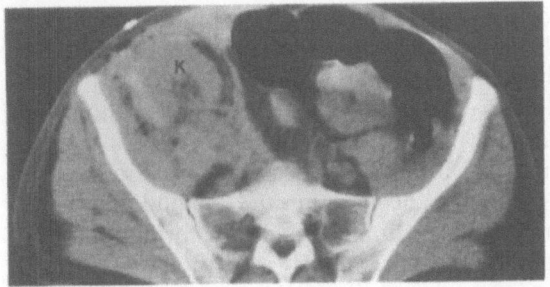

Fig. 7.7a,b. CT scan 3 days following renal transplant demonstrates a large fluid collection (*arrows*) with increased attenuation around the kidney (*K*). The hematoma compresses the kidney and the psoas muscle, and extends along the sacrum.

[3]. A urinoma is generally a well defined, fluid-density mass on CT scan and is most often located in the perirenal space. The kidney may be displaced superiorly or laterally, and there may be associated hydronephrosis. With extravasation of the urine, there is a resultant lipolysis of the perirenal fat, and a pseudocapsule is often formed [1]. The diagnosis may be suggested by CT or ultrasound, but often cannot be distinguished from abscess or hematoma.

Retroperitoneal hemorrhage is most often secondary to trauma but may be seen with a bleeding diathesis, anticoagulant therapy, or spontaneous adrenal or renal bleeding. The latter is usually caused by a tumor, especially renal cell carcinoma or angiomyolipoma. The hematoma is usually seen as a soft tissue mass on CT with attenuation values of 20–80 HU; the higher numbers are present during the more acute phase of bleeding [29] (Fig. 7.7). In the acute stages, the hemorrhage may have the same density as the surrounding tissues without contrast injection. Following injection of iodine contrast, the hematoma is obvious, as it does not enhance. However, over time the attenuation values of the hematoma gradually decrease, and the collection may even appear cystic.

Results

The results of CT-directed percutaneous abscess drainage have been very gratifying. Overall, throughout the abdomen, the success rate has been from 75% to 90% [9, 10, 13, 17, 35]. The complication rate from these reports has been 0%–15% with reduced morbidity and virtually no mortality in the more recent literature. The results are even better with renal, perinephric, and other retroperitoneal abscesses [18]. Although occasionally there will be an abscess that will not resolve with percutaneous drainage, there are several advantages over surgical drainage [11]: (1) avoidance of surgery and general anesthesia and their associated complications, (2) earlier diagnosis and treatment, (3) reduction of time and expense of treatment, (4) better patient acceptance, (5) easier nursing care, and (6) better infection control with the closed drainage system. Johnson et al. reported comparative evaluation of operative drainage versus percutaneous catheter drainage and found that complications, inadequate drainage, and duration of drainage were less in the percutaneous group than in the operative group [16]. More recently, Gerzof has stated that only those patients not amenable to percutaneous drainage or those in whom that procedure has failed should be drained surgically [7]. There are some who prefer a combination of (a) CT for anatomic localization and determination of the extent of the abscess followed by (b) ultrasonographic guidance for puncture and/or catheter placement. Gronvall reports 50 abdominal abscesses treated by ultrasonically guided drainage with irrigation of the cavity and local injection of antibiotics [12]. Twenty-eight had only needle aspiration, and 22 had catheter placement, with an overall success rate of 90%.

A more simplified technique may be utilized for percutaneous drainage of noninfected fluid collections, i.e., urinoma, hematoma, and lymphocele. These should not be left to long-term drainage, which might cause the formation of an abscess in a benign collection. Without infection, complete aspiration is performed at the initial session, and no further catheters are inserted.

Renal Transplants

The urologic complications following renal transplantation are generally related to extravasation of urine, urinary or vascular obstruction, and extraurinary fluid collections. These latter complications are generally in the form of abscess, hematoma, lymphocele, or urinoma. In the early post-transplant period, the development of a soft tissue mass around the kidney, ureter, or bladder is usually the result of urinoma, hematoma, or abscess. The most common post-transplant fluid collection, lymphocele, generally occurs late, with the reported incidence varying from 1% to 15% [2]. Radionuclide scanning may be helpful in the diagnosis of urinoma. If there is no evidence of a fluid leak, the collection is more likely hematoma, lymphocele, or abscess. These extraurinary fluid collections may deviate or compress the transplanted kidney, as well as obstruct the ureter. Gallium scanning may be helpful if abscess is suspected clinically, although the results are nonspecific, especially in the early postoperative period. Cross-sectional imaging with CT or ultrasound is generally quite helpful in evaluation of the suspected post-transplant fluid collection.

Ultrasound may not be able to differentiate pus, blood, lymph, and urine, but certain characteristics may be helpful. Perinephric hematoma is usually seen in the early postoperative period and may present as a palpable mass or enlargement of the transplant with or without associated pain and tenderness or falling hematocrit [22]. The ultrasound pattern tends to vary with the age of the hematoma; those in the early and late stages appear as well defined echo-free masses, while the intermediate aged hematomas usually are more complex, with a varying amount of low-level echoes [37]. CT scan may demonstrate increased attenuation values in the peritransplant fluid collection during the acute phase of hemorrhage (Fig. 7.7). Urinoma usually presents with localized swelling and tenderness and decreased urine output in the first 2 weeks after renal transplant. The ultrasound pattern is generally that of a sonolucent mass which is difficult to separate from other fluid collections, especially lymphocele (Fig. 7.8). Abscess usually occurs in the early postoperative period, although it has been reported to occur months later [32]. Ultrasound will usually demonstrate a relatively echo-free or a complex mass with ill-defined borders. Lymphocele usually presents from 2 weeks to 6 months after transplant and is seen as a single, sonolucent mass with well defined borders on ultrasound. Lymphoceles may be followed by serial ultrasound studies unless there

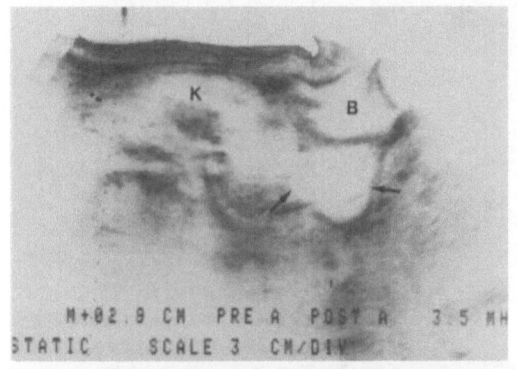

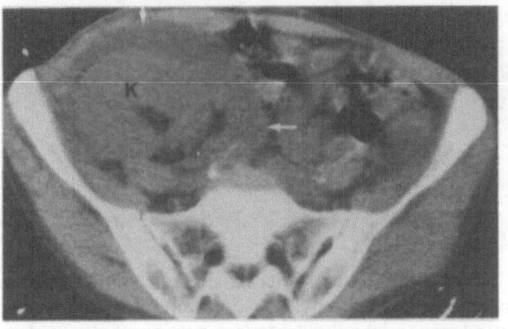

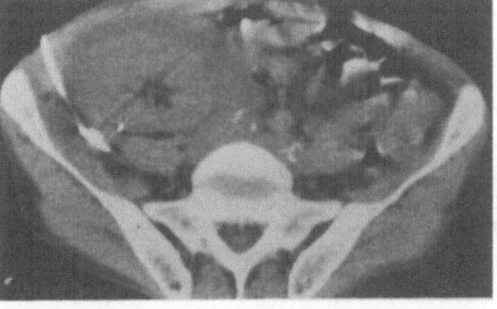

Fig. 7.8. a Longitudinal ultrasound scan 24 days following renal transplant demonstrates a cystic fluid collection (*arrows*) posterior and superior to the bladder (*B*) and adjacent to the kidney (*K*). **b** CT scan demonstrates the fluid collection (*arrows*) surrounding the transplanted kidney (*K*).
c CT-guided percutaneous drainage was done with a 12-F nephrostomy catheter into the urinoma, which resulted from a leak in the bladder.

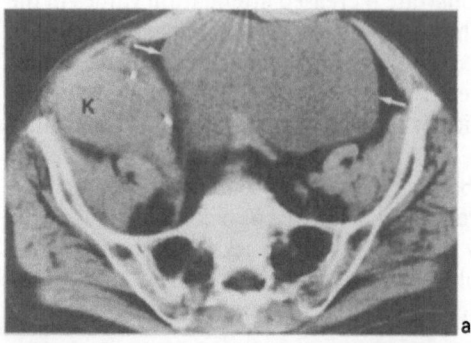

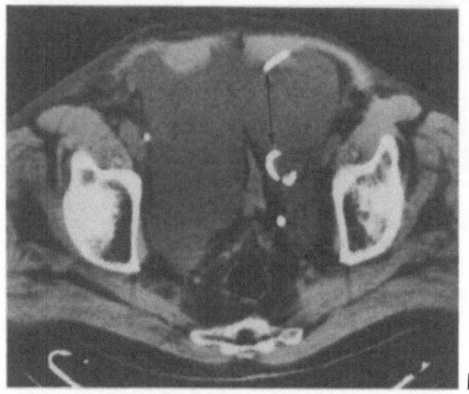

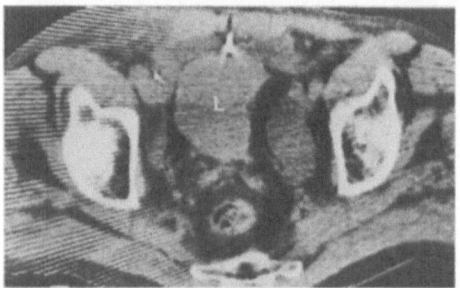

Fig. 7.9. a CT scan 6 weeks after renal transplant demonstrates a large fluid collection (*arrows*) in the pelvis adjacent to kidney (*K*). **b** Following percutaneous insertion of an 8-F nephrostomy pigtail catheter (*arrows*) into the dependent portion of the fluid collection, 2000 cc clear yellow fluid was removed. **c** Follow-up CT scan shows a marked decrease in the size of lymphocele (*L*).

is some additional complication which reduces renal function or urine output. They generally remain stable in size for some time and then gradually get smaller. With an enlarging lymphocele, drainage may be necessary, but the fluid may also reaccumulate after needle aspiration (Fig. 7.9).

Silver et al. reported the occurrence of peritransplant fluid collections in approximately 50% of 100 transplant patients studied. Of these, 23 required drainage, either aspiration or surgical [31]. The location, size, and shape of the fluid collections were not helpful, and there was considerable overlap in the ultrasound pattern. Differentiation of the type of fluid collections may be enhanced in the post-transplant patient by CT. This modality is, of course, known to be helpful in differentiating between patients with acute rejection and those with obstructive uropathy, urinary fistula, or significant perinephric collections [26]. As with fluid collections in other locations, CT guidance may be useful for needle aspiration or catheter drainage of fluid or abscess in the renal transplant patient (Fig. 7.10). With location of the transplanted kidney in the pelvis, the usual retroperitoneal approach to perinephric fluid collections cannot be utilized. In addition, selection of the route to use for drainage may be complicated by the presence of bowel interposed between the renal transplant and the anterior abdominal wall. Thus, caution should be used when determining a drainage access route for peritransplant fluid collections.

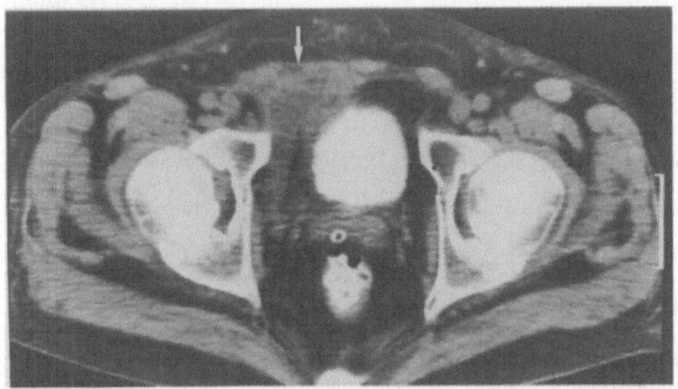

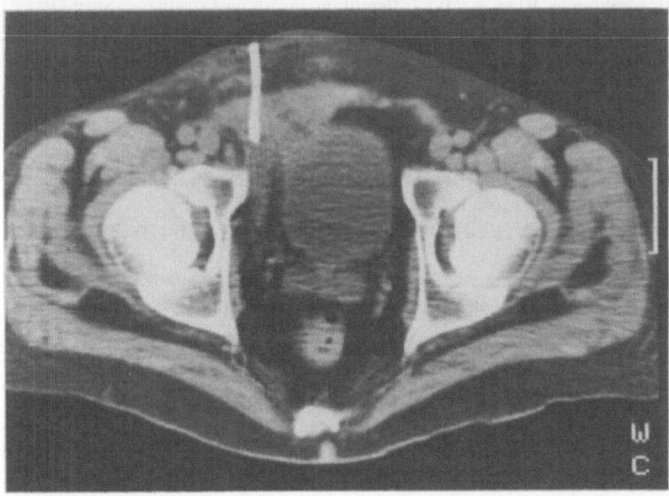

Fig. 7.10. a CT scan 8 weeks following renal transplant demonstrates irregular soft tissue density with central area of diminished attenuation (*arrow*), suggesting abscess anterolateral to the bladder. **b** The following day, percutaneous drainage with CT guidance yielded pus which cultured *Staphylococcus aureus*. The catheter was connected to closed drainage, and appropriate antibiotics were continued.

References

1. Alexander ES, Colley DP, Clark RA (1981) Computed tomography of retroperitoneal fluid collections. Semin Roentgenol 16:268–276
2. Becker JA, Kutcher R (1978) Urologic complications of renal transplantation. Semin Roentgenol 13:341–351
3. Bernardino ME, McClennan BL (1976) High dose urography: Incidence and relationship to peripelvic extravasation. AJR 127:373–375
4. Bernardino ME, Berkman WA, Plemmons M, Sones PJ, Price RB, Casarella WJ (1984) Multiseptated hepatic abscess drainage. J Comput Assist Tomogr 8:38–41
5. Connell TR, Stephens DH, Carlson HC, Brown ML (1980) Upper abdominal abscess: A continuing and deadly problem. AJR 134:759–765
6. Ferrucci JT, van Sonnenberg E (1981) Intraabdominal abscess—radiological diagnosis and treatment. JAMA 246:2728–2733
7. Gerzof SG (1981) Percutaneous drainage of renal and perinephric abscess. Urol Radiol 2:171–179
8. Gerzof SG, Gale ME (1982) Computed tomography and ultrasonography for diagnosis and treatment of renal and retroperitoneal abscesses. Urol Clin North Am 9:185–193
9. Gerzof SG, Robbins AH, Birkett DH et al. (1979) Percutaneous catheter drainage of abdominal abscesses guided by ultrasound and computed tomography. AJR 133:1–8
10. Gerzof SG, Robbins AH, Johnson WC et al. (1981) Percutaneous catheter drainage of abdominal abscesses: A five-year experience. N Engl J Med 305:653–657
11. Gerzof SG, Spira R, Robbins AH (1981) Percutaneous abscess drainage. Semin Roentgenol 16:62–71
12. Gronvall S, Gammelgaard H, Hanbek A et al. (1982) Drainage of abdominal abscess guided by sonography. AJR 138:527–529
13. Haaga JR, Weinstein AJ (1980) CT-guided percutaneous aspiration and drainage of abscesses. AJR 135:1187–1194
14. Halber MD, Daffner RH, Morgan CL et al. (1979) Intraabdominal abscess: Current concepts in radiologic evaluation. AJR 133:9–13
15. Hoddick W, Jeffrey RB, Goldberg HI et al. (1983) CT and sonography of severe renal and perirenal infections. AJR 140:517–520
16. Johnson WC, Gerzof SG, Robbins AH, Nasbeth DC (1981) Treatment of abdominal abscesses: Comparative evaluation of operative drainage versus percutaneous catheter drainage guided by computed tomography or ultrasound. Ann Surg 194:510–520
17. Karlson KB, Martin EB, Fankuchen EI et al. (1982) Percutaneous abscess drainage. Surg Gynec Obstet 154:44–48
18. Korobkin M, Callen PW, Filly RA et al. (1978) Comparison of computed tomography, ultrasonography and gallium-67 scanning in the evaluation of suspected abdominal abscess. Radiology 129:89–93
19. Kressel HY, Filly RA (1978) Ultrasonographic appearance of gas containing abscesses in the abdomen. AJR 130:71–73
20. Lee JKT, McClennan BL, Melson GL, Stanley RJ (1980) Acute focal bacterial nephritis: Emphasis on gray scale sonography and computed tomography. AJR 135:87–92
21. Love L, Meyers MA, Churchill RJ et al. (1981) Computed tomography of extraperitoneal spaces. AJR 136:781–789
22. Maklad NF (1981) Ultrasonic evaluation of renal transplants. Semin Ultrasound 2:88–96
23. Mendez G, Isikoff MB, Morillo G (1979) Role of computed tomography in diagnosis of renal and perirenal abscesses. J Urol 122:582–586
24. Meyers MA (1975) Uriniferous perirenal pseudocyst: New observations. Radiology 117:539–545
25. Meyers MA (1976) Dynamic radiology of the abdomen. Springer, New York
26. Novick AC, Irish C, Steinmuller D et al. (1981) The role of computerized tomography in renal transplant patients. J Urol 125:15–18
27. Rauschkolb EN, Sandler CM, Patel S, Childs TL (1982) Computed tomography of renal inflammatory disease. J Comput Assist Tomogr 6:502–506
28. Rosenfield AT, Glickman MG, Taylor KJW et al. (1979) Acute focal bacterial nephritis (acute lobar nephronia). Radiology 132:553–561
29. Sagel SS, Siegel MJ, Stanley RT et al. (1977) Detection of retroperitoneal hemorrhage by computed tomography. AJR 129:403–407
30. Salvatierra O, Bucklew WB, Morrow JW (1967) Perinephric abscess: A report of 71 cases. J Urol 98:296–302

31. Silver TM, Campbell D, Wicks JD et al. (1981) Peritransplant fluid collections—ultrasound evaluation and clinical significance. Radiology 138:145–151
32. Smith EH, Bartrum RJ (1974) Ultrasonically guided percutaneous aspiration of abscesses. AJR 122:309–312
33. Somogyi J, Cohen WN, Omar MM, Makhuli Z (1979) Communication of right and left perirenal spaces demonstrated by computed tomography. J Comput Assist Tomogr 3:270–273
34. Stevenson EOS, Ozeran RS (1969) Retroperitoneal space abscesses. Surg Gynec Obstet 128:1202–1208
35. van Sonnenberg E, Ferrucci JT, Mueller PR et al. (1982) Percutaneous drainage of abscesses and fluid collections: Technique, results and applications. Radiology 142:1–10
36. Wadsworth DE, McClennan BL, Stanley RJ (1982) CT of the renal mass. Urol Radiol 4:85–94
37. Wicks JD, Silver TM, Bree RL (1978) Gray scale features of hematomas: An ultrasonic spectrum. AJR 131:977–980
38. Wolverson MK, Jagannadharao B, Sundaram M et al. (1979) CT as a primary diagnostic method in evaluating intraabdominal abscess. AJR 133:1089–1095

Chapter 8

Fine Needle Aspiration Biopsy for Metastatic Tumors of the Kidneys and Urogenital Tract

Klemens H. Barth

Introduction

Metastatic tumors of the kidneys and urogenital tract are subject to palliative therapy in the form of resection, radiation and/or chemotherapy. Prior to such treatment, definitive cytopathologic or histologic identification is essential; however, this should be achieved with minimal invasion. Fine needle aspiration biopsy fulfills this prerequisite to a large extent as it represents a safe and sensitive diagnostic technique.

Technical Principles

"Fine needle" refers to all biopsy needles of 20 to 33 gauge [22]. The biopsy specimen is obtained from an area deep to the needle entry and usually recovered by suction applied to the needle hub: hence the term "aspiration biopsy." Since most such aspirations are carried out by a percutaneous approach, the term "percutaneous fine needle aspiration biopsy" serves as a correct description but the short form "needle biopsy" will generally be used. Aspiration is not the only mechanism by which biopsy material is recovered. Other mechanisms are coring by advancing cutting or slotted needles through the lesion, or by using a screw-type biopsy stylet [14]. Commonly used needle configurations are shown in Fig. 8.1. It should be noted that there is no convincing evidence that any of these needles is consistently superior in its diagnostic yield [27]. The most important determinant of a successful fine needle biopsy remains operator skill, particularly precision of needle direction to the target.

Biopsies are performed under guidance by fluoroscopy, ultrasound (US) or computed tomography (CT). Orthogonal biplane fluoroscopy provides excellent guidance for lung biopsies. US is most frequently used for abdominal biopsies.

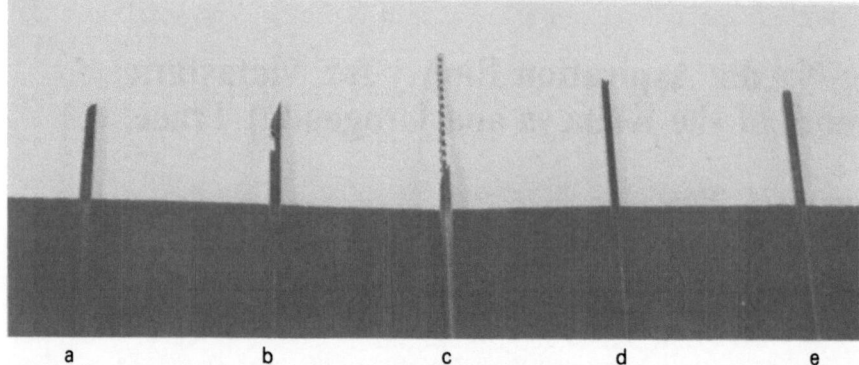

Fig. 8.1a–e. Needles frequently used for fine needle aspiration biopsies. **a** *Turner needle* (20–22 gauge); cutting edge; 45° bevel allows better needle direction than the 25° bevel of the Chiba needle; general purpose needle. **b** *Westcott needle* (20 gauge) slotted; designed for lung biopsy; often adequate for core biopsy. **c** *Rotex needle* (20 gauge); screw biopsy needle for cytopathology, screw not suitable for histologic biopsy; needle can be used for coring. **d** *Franseen needle* (20–22 gauge); serrated tip with diamond stylet; good for small targets (lymph nodes); limits as discussed. **e** *Greene needle* (20–22 gauge); nonbeveled; cutting edge; general purpose needle.

```
                    ASPIRATE
                         \
                          \
                           \--------------------- Suspension
                            \                          |
                             \                         |
                              \               Filtration, cell block
                               v
    Air dried ——— Slides ———————————— Immediate alcohol fixation
        |                                         |
        |                                         |
  Giemsa stains                                   |
   for small                                      |
     cells                                        |
                                                  |
                                         Modif. Pap. stain
                                        /        |        \
                                       /         |         \
                              Definitely    Indeterminate   Nonmalignant
                              malignant,          \            /
                              cell type            \          /
                                                    \        /
                                                 Repeat biopsy:
                                                 Core biopsy
                                                 Gram stains, ——Histology
                                                   AFB-
                                                 fungus stains
```

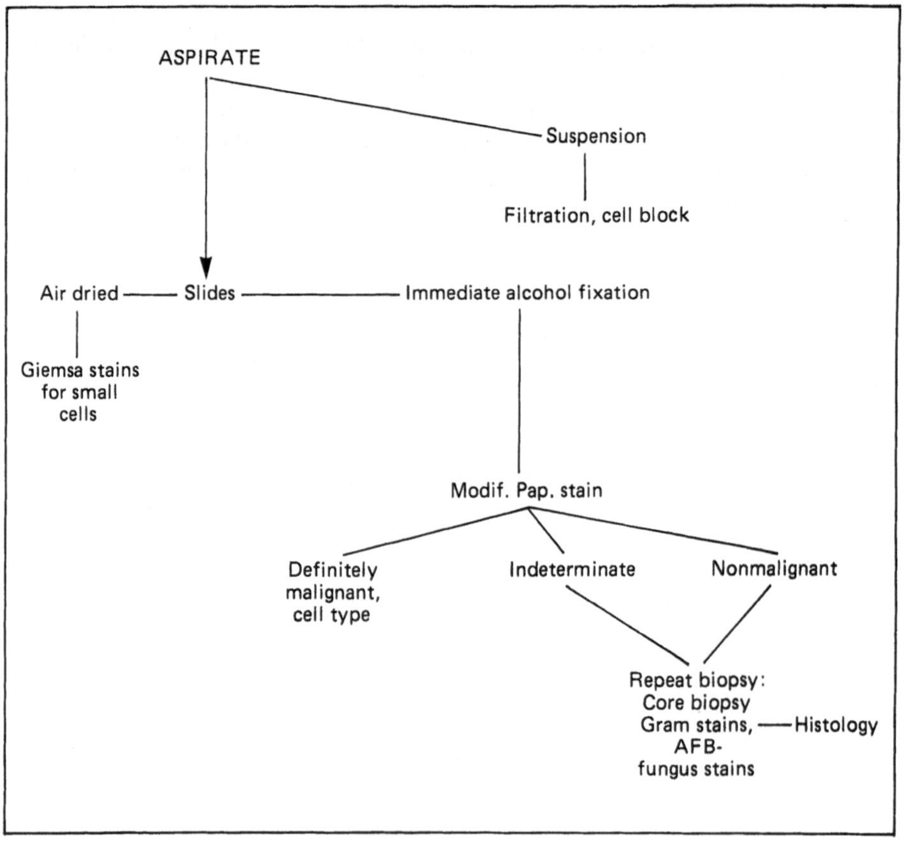

Fig. 8.2. Workup of cytopathologic specimens.

Due to its better spatial resolution and tissue discrimination with the aid of vascular contrast, CT guidance is preferred for biopsy of large lesions with expected extensive necrosis or where a high risk of large vessel hemorrhage or nerve injury is present, as in the spinal or paraspinal areas as well as in the mediastinum and the pulmonary hilum [2]. Once lymph nodes are opacified by contrast material, fluoroscopy is the guidance of choice for biopsy [12, 17, 24].

Ultrasound guidance uses real-time image display to monitor the advancing needle tip or needle shaft echo. Specially designed transducers allow attachment of the needle obliquely to the central echo and adjustment of the needle angle so that the needle trajectory intersects with the central echo in the target area [4, 7, 15]. US allows multiangled needle direction with great ease, the circumstances being especially important for liver biopsies through intercostal or subcostal approaches.

As a general rule, no needle biopsy is undertaken in patients with clotting deficiencies. Prothrombin time, partial thromboplastin time and platelet count are routinely obtained from patients considered for biopsy. Any anticoagulation is discontinued, including ASA, and clotting function is restored prior to biopsy. Seeding of malignant cells along the needle tract after fine needle biopsy is by all available experience extremely rare [6, 20, 22]. A projected incidence might be one in 2–3000 [5]. Almost all percutaneous biopsies are performed under local anesthesia. Patients for vertebral biopsies may have to undergo general anesthesia or heavy sedation [22]. Fine needle biopsies do not require hospitalization of patients except for lung biopsies of patients with known emphysema and biopsies of the mediastinum and the vertebral bodies.

Processing of Biopsy Material

Fine needle aspiration biopsies are most frequently used for cytopathology following the procedure outlined in Fig. 8.2. Cytopathologic criteria are quite specific for identification of malignant cells of epithelial origin. In some instances they are adequate to identify the tissue of origin, e.g., clear cell tumors, adenocarcinomas, transitional cell carcinomas, and squamous cell carcinomas. Therefore, metastatic lesions of tumors of the kidneys and urogenital tract should be identifiable by cytopathology with a high degree of accuracy.

Adequacy of an aspiration biopsy in terms of material recovered can be determined with fair accuracy at the time of biopsy after spreading the aspirate on glass slides. Needle aspiration should be continued until enough material has been recovered to cover at least two slides. Adequacy of aspiration in terms of geographic accuracy is a question of needle guidance, as mentioned above. It is important to work quickly between removing the needle or stylet and spreading the material on glass slides. The slides are immediately immersed into alcohol fixation. Slides should not be air dried unless used for special stains, as indicated in Fig. 8.2. Giemsa staining of air-dried slides is used primarily for identification of small cells of lymphomas and leukemias, not subject to this discussion. Slide separation with mucin or albumin is only required for liquid aspirates. Modified Papanicolaou stains, the routine cytologic stains, can be processed and reviewed within a few hours. A quick staining technique is available for preliminary diagnostic assessment, while the biopsy procedure is ongoing, similar to frozen sections. This may be useful in cases where the adequacy of the obtained material remains in question [8]. It is important to communicate with the cytopathologist and the cytopathology technologist before biopsy so that appropriate processing can be determined.

In addition to the direct slide technique it is advisable to rinse the aspiration needle in a balanced salt solution for filtration and cell block techniques [8] (Fig. 8.3).

Histologic processing of the aspirate is most desirable when a benign lesion is suspected or cytopathology is inconclusive. Frequently the latter will be subject to repeat biopsy (Fig. 8.2). Inflammatory lesions and most benign tumors can only be diagnosed with confidence by reviewing a histologic specimen since cell characteristics are non-specific. Fine needles are capable of recovering small tissue cylinders for histologic interpretation.

Several needles have been designed to improve the yield of histologic biopsies (Fig. 8.1). However, no particular one has achieved exclusive use, as stated in the foregoing section. If a core of tissue is recovered, it is advantageous to expel the cylinder onto a small piece of filter paper to keep it from coiling up. The paper with the tissue adherent is then suspended in buffered formalin, to which some eosin has been added for better specimen identification in the paraffin block. Histologic processing will normally take at least 24 h.

It should be noted that histology is not necessarily superior to cytology. The low risk thin needle aspiration biopsy coupled with the interpretive skill of a cytopathologist has a high degree of accuracy for epithelial tumors. The yield of adequate histologic material with fine needle biopsies is lower than that for cytology [9]. Since histology may increase the diagnostic yield in some cases, core biopsies should be attempted in all cases in which cytology is negative or indeterminate (Fig. 8.2). Depending on individual circumstances, the benefit of a histologic biopsy may well offset the higher risks associated with using larger caliber biopsy needles [11, 22].

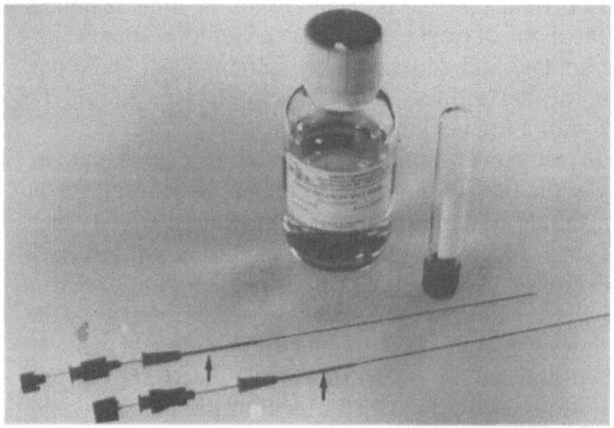

Fig. 8.3. Needle setup for transabdominal biopsies and suspension solution for aspirate. The biopsy needle is advanced through an 16–18 gauge injection needle (*arrows*) which extends through the abdominal wall. This coaxial technique increases the directability of the biopsy needle. Balanced salt solution is aspirated out of a sterile container and the needle contents rinsed into a sterile test tube for processing. Sterile technique allows repeated use of the same biopsy needle.

Specific Applications

Biopsy of Pulmonary Lesions

Biplane fixed or single plane rotational fluoroscopy is the guidance of choice [3, 11]. Difficulty with fluoroscopy may be encountered with lesions less than 2 cm in size, lesions with irregular margins, or lesions that are pleural or mediastinal based. Apical lesions may be poorly visible on lateral fluoroscopy owing to soft tissue and bone in the shoulder regions. Oblique patient position or bilateral oblique fluoroscopy [21] can help in these instances. The same maneuver may be applied to small lesions or in the presence of multiple lesions where lateral fluoroscopy does not allow adequate discrimination. Recent chest X-rays are the best guide to determine whether a lesion will be identifiable fluoroscopically. If the lesion cannot be seen definitively on either frontal or lateral films, it is likely that fluoroscopy will not be adequate. In such cases, it is better to plan biopsy under CT guidance (Fig. 8.4). The disadvantage of CT is the fact that it is not a real-time technique. Hence, respiratory motion between localization and needle advancement induces uncertainty of needle position. This is, of course, most critical in lesions less than 2 cm in diameter. CT-guided lung biopsies under contrast enhancement have been advocated for large lesions where a great deal of necrotic material is suspected [16]. However, as a general rule, biopsy material should be obtained from the periphery of any lesion. Therefore, we do not consider CT a prerequisite for biopsy of large pulmonary lesions with good contrast to surrounding lung tissue. Biopsy of lesions in critical areas such as the middle mediastinum or the immediate vicinity of the

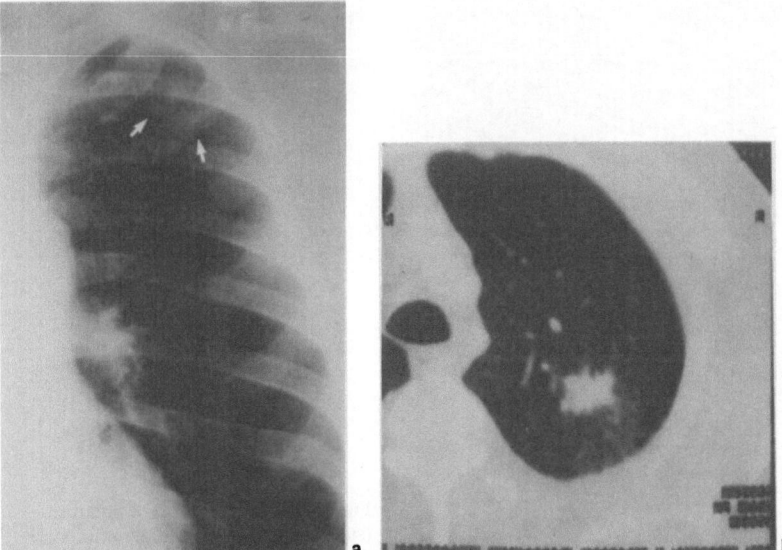

Fig. 8.4. a Poorly marginated adenocarcinoma in left pulmonary apex (*arrows*) on PCA chest X-ray. Lesion not seen on lateral chest X-ray. **b** CT shows excellent delineation of the spiculated mass. Aspiration biopsy was and should be performed under CT guidance.

hilum, should be performed exclusively under CT guidance with clear identification of the aorta because of the reported risk of major hemorrhage including cardiac tamponade [10, 18].

Our preference for cytopathologic aspiration biopsies is the 20 gauge screw biopsy needle (Rotex needle, Surgimed Inc., Summerville, S.C. 29483). The screw stylette has an excellent recovery rate, but the material is not useful for histologic workup. The most important reason for its use is that the stylet recovers the biopsy material and can be inserted repeatedly through the needle after a single transpleural needle pass (Fig. 8.5). At the end of the procedure direct aspiration through the needle is performed and may be used for histologic processing. Core biopsies can be obtained with the 20 gauge Westcott needle (Becton-Dickinson, Inc., Rutherford, N.J. 07070) as well as with the Surecut needle (Surgimed Inc., Summerville, S.C. 29483). The latter needle has its own aspiration syringe permanently attached.

A high number of diagnostic biopsies are obtained, ranging from 80% to 90%. Pneumothorax is the only significant risk of lung biopsies outside the hilum and the mediastinum [3, 11, 26, 28]. Small pneumothoraces (20%) occur in about 25% of biopsies [3, 11]. Larger pneumothoraces requiring evacuation occur in approximately 5% [11, 22]. Patients at high risk for a large pneumothorax are those with parenchymal lung disease, particularly obstructive pulmonary disease. Routinely,

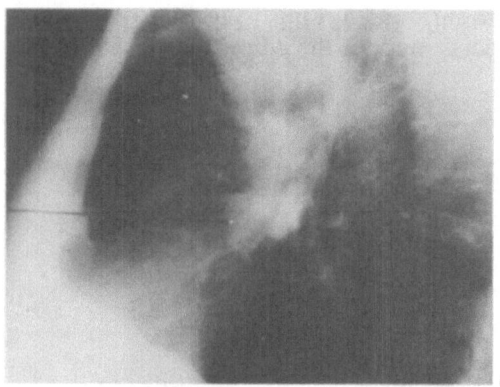

a

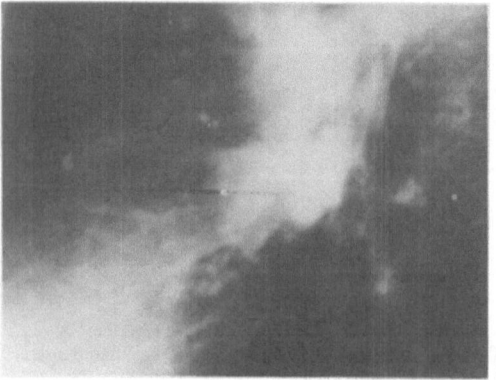

Fig. 8.5a,b. Screw biopsy technique: (superimposition on radiograph). **a** 20-gauge cannula (screw stylet retracted) advanced into periphery of mass under biplane fluoroscopy. **b** Stylet advanced 1–2 cm, to obtain specimen.

b

inspiration and expiration chest X-rays are obtained after completion of lung biopsies. Evacuation of the pneumothorax is best performed by a chest tube placed by a pulmonary specialist or a chest surgeon. The radiologist may use the Heimlich valve as temporary relief of an enlarging pneumothorax [11]. However, this treatment should not be considered definitive in patients with emphysema.

Biopsy of Suspected Liver Metastases

Ultrasound or CT provides appropriate guidance. As a general rule and for logistic reasons, US guidance is the first choice [19]. Real-time linear or phased array transducers allow needle direction towards the lesion as previously described (Fig. 8.6). The most suitable needle entry can be selected avoiding passage through the pleural recess. US may fail as a guidance for liver biopsy due to lack of discrimination between liver tissue and liver mass or whenever interposed ribs, bowel gas or lungs prevent US penetration. These limitations for US should not be a barrier to successful CT-guided biopsy, particularly when contrast is used (Fig. 8.7). For suspected malignant lesions, 20- to 22-gauge needles are adequate. Those

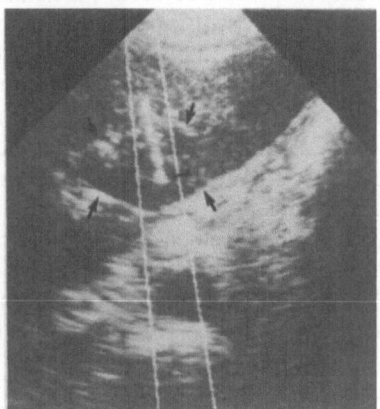

Fig. 8.6. US-guided fine needle aspiration biopsy of metastatic adenocarcinoma to right lobe of the liver (*arrows*). Guidance trajectories superimposed on CRT display. Needle echoes visible with needle tip deep in lesion (*arrowhead*).

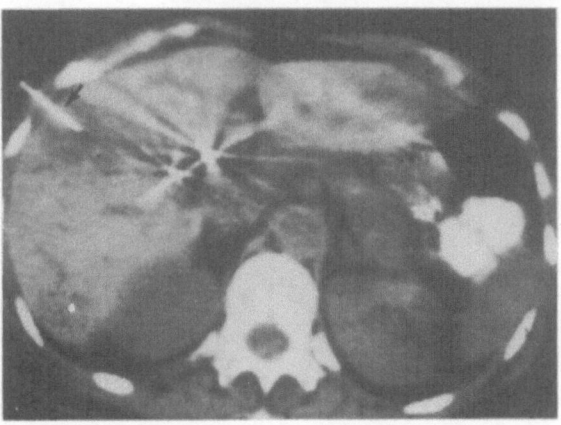

Fig. 8.7. CT-guided fine needle aspiration biopsy of superficial metastatic ovarian carcinoma to liver after intravenous contrast enhancement. Biopsy needle easily identifiable (*arrow*).

needles with a cutting edge can be used to obtain core biopsies by advancing the open needle through the lesion under suction which is maintained during needle retrieval. Again, aspiration is repeated until sufficient material has been obtained, as described initially.

Biopsy of Paraaortic and Pelvic Lymph Nodes

Ultrasound is the guidance of first choice for clearly identifiable nodal masses using the anterior approach (Fig. 8.8). Borderline enlarged lymph nodes are approached under CT guidance.

With the high incidence of subclinical nodal metastases in carcinoma of the prostate, routine staging lymphography is advocated for stage C tumors [12, 17, 24]. Lymphography remains superior to CT and US in assessment of structural lymph node abnormalities, independent of nodal enlargement [17]. Fluoroscopically guided needle biopsy by anterior approach is a well established method to confirm lymphographically suspected nodal metastases (Fig. 8.9). True positive biopsies with this technique can be obtained in approximately 75%–80% of cases [17]. A negative aspiration should not alter further clinical workup, including node dissection. Biplane fluoroscopy is again the optimum set-up; however, rotational fluoroscopy can be used, particularly in the region of the pelvis, where adequate lateral fluoroscopy might be impossible. Bilateral 40° angulation of the fluoroscopic unit will allow triangulation of the needle tip position [21]. Since the target is small and usually deep to the area of entry, utmost care in needle guidance is essential. Biopsy of deep-seated lymph nodes requires the stiffness of a 21- or at least 22-gauge needle. 23-gauge needles are difficult to direct in our experience, contrary to Wein et al. [25]. Further directional support is given by a 16- or 18-gauge injection needle inserted first through the abdominal wall followed by coaxial advancement of the biopsy needle (Fig. 8.3).

We have found the 22-gauge Franzén needle (Cook Inc., Bloomington, Ind. 47402) advantageous for aspiration of small retroperitoneal lymph nodes since the serrated tip always recovers tissue. Large tissue cylinders cannot be aspirated since this tip frequently prevents a tissue particle from entering the needle shaft. Several passes may be performed safely with any needle.

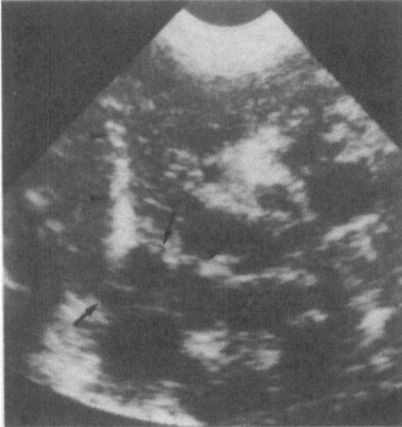

Fig. 8.8. US-guided biopsy of poorly differentiated adenocarcinoma to retroperitoneal lymph nodes (*arrows*). Needle echoes of 22-gauge needle well seen (*arrowheads*) as it traverses the left lobe of the liver.

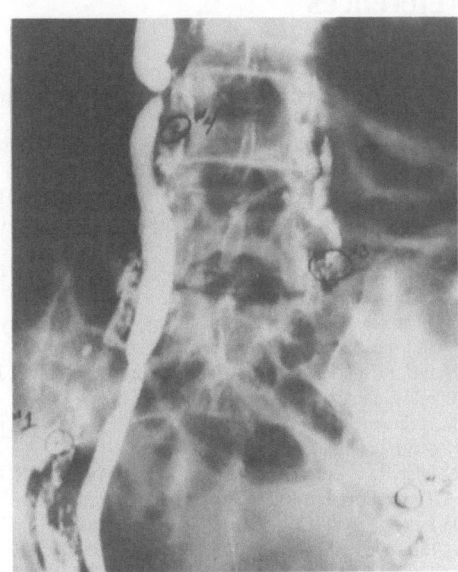

Fig. 8.9. Metastatic carcinoma of cervix to pelvic and paraaortic lymph nodes. Needle aspirates with 27-gauge needle have been obtained under rotational fluoroscopy from nodes marked on lymphogram.

Complications of retroperitoneal lymph node biopsy are few and essentially represent hemorrhage from neighboring arteries. Bleeding is self limited unless a clotting deficiency is present.

Biopsy of Bone Metastases

Renal cell carcinomas and adenocarcinomas of the prostate metastatic to bone are the tumors considered in this discussion. While the former are purely osteolytic, the latter are frequently osteoblastic. Both types of lesion are well amenable to percutaneous biopsy, both in the axial skeleton and in the extremities.

Traditionally, bone biopsies have been performed with large caliber needles (10–18 gauge) owing to resistance of cortical bone [5, 13]. Osteolytic lesions can be successfully biopsied with fine needles [1, 23]. A coaxial needle with an outer needle penetrating the cortex and the inner fine needle aspirating the marrow can reduce the biopsy-related bleeding [5]. All techniques have been adequately described and will not be reviewed here in detail [1, 5].

Biplane fluoroscopy is again the guidance of choice in the pelvis, the shoulders, the ribs, and the extremities. Spinal biopsies are performed with increasing frequency under CT guidance, which allows a more precise determination of the oblique needle direction. In tubular bones, the needle is directed perpendicular to the bone surface. Flat bones like ribs, scapula, and ilium are entered at lesser angles to achieve better sampling in the marrow.

Reviewing 1000 cases, Murphy found an overall accuracy for needle biopsy of spinal metastases of 95%. Complications, particularly hemorrhage, were in the order of 0.2% [13]. The only significant risk of bone biopsy is spinal cord damage during spinal biopsy [28]. Needle passage through larger arteries, particularly in spinal, shoulder and hip biopsies, should be avoided by proper approach, which is anterior or lateral for the latter two areas.

References

1. Adler O, Rosenberger A (1979) Fine needle aspiration biopsy of osteolytic metastatic lesions. AJR 133:15–18
2. Adler OB, Rosenberger A, Peleg H (1983) Fine-needle aspiration biopsy of mediastinal masses: evaluation of 136 experiences. AJR 140:893–896
3. Bernardino ME (1984) Percutaneous biopsy. AJR 142:41–45
4. Buonocore E, Skipper GJ (1981) Steerable real-time sonographically guided needle biopsy. AJR 136:387–392
5. deSantos LA, Lukeman JM, Wallace S, Murray JA, Ayala AG (1978) Percutaneous needle biopsy of bone in the cancer patient. Am J Roentgenol 130:641–649
6. Ferrucci JT, Wittenberg J, Margolies MN, Carey RW (1979) Malignant seeding of the tract after thin-needle aspiration biopsy. Radiology 130:345–346
7. Grant EG, Richardson JD, Smirniotopoulos JG, Jacobs NM (1983) Fine-needle biopsy directed by real-time sonography. AJR 141:29–32
8. Heaston DK, Handel DB, Ashton PR, Korobkin M (1982) Narrow gauge needle aspiration of solid adrenal masses. AJR 138:1143–1148
9. Isler RJ, Ferrucci JT, Wittenberg J, Mueller PR, Simeone JF, van Sonnenberg E, Hall DA (1981) Tissue core biopsy of abdominal tumors with a 22 gauge cutting needle. AJR 136: 725–728
10. Kucharczyk W, Weisbrod GL, Cooper JD, Todd T (1982) Cardiac tamponade as a complication of thin-needle aspiration lung biopsy. Chest 82:120–121
11. Lalli AF, McCormack LJ, Zelch M, Reich NE, Belovich D (1978) Aspiration biopsies of chest lesions. Radiology 127:35–40
12. Liebner EJ, Stefani S (1980) An evaluation of lymphography with nodal biopsy in localized carcinoma of the prostate. Cancer 45:728–734
13. Murphy WA, Destouet JM, Gilula LA (1981) Percutaneous skeletal biopsy 1981: A procedure for radiologists—results, review, and recommendations. Radiology 139:545–549
14. Nordenstrom B (1975) New instruments for biopsy. Radiology 117:474–475
15. Ohto M, Karasawa E, Tsuchiya Y, Kimura K, Saisho H, Ono T, Okuda K (1980) Ultrasonically guided percutaneous contrast medium injection and aspiration biopsy using a real-time puncture transducer. Radiology 136:171–176
16. Pinstein ML, Scott RL, Salazar J (1983) Avoidance of negative percutaneous lung biopsy using contrast-enhanced CT. AJR 140:265–267
17. Prando A, Wallace S, Von Eschenbach AC, Jing BS, Rosengren JE, Hussey DH (1979) Lymphangiography in staging of carcinoma of the prostate. Radiology 131:641–645
18. Rosenberger A, Adler O (1978) Fine needle aspiration biopsy in the diagnosis of mediastinal lesions. Am J Roentgenol 131:239–242
19. Schwerk WB, Schmitz-Moormann P (1981) Ultrasonically guided fine-needle biopsies in neoplastic liver disease: cytohistologic diagnoses and echo pattern of lesions. Cancer 48:1469–1477
20. Sinner WN, Zajicek J (1975) Implantation metastasis after percutaneous transthoracic needle aspiration biopsy. Acta Radiol [Diagn] 17:473–480
21. Smith DF, Doust BD (1982) Angulated fluoroscopy for needle biopsy localization. AJR 138:765–767
22. Tao LC, Pearson FG, Delarue NC, Langer B, Sanders DE (1980) Percutaneous fine-needle aspiration biopsy. Cancer 45:1480–1485
23. Tehranzadeh J, Freiberger RH, Ghelman B (1983) Closed skeletal needle biopsy: review of 120 cases. AJR 140:113–115
24. Wajsman Z, Gamarra M, Park JJ, Beckley S, Pontes JE (1982) Transabdominal fine needle aspiration of retroperitoneal lymph nodes in staging of genitourinary tract cancer (correlation with lymphography and lymph node dissection findings). J Urol 82:1238–1240
25. Wein AJ, Ring EJ, Freiman DB, Oleaga JA, Carpiniello VL, Banner MP, Pollack HM (1979) Applications of thin needle aspiration biopsy in urology. J Urol 121:626–629
26. Westcott JL (1980) Direct percutaneous needle aspiration of localized pulmonary lesions: results in 422 patients. Radiology 137:31–35
27. Wittenberg J, Mueller PR, Ferrucci JT, Simeone JF, van Sonnenberg E, Neff CC, Palermo RA, Isler RJ (1982) Percutaneous core biopsy of abdominal tumors using 22 gauge needles: further observations. AJR 139:75–80
28. Zornoza J (1982) Needle biopsy of metastases. Radiol Clin North Am 20:569–590

Chapter 9

Diagnosis and Management of Renal Cysts

Erich K. Lang

Introduction

Cystic lesions are one of the most common abnormalities of the kidney [19, 22, 23, 26]. Although some cystic lesions of the kidney are associated with devastating medical disease and present with severe symptoms, e.g., uremic medullary cystic disease, the majority of renal cystic lesions are asymptomatic and discovered incidentally on intravenous urograms or computed tomograms performed for other reasons [19, 20, 23, 26, 28]. However, an incidence of malignancies of approximately 5.5% in the group of patients discovered to harbor an asymptomatic space-occupying lesion mandates investigations to establish the diagnosis with acceptable accuracy [19, 23, 26].

This treatise will attempt to outline the state of the art approach to the assessment of both solitary and multiple renal mass lesions. The diagnostic approach takes into consideration the probability of occurrence of certain mass lesions, the differing diagnostic capability of the discovering examination, and above all the clinical scenario, specifically whether presenting as a symptomatic or asymptomatic renal mass.

Localized Cystic Lesions of the Kidney

Until the early 1960s, renal cysts were diagnosed only rarely, although they were known from pathologic material to occur rather frequently. Once the presence of a space-occupying lesion of the kidney was suggested, surgical exploration was performed almost always, to establish the definitive diagnosis [19]. The then available diagnostic examinations, including arteriography, were not credited with establishing the diagnosis with acceptable confidence.

The introduction of ultrasonography and guided cyst puncture and aspiration greatly changed concepts of diagnosis and management of renal cysts [19, 23, 37]. Algorithms for the workup of asymptomatic space-occupying lesions of the kidney

Table 9.1. Diagnostic examination establishing the etiologic diagnosis of renal mass lesions discovered on computed tomograms

Pathologic condition	Total no. of patients	Definitively diagnosed by				
		CT	PAB	Arteriogram	Nuclear medicine	Ultrasound
Benign cyst	503	482	12	—	—	9
Septated cyst	63	38	10	—	—	15
Multilocular cyst	7	2	4	1	—	(4)
Inflammatory cyst	21	4	16	1	—	—
Hemorrhagic cyst	27	5	20	2	—	—
Calcified cyst	4	4	(4)	(3)	—	(4)
Cystic, dysplastic	3	2	(1)	(1)	—	1
Polycystic disease	6	5	1	—	—	—
Parapelvic cyst	6	4	2	(1)	—	—
Renal cell carcinoma	12	10	1	1	—	—
Metastatic carcinoma	11	2	7	1	1	—
Lymphoma	4	2	2	1	—	—
Wilms' tumor	1	—	—	1	—	—
Capsular sarcoma	2	1	—	1	—	—
Transitional cell carcinoma	6	2	3	1	—	—
Adenoma[b]	2	—	1	—	—	—
Fibroma[b]	2	—	1	—	—	—
Angiomyolipoma	4	4	—	—	—	(4)
Hamartoma[b]	1	—	—	—	—	—
Tumefactive xanthogranulomatous pyelonephritis	3	2	—	1	—	—
Renal infarct	6	5	—	1	—	—
Abscess	11	4	7	—	(2)	—
Pyonephrosis	9	1	8	—	(1)	—
Focal lobar nephronia	36	25	1	(1)	10	—
Hematoma	15	11	4	2	—	—
AV fistula	2	—	—	2	—	—
Pseudotumor	22	8	—	—	14	—

[a]PAB, puncture, aspiration, and biopsy
[b]Some refractory to radiologic diagnosis

Table 9.2. Diagnostic examination establishing the etiologic diagnosis of renal mass lesions identified on intravenous urograms

Pathologic condition	Total no. of patients	Examination establishing the diagnosis					
		IVU	Ultrasound	CT	PAB[a]	Arteriogram	Nuclear medicine
Benign cyst	552	34	431	44	42	1	—
Septated benign cyst	22	—	15	4	3	—	—
Multilocular cyst	5	—	1	2	2	(1)	—
Inflammatory cyst	19	—	—	1	17	1	—
Hemorrhagic cyst	15	—	—	—	14	1	—
Calcified cyst	2	1	—	1	1	(1)	—
Cystic, dysplastic	1	—	1	—	—	—	—
Polycystic disease	20	19	1	—	—	—	—
Parapelvic cyst	7	3	—	—	—	—	—
Renal cell carcinoma	8	—	—	2	2	6	—
Metastatic carcinoma[b]	7	—	—	2	2	2	—
Lymphoma[b]	1	—	—	—	—	—	—
Transitional cell carcinoma	20	—	—	(2)	18	1	—
Adenoma[b]	1	—	—	1	—	—	—
Angiomyolipoma	3	—	2	—	—	1	—
Xanthogranulomatous pyelonephritis[b]	3	1	—	2	—	—	—
Abscess	4	—	—	2	2	(1)	—
Pyonephrosis	13	—	—	1	7	3	2
Focal lobar nephronia[b]	27	—	—	10	—	6	10
Hematoma	4	—	—	1	3	—	—
Pseudotumor[b]	71	—	—	—	—	3	67

[a]PAB, puncture, aspiration, and biopsy
[b]Some refractory to radiologic diagnosis

became fashionable. However, computed tomography, being responsible for the discovery of about one-half of all space-occupying lesions of the kidney, had an even more profound impact on the diagnostic workup [33, 38].

Today, almost 20% of all patients over the age of 55 and examined by computed tomography or intravenous urography are found to have an asymptomatic renal mass lesion [19, 23, 26]. Sixty-six percent of all renal mass lesions prove to be benign renal cysts, 9% atypical renal cysts, 18% inflammatory renal mass lesions, pseudotumors, and benign renal tumors, and only about 7% malignancies, abscesses, consequential inflammatory mass lesions, or vascular malformations requiring treatment [26] (Table 9.1).

The magnitude of the workup considered necessary is therefore determined to a large degree by the well-known rate of occurrence of etiologically different lesions and the sensitivity, specificity, and accuracy of the various diagnostic examinations [26].

The diagnostic approach to symptomatic and asymptomatic renal mass lesions is obviously different. Likewise, the disparity of diagnostic capability of the discovering examination, the intravenous urogram and the computed tomogram, calls for different algorithms to be followed when working up such lesions.

In general, the computed tomogram can establish the definitive diagnosis of benign renal cyst, septated renal cyst, renal cell carcinoma, cystic renal cell carcinoma, renal infarct, column of Bertin, angiomyolipoma, focal bacterial nephritis, and pyonephrosis with confidence [6, 11, 24, 25, 27, 34, 38, 41, 45, 48]. Thus 79% of all asymptomatic lesions discovered on computed tomograms are also diagnosed by this examination with acceptable confidence.

Conversely, the intravenous urogram often merely indicates the presence of a space-occupying lesion. A definitive diagnosis is made in less than 5% of the patients on the basis of the intravenous urogram. However, the ultrasonogram, usually advocated for the next examination, can establish a definitive diagnosis in about 90% of all benign simple renal cysts [38]. Since this lesion occurs at an incidence rate of about 70%, 63% of the asymptomatic space-occupying lesions of the kidney discovered on intravenous urograms are then definitively diagnosed by the ultrasonogram [38]. In our own series, 66% of all asymptomatic space-occupying lesions proved to be benign cysts, which with the sensitivity and specificity of our ultrasound diagnosis, diagnosed with definitude 56% of these lesions (Table 9.2).

At this point in time, in the algorithmic pathway started either with the computed tomogram or the intravenous urogram, cyst puncture and aspiration, double contrast cyst study, guided thin needle biopsy, computed tomography with dynamic phase recording, radionuclide scintiscanograms and rarely arteriography may be advocated to establish the diagnosis with an acceptable confidence level [2, 8, 10, 18, 19, 21, 23–26, 32, 38, 43, 47, 49; H. Hricak, personal communications]. In general, an acceptable diagnostic confidence level is established if all criteria defining a specific lesion are met and if these criteria have been proven to be of acceptable specificity.

Benign Renal Cysts

On intravenous urograms and tomograms performed during the nephrographic phase of intravenous urography, benign renal cysts present as a more or less

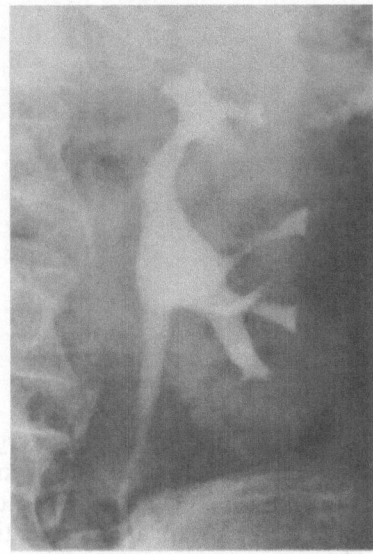

Fig. 9.1. Fifteen-minute intravenous urogram showing stretch effect of the infundibula of the midcalyceal group. The presence of a space-occupying lesion is suggested.

spherical mass lesion, sharply defined against adjacent renal parenchyma, lacking enhancement and, if extending to the cortical margins, causing "cortical spurs." Extrarenal components of such cysts are characterized by an infinitely thin wall [19]. Dependent on their location, displacement and even clubbing of calyces and infundibula may result (Fig. 9.1).

On ultrasonograms, benign renal cysts are depicted as sharply defined, more or less spherical mass lesions, featuring a characteristic absence of echoes from within the cyst. Most important, transmission through the cystic lesion should be significantly greater than through adjacent renal parenchyma [38]. Therefore, the far wall of the cyst should be seen as a smooth curved line, seemingly accentuated by the improved transmission of ultrasound echoes through the renal cyst (Fig. 9.2). Not infrequently, reverberation echoes may be seen close to the near wall of the cyst.

The resolution of the system must take into consideration the depth of the mass and adapt transducer frequency accordingly. Some deep cysts may be difficult to

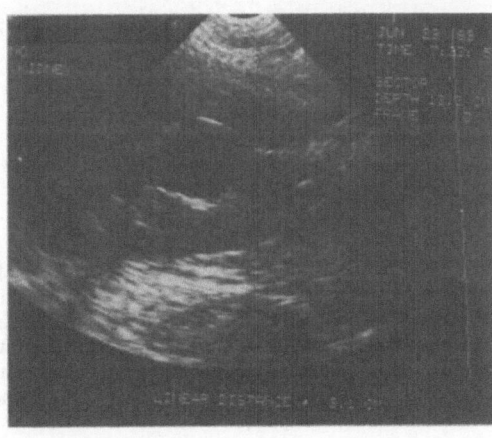

Fig. 9.2. An ultrasonogram demonstrating a sharply defined spherical anechoic mass in the kidney. Echoes from the far wall are seemingly accentuated, suggesting excellent transmission of ultrasound echoes and therefore a fluid content. The appearance is characteristic for a benign renal cyst.

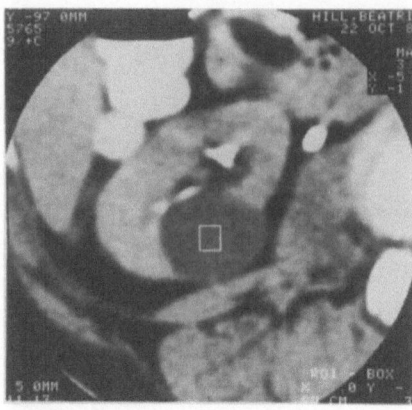

Fig. 9.3. A computed tomogram obtained after administration of intravenous contrast medium, demonstrating a sharply delineated, round mass in the posterior aspects of the mid-section of the right kidney. The attenuation coefficient measured over the lesion remains 6.77, unchanged from the pre-enhancement values. The findings are characteristic for a benign renal cyst.

diagnose because of beam divergence. If the width of the beam exceeds the diameter of the mass, echoes from adjacent structures may appear to originate from within the mass [38]. Even the use of lower frequency transducers cannot overcome the loss of lateral resolution, which is inversely proportional to the beam width.

Since all criteria are based on a fluid content of the intrarenal mass, it is obvious that arteriovenous fistulas cannot be differentiated from benign renal cysts unless pulsed Doppler is available to record flow within the lesion [38].

Ninety-eight percent of all cystic lesions greater than 0.5 cm in diameter can be identified on ultrasonograms and 95% of these are correctly diagnosed as cysts [38].

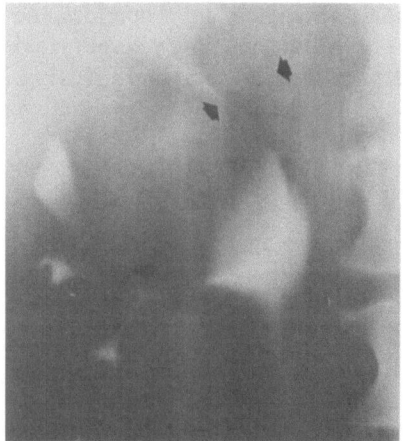
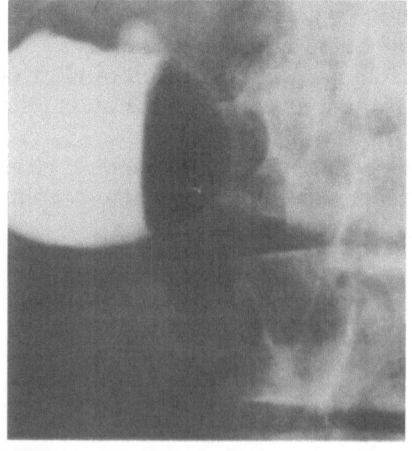

a   b

Fig. 9.4. a A tomographic cut obtained during the intravenous urogram demonstrating splaying and compression of the infundibula of the superior and mid-calyceal groups (*arrows*). **b** A subsequent double contrast cyst study replacing the aspirate with an aliquot of contrast medium and air demonstrates smooth contours of all inner surfaces of the cyst in multiple decubitus positions. The lesion proved perfectly superimposable upon the negative defect demonstrated on the intravenous urogram. These findings, together with the biochemical and cytologic data, affirmed the diagnosis of a benign renal cyst. [By courtesy of Lang E. K. and Skinner-DeKernion (1978) Genitourinary cancer. W. B. Saunders, Philadelphia]

Benign renal cysts present on computed tomograms as sharply delineated, elliptical or round masses with smooth border. Attenuation coefficients of − 10 to + 10 are encountered in 95% of the benign renal cysts on the pre-enhancement, dynamic phase, and postenhancement studies [33]. Following administration of intravenous contrast medium, there should be no change in the attenuation coefficient obtained over the cyst (Fig. 9.3).

Guided cyst puncture and aspiration yields crystal-clear fluid with low lactic acid dehydrogenase, fat, and protein contents and negative cytologic examination [18, 19]. A double contrast study produced by introducing contrast medium and air into the partly evacuated cyst should demonstrate smooth contours of all inner surfaces of the cyst (Fig. 9.4). Moreover, the thus demonstrated lesion should be perfectly superimposable upon the negative defect demonstrated previously on conventional tomograms or computed tomograms. There should be no unexplained deficit between the mass on preliminary examination and the lesion documented by double contrast study [18, 19, 22, 23].

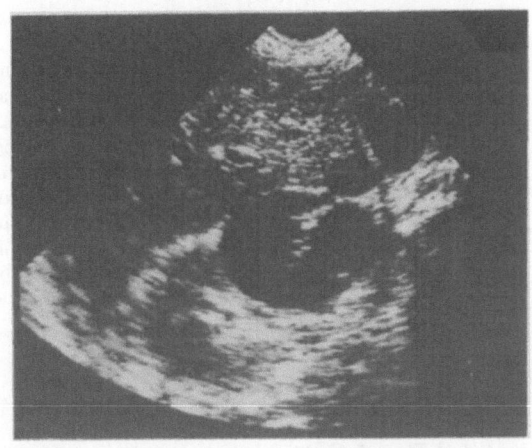

Fig. 9.5. Sonogram demonstrating a largely hyperechoic renal mass lesion. However, clusters of echoes are documented near the far wall of this cystic lesion that cannot be explained as reverberation echoes. This assigns the lesion to the group of "complex cysts." Fibrous septa within the cyst proved responsible for the appearance.

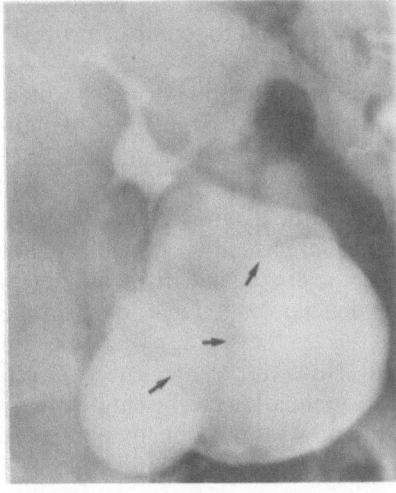

Fig. 9.6. A double contrast cyst study demonstrating multiple septa partially subdividing a lobulated cystic lesion in the lower pole of the left kidney. Uninhibited diffusion of contrast medium through all compartments attests to free interchange and incomplete division of the cyst by septa. Histochemical and cytologic examinations affirm the diagnosis of a benign cyst [By courtesy of Radiology]

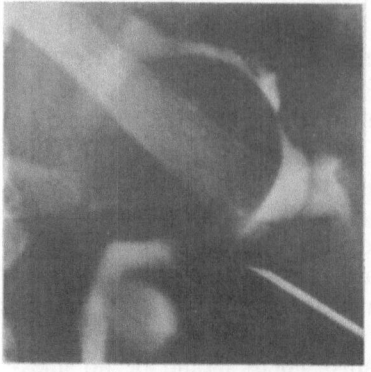
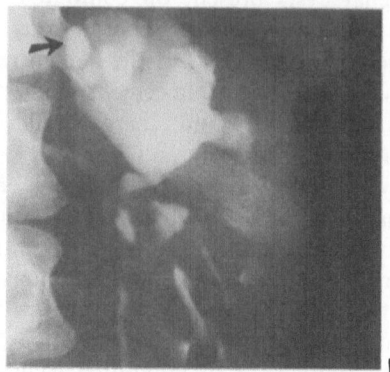
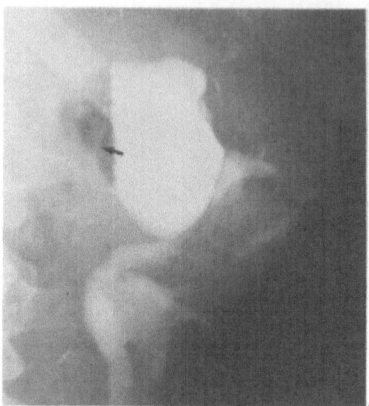

Fig. 9.7.a Under fluoroscopic guidance, a direct puncture of a cystic lesion in the upper pole of the left kidney is carried out. b The double contrast study demonstrates multiple lobulated components of this cyst (*arrow*). Though septation is readily demonstrated, all compartments intercommunicate freely. c A lateral decubitus projection allows air to gravitate into the lobulated section of this cyst and demonstrates the thin septa to great advantage. [By courtesy of Radiology]

Septated Renal Cysts

Septated renal cysts are benign cysts divided by fibrous septa, completely or incompletely, into compartments. The septation has no special pathological significance.

The ultrasonogram demonstrates a mass lesion with sound transmission characteristics of a cyst. Sometimes, septations may be clearly delineated ultrasonically. However, at times, the internal echoes elicited from the septa may force assignment to the group of "complex cysts" and further evaluation may be deemed necessary to affirm the diagnosis [38] (Fig. 9.5).

Septa are usually readily identifiable on computed tomograms. The appearance is characteristic and permits differentiation against multiple contiguous cysts or multilocular cysts. Depending on the thickness of the mesenchymal components making up the septa, dynamic computed tomograms may show some enhancement. However, readings over the central areas of the cyst will fail to show a step-up in attenuation coefficients. Moreover, the attenuation coefficients obtained over the cystic areas of a noncomplicated septated cyst tend to be in the range of − 10 to + 10 IU.

Most recently, magnetic resonance imaging has been shown to provide criteria for tissue characterization of the make-up of such septa [44].

Cyst puncture and aspiration will eliminate any remaining doubt as to the precise nature of such a lesion. Histochemical and cytologic assessment of the aspirate provides pristine criteria for elimination of associated neoplastic disease, inflammation, or hemorrhage into such cysts [18, 19, 23, 26] (Figs. 9.6, 9.7).

Infected (Inflammatory) Cysts

Inflammatory cysts result when simple benign renal cysts become infected. The walls of such cysts are thickened; histologically a round cell infiltrate is appreciated beneath the cuboidal lining of the cyst. Longstanding inflammatory process gives rise to inflammatory neovascularity which converts the extremely thin wall of a benign cyst into a thick inflammatory rind [18, 19, 23].

On ultrasonograms, inflammatory cysts tend to present with a complex pattern. The presence of particulate material floating in the cyst gives rise to internal echoes (Fig. 9.8). At times, rescanning in lateral decubitus positions will identify debris-free segments within the cavity created by the layering effect which reflects the specific gravity of the debris and that of the cyst fluid. Occasionally, echogenic mural masses may be shown simulating a necrotic tumor. Although these are due to exudate adherent to the cyst wall, the ultrasonogram does not provide any criteria for differentiation of these two conditions.

Computed tomograms readily identify the thickened cyst walls. Dynamic phase recordings may show a characteristic enhancement of the wall consistent with inflammatory hyperemia [24] (Fig. 9.9a). A characteristic step-up pattern of attenuation coefficients recorded over the wall of the lesion during the phases of transit of contrast medium (graph of attenuation coefficients) often makes possible differentiation of an inflammatory pattern against a necrotic tumor. Moreover, there do not tend to be enhancing mass components such as are characteristically seen with necrotic neoplasms [25]. A "senechial pattern" in the abutting perirenal space favors inflammatory neovascularity and edema but admittedly is difficult to differentiate against lymphatic spread of a neoplasm [24, 25] (Fig. 9.9b). The relatively high attenuation values recorded over the cyst in particular cause diagnostic confusion and often result in assigning the lesion to an indeterminate

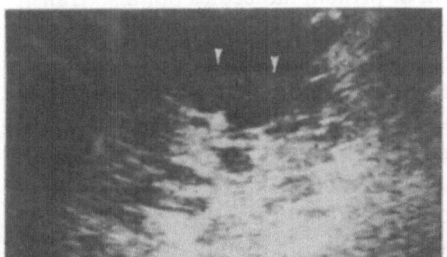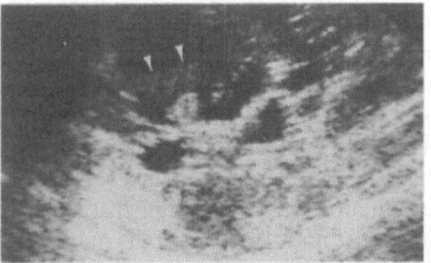

a   b

Fig. 9.8 a,b Layering of echogenic material is suggested in what otherwise qualifies sonographically for a benign renal cyst. The appearance strongly suggests particulate debris of a different specific gravity and therefore heralds an inflammatory cyst.

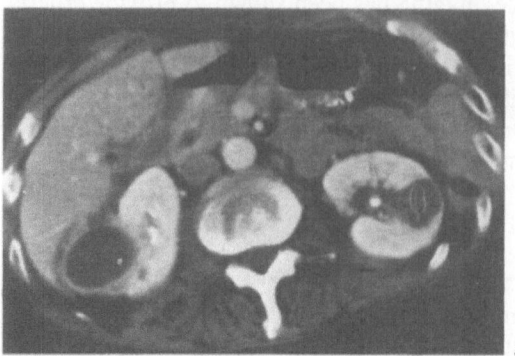

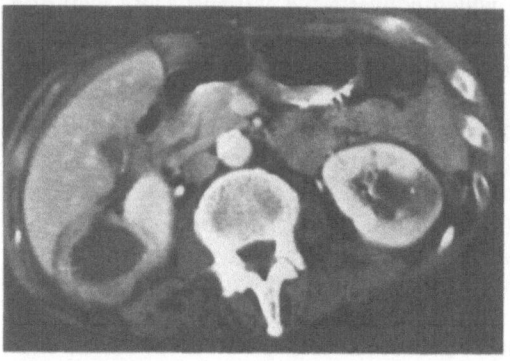

Fig. 9.9. a Dynamic phase computed tomogram demonstrating marked enhancement of the wall of a mass that would otherwise qualify for a benign cyst in the mid-pole of the right kidney. Note the lack of any enhancing wall of a typical benign cyst in the mid-pole of the left kidney. **b** A "synechial pattern" in the abutting perirenal space is compatible with inflammatory edema; however, lymphangitic neoplastic spread could present in an identical fashion. [By courtesy of Radiology]

group [2, 8, 10, 44, 47]. A number of explanations have been advanced for hyperdense renal cysts. Hemorrhage or high protein content may certainly cause a high CT number [10, 46, 47]. Necrotic debris will increase the protein content; an inflammatory rind may likewise cause protein transudate to leak into the cyst.

Alteration of the permeability of a cyst wall attendant upon inflammatory disease may encourage not only transmission of protein molecules but also transit of contrast medium. This may explain why sometimes a step-up of CT numbers may be recorded over inflammatory renal cysts hours after urography or arteriography [44] (Fig. 9.10). Most often, however, inflammatory debris in a benign cyst is characterized by inhomogeneous attenuation coefficients reflecting the divergent chemical compositions of material contained in such debris. Moreover, in the vast majority of inflammatory cysts, there prevails a characteristic absence of step-up of attenuation coefficient after intravenous administration of contrast medium.

Rarely, mural calcifications may develop in the walls of inflammatory cysts (Fig. 9.11). Despite some assertions in the literature that exclusive localization of shell-like calcifications in the rim of the lesion, low attenuation coefficient readings over the center of the lesion, and absence of a discernible soft tissue mass in the rim of

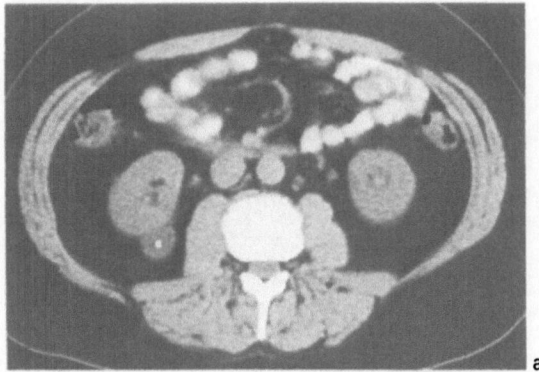

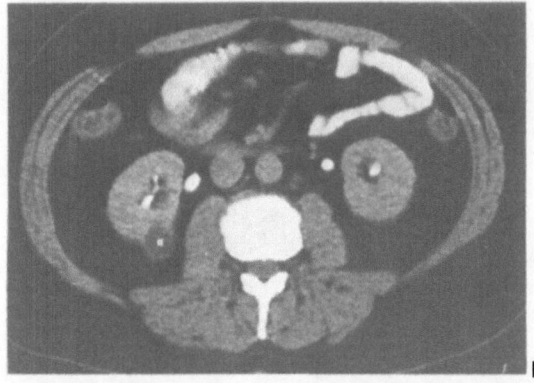

Fig. 9.10 a,b A significant step-up in attenuation coefficients from -13 to $+27$ occurred within 20 min after administration of intravenous contrast medium in a lesion otherwise meeting all CT criteria for benign renal cyst. It is postulated that this phenomenon reflects increased permeability of the cyst wall. Cyst puncture and aspiration and histochemical and cytologic examination confirmed the presence of a benign renal cyst.

the lesion represent a reliable criteria constellation for the diagnosis of calcifications in a benign cyst, many documented exceptions have invalidated such claims [16, 50].

Guided cyst puncture and aspiration and histochemical and cytologic assessment of the aspirate remains the procedure of choice in equivocal cases [18, 19, 23, 26]. A relatively low fat content of the aspirate and a lactic acid dehydrogenase (LDH) value of less than 250 IMU per milliliter make possible differentiation of an inflammatory exudate against the debris resulting from necrotic neoplasms, despite the common denominator of a very high protein content [19, 23, 26]. Absence of neoplastic cells on cytologic examination and of any cells graded higher than grade IV eliminates necrotic and cystic neoplastic lesions from differential diagnostic consideration.

Double contrast cystograms performed by replacing the aspirate with an aliquot of contrast medium and air should demonstrate absence of tumor masses protruding into the lumen of the cyst. This observation needs to be confirmed in

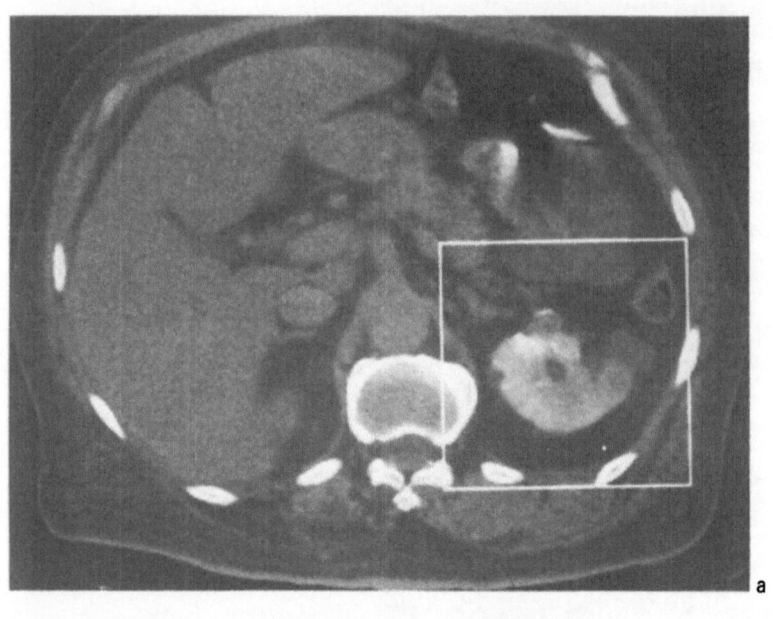

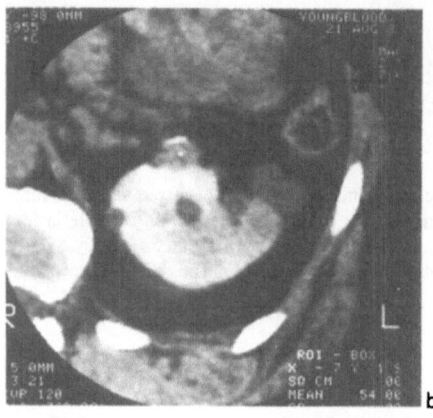

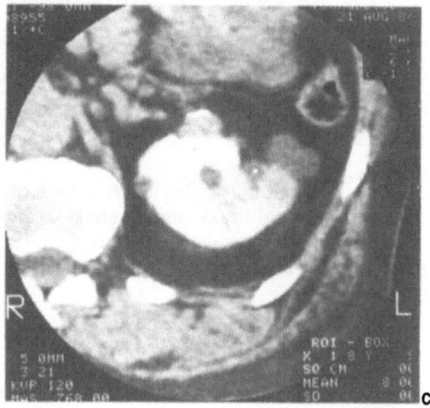

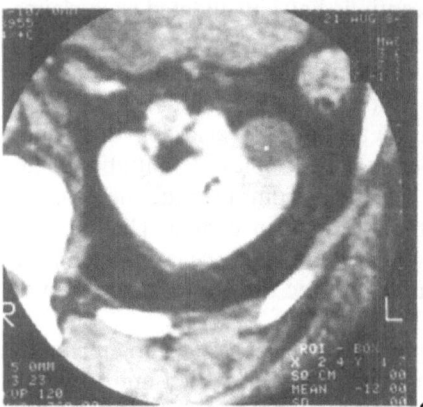

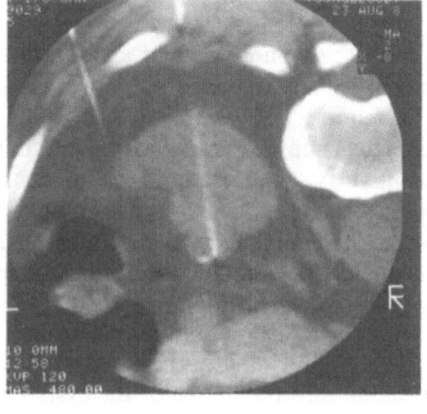

◄ **Fig. 9.11. a** A faint shell-like rim calcification is demonstrated in the anterior wall of a cystic lesion projecting from the mid-pole of the left kidney. **b–d** Attenuation coefficient readings over the center of the lesion featuring this shell-like calcification are in the mid 50s, but there is no step-up after administration of intravenous contrast medium. Conversely, attenuation coefficients recorded over multiple cystic appearing lesions originating from the lateral circumference of the mid-pole of the left kidney are in the range of benign renal cysts and again show no evidence of step-up after administration of intravenous contrast medium. The dynamic phase study shows no evidence of an enhancing soft tissue mass associated with the perimeter of the suspect cystic lesion. **e** Despite the above findings suggesting an inflammatory or hemorrhagic cyst with calcifications, CT-guided cyst puncture and aspiration was carried out on the anterior suspect lesion as well as one laterally located cyst. Biochemical and cytologic findings affirmed the diagnosis of a benign hemorrhagic cyst for the anteriorly located lesion and benign renal cyst for the laterally located lesion. [By courtesy of Radiology]

---

multiple decubitus and upright positions to document properly all perimeters of the cyst wall [18, 19] (Fig. 9.12). Necrotic exudate adherent to the cyst wall, however, can at times mimic a tumor nodule and may be impossible to differentiate on the basis of the double contrast study alone. In our experience, cytologic and histochemical examinations have proven to be the gold standard for differentiating inflammatory cysts from cystic necrotic neoplasms or neoplasms arising in the cyst wall [1, 15, 18, 19, 22, 23].

Hemorrhagic Cysts

Bleeding into benign renal cysts attendant upon trauma, bleeding diathesis, or factors of unknown etiology may occur in perhaps 6% of all renal cysts [5].

Hemorrhagic renal cysts usually present with a complex pattern on ultrasonograms. The appearance is indistinguishable from inflammatory renal cysts. At times, echoes may be elicited from liquifying blood clots adherent to the cyst wall.

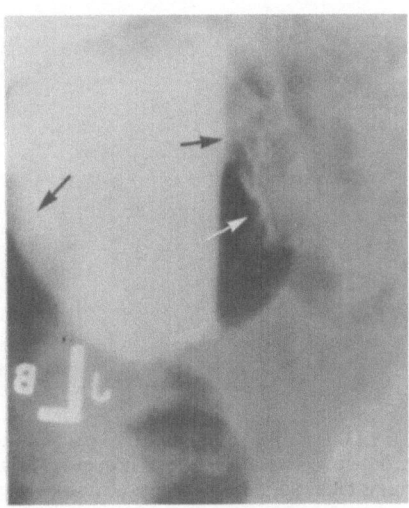

Fig. 9.12. A double contrast cyst study demonstrating mural masses protruding into the lumen of the cyst. This is considered characteristic for a hypernephroma arising from the cyst wall or a cystic and necrotic tumor. Moreover, the murky appearing aspirate revealed a high fat and lactic acid dehydrogenase content and readily identified neoplastic cells on cytologic examination. Thus the diagnosis of a tumor within the cyst causing a hemorrhagic exudate was readily established. [By courtesy of Radiology]

Clots immersed in a liquid medium offer an acoustic interface which causes the complex pattern. As fragmentation of clots increases, the number of echoes increases. However, serosanguinous fluid without formed blood clots appears on ultrasonograms like a benign renal cyst.

Hemorrhagic cysts are characterized by a high CT number. The attenuation value reflects the high hemoglobin and/or iron content in such hemorrhagic cysts [8, 46, 47, 50] (Fig. 9.11). Enhancement of the wall of hemorrhagic cysts is often observed on dynamic CTs during the late capillary phase of contrast medium transit. The enhancement reflects inflammatory neovascularity in the wall of such cysts provoked by the blood content [24]. Once again, the enhancement pattern is identical to that of inflammatory cysts, since in effect the pathophysiologic mechanism is the same.

Cyst puncture and aspiration are resorted to as the ultimate arbiter between a benign hemorrhagic cyst and hemorrhage into a cyst caused by an obscure tumor within a cystic lesion [5]. A relatively low fat and LDH content below 250 IMU per milliliter, cholesterol clefts in the aspirate, and an absence of neoplastic cells or grade IV or higher grade cells on cytologic examination suggest a benign etiology of a hemorrhagic aspirate [15, 19, 23] (Fig. 9.13).

Acute hemorrhage attendant upon a traumatic puncture is readily differentiable against the aspirate obtained from a hemorrhagic cyst. The former is characterized by changing blood content while aspirating the fluid whereas the latter is characterized by a murky but more or less homogeneous aspirate.

Magnetic resonance imaging can differentiate benign from hemorrhagic cysts [14; H. Hricak, personal communications] (Fig. 9.14). However, an overlap of T-1 and T-2 values exists between hemorrhagic cysts and solid tumors, making this differentiation difficult.

Calcified Cysts

Mural calcifications occur in approximately 1% of simple serous cysts and more frequently in inflammatory or hemorrhagic cysts. The calcifications in simple

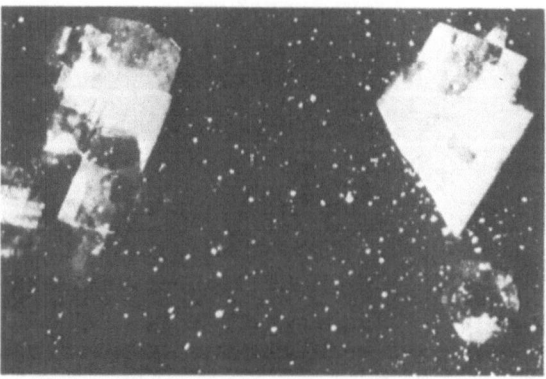

Fig. 9.13. Dark field examination of the aspirate from a hemorrhagic cyst revealing the characteristic cholesterol crystals. Absence of neoplastic cells or grade IV cells or higher on cytologic examination affirms the diagnosis of a benign hemorrhagic cyst.

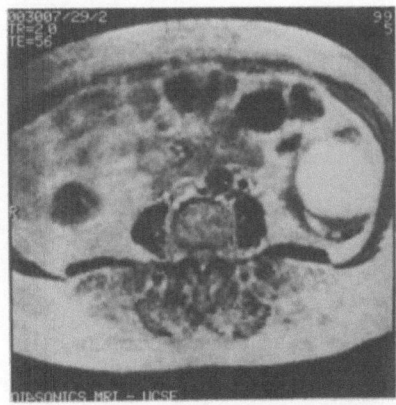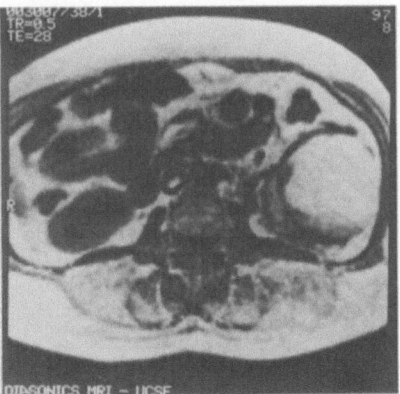

Fig. 9.14. The T-1 and T-2 values for hemorrhagic cysts are variable but much shorter than those for simple cysts. Thus recording at SE 500/28 and, for example, SE 1000/56 will document a marked intensity change. [By courtesy of Dr. H. Hricak and Radiology]

serous cysts are characterized as a "thin eggshell layer of calcifications in the cyst wall." Conversely, calcifications in a tumor are of the dystrophic variety and occur throughout the necrotic tumor elements. Inflammatory calcifications or calcifications in hemorrhagic cysts also occur as an eggshell calcification but often appear to be thicker and irregular [50].

Ultrasonograms offer few criteria for the differentiation of these conditions. Calcium in the wall of the cyst significantly reduces sound transmission and may in fact mimic a solid mass. Sometimes, the ultrasonogram will suggest a solid mass for the component of the cyst that features calcifications and a benign cyst for the remainder of the lesion. Only collation to radiographs makes possible the diagnosis.

Although it has been suggested that if all calcifications are thin and in the rim of the lesion, the CT number over the center of the lesion is low, and there is no associated soft tissue mass at the perimeter of the lesion, one can diagnose a benign cyst, these criteria have not held up to the test of time [16, 50] (Figs. 9.11, 9.15).

Guided cyst puncture and aspiration is the procedure of choice for the diagnosis of all lesions presumed to be cystic in nature but featuring calcifications. Histochemical and cytopathological criteria are considered much more reliable than criteria derived from imaging studies [19, 23, 26]. If, however, there remains doubt as to the etiology of such calcified cysts, e.g., as is cast by a grade IV or higher grade cytology, then exploration is strongly advocated so as not to miss an occult neoplastic lesion [1, 5, 16].

Multilocular Cystic Nephroma

Multilocular cystic nephroma may involve a portion of a kidney whereas involvement of the entire kidney is usually referred to as multicystic dysplastic kidney [12, 30, 31]. Etiologically, this malformation most likely results from congenital ureteric atresia. Nephrons obstructed during this development then form cysts. Microdissection studies by Madewell et al. appear to bear out this hypothesis [30].

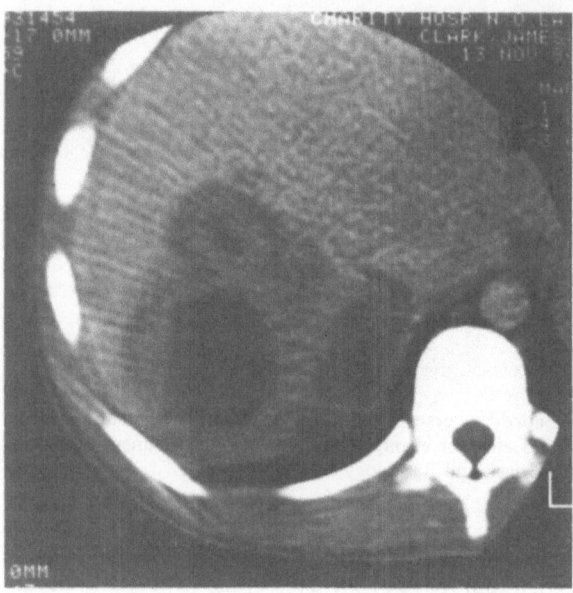

Fig. 9.15. Computed tomogram demonstrating multilobulated cystic masses in the retroperitoneal space of the left upper abdominal quadrant. There were no demonstrable elements of functioning renal parenchyma. The appearance strongly suggests a cystic dysplastic element created by pelvoinfundibular atresia.

The ultrasonogram usually demonstrates a cystic or complex pattern. The presence of clusters of cysts partially or completely separated by septa may occasion a hyperechoic pattern.

On computed tomograms, multilocular cystic nephroma usually presents as a well margined, rounded or polycyclic cortical mass [3, 6, 31, 34]. Cysts of varying size, separated by septa of variable wall thickness, are readily identified. The attenuation coefficients obtained over these cysts may vary markedly. Since calcifications in the cyst walls are frequently present, partial volume pixels suggest abnormally high attenuation coefficients [34] (Figs. 9.11, 9.15).

Although the diagnosis may be suggested on computed tomogram, confirmation by cyst puncture and aspiration may be required [43]. Often the aspirate has a crankoil consistency, with high protein content. Contrast studies of the aspirated lesions demonstrate single or multiple cysts communicating by tubular structures. The cysts may or may not feature calcifications in their wall [34] (Fig. 9.16). Opacification of tubules leading from cysts or interconnecting cysts is considered by many to be the ultimate arbiter in cases of doubt [43]. The arteriogram, though advocated in the past, offers no specific criteria for affirming the diagnosis but merely suggests the presence of multiple avascular or cystic lesions.

Lesions in Differential Diagnosis

Intrarenal abscesses, intrarenal or subcapsular hematomas, and the entire spectrum of solid mass lesions enter into the differential diagnosis. With the notable exception of abscesses and some fresh hematomas, the ultrasonogram should suggest solid or complex mass lesions for these pathologic entities.

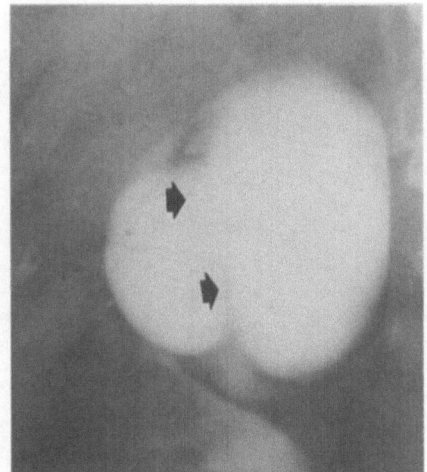

Fig. 9.16. Cyst puncture and aspiration of a calcified cystic mass in the right retroperitoneal space yielded a yellowish–brownish crankoil aspirate. The appearance on the double contrast study is consistent with a cystic dysplastic renal moiety. There was no evidence of any functioning renal parenchyma on the right side nor in a pelvic location. [By courtesy of Radiology]

Renal Abscess and Pyonephrosis

Ultrasonograms may suggest a cystic or multicystic pattern. However, the lesions are only rarely completely echo free. In general, debris produces numerous acoustic interfaces. Moreover, chronic abscesses may demonstrate internal septa. Abscesses associated with gas-forming organisms demonstrate characteristic acoustic shadowing due to the microbubbles contained in such lesions [17].

On computed tomograms, abscesses tend to present as a cyst-like structure but usually with irregular walls. Attenuation coefficients obtained over the center of the cystic area tend to be in a range from $+10$ to $+30$, characterized by inhomogeneity reflecting the presence of debris [24]. Since the center of the abscess contains liquified material, there is no enhancement following administration of contrast medium. However, dynamic computed tomograms may demonstrate a densely enhancing abscess wall reflecting inflammatory neovascularity in the rind of such an abscess [24] (Fig. 9.17). Pyonephrotic kidneys present in a similar fashion with the exception that the multiple cyst-like structures are found in the general location of calyces (Fig. 9.18).

Intrarenal and Subcapsular Renal Hematomas

Intrarenal hematomas result from a variety of causes. Spontaneous intrarenal or subcapsular hematomas are not infrequently the consequence of bleeding from a small renal cell carcinoma or angiomyolipoma or arteriovenous malformation [5, 13, 42]. Meticulous assessment is therefore necessary, particularly in the group of patients featuring spontaneous hematomas.

The ultrasonographic characteristics vary with the physical state of the hematoma, which is age dependent [38]. Fresh hematomas behave like a cystic lesion whereas older hematomas feature clots which elicit internal echoes. These increase as fragmentation of the clot occurs. Chronic hematomas may show calcifications with attendant attenuation of sound transmission.

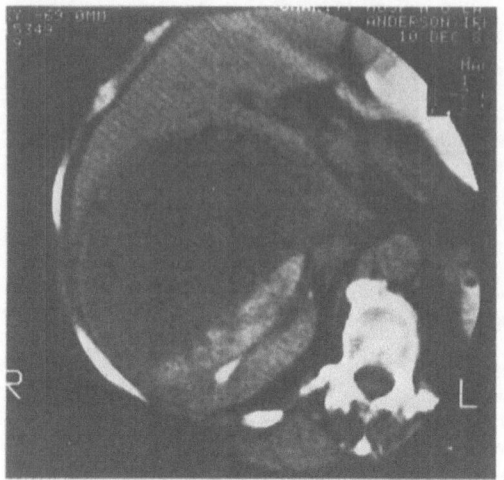

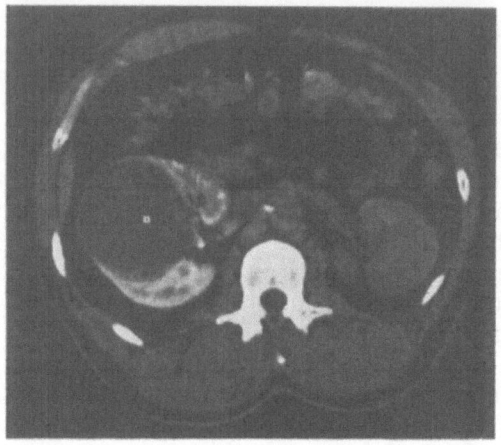

Fig. 9.17. a A relatively sharply demarcated mass is demonstrated in the mid-pole of the right kidney. Gas bubbles are identified both within this mass as well as in the perirenal space. A moth-eaten appearance of the abutting cortex suggests the presence of microabscesses in the cortex. **b** A dynamic CT demonstrating enhancement of the capsule of this intrarenal abscess. Attenuation coefficient readings over the abscess are inhomogeneous, varying from $+10$ to $+36$, reflecting the presence of debris. Pixel readings obtained over the gas bubbles rendered readings in the -300 to -400 range. The appearance is considered characteristic for a gas-forming abscess.

On computed tomograms, fresh intrarenal hematomas are usually recognized on the basis of the high attenuation coefficient of blood [9, 42]. Depending on the age of the hematoma, attenuation coefficients from $+10$ to $+65$ units may be encountered. There is, therefore, an obvious overlap with those of neoplasms. However, in contradistinction to solid tumors, hematomas do not enhance after administration of intravenous contrast medium. A rim enhancement may be present, particularly on dynamic phase computed tomograms, and reflects inflammatory neovascularity in the rind delineating an older hematoma [24]. In some old hematomas, layering may occur, with the less attenuating plasma on top and the more attenuating cellular debris in a dependent position [42].

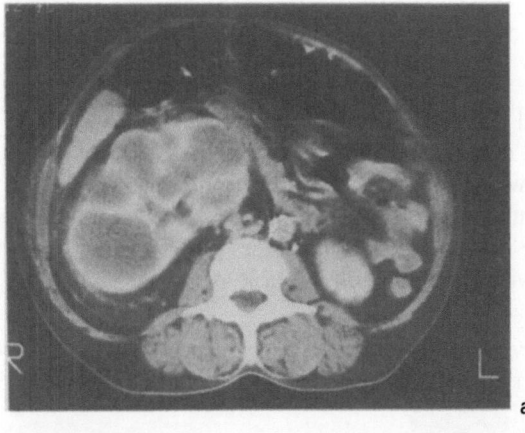

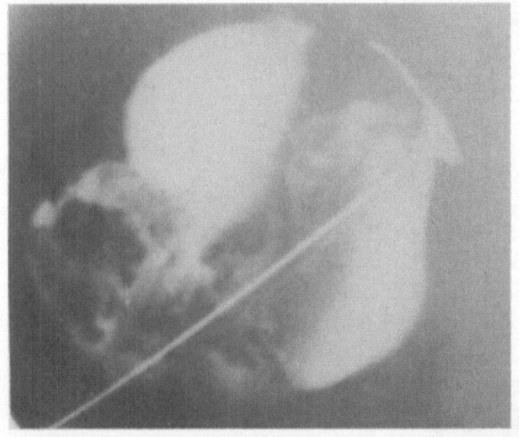

Fig. 9.18. a Dynamic computed tomogram demonstrating multiple interconnected or separated low density masses throughout the kidney. A rim stain suggests an inflammatory rind. The location of some of the seemingly interconnected low density masses suggests dilated calyces and therefore the diagnosis of pyonephrosis. Isolated interspersed cortical abscesses may be responsible for the seemingly nonconnected mass lesions. **b** Guided puncture and aspiration yielded creamy pus and the double contrast study documented abundant debris in hugely dilated calyces. [By courtesy of Radiology]

Aneurysms and Arteriovenous Malformations

On ultrasonograms, aneurysms and arteriovenous malformations usually present as cystic lesions. Real-time ultrasound may identify pulsations and thus suggest the correct diagnosis [38].

On computed tomograms, the nature of this otherwise cystic appearing lesion may be suggested by high attenuation coefficients consistent with blood. A definitive diagnosis is possible on dynamic computed tomograms, which on appropriate phase demonstrate dense opacification of the lesion [24]. More recently, magnetic resonance scanning has also provided definitive criteria (lack of or decreased signal intensity attendant upon a moving blood column) for identification of such lesions [14; H. Hricak, personal communications].

Solid Tumors

Renal Cell Carcinoma

On ultrasonograms, nearly all renal cell carcinomas are characterized as a solid mass. Necrotic and cystic renal cell carcinomas may occasionally present with a complex pattern. Irregularity of the wall contours, however, should raise suspicion of a neoplastic lesion. Tubular adenocarcinomas, featuring a sparse vascularity, tend to be hypechoic since there are fewer reflecting interfaces [38]. Papillary cyst adenocarcinoma likewise presents with a relatively hypechoic pattern.

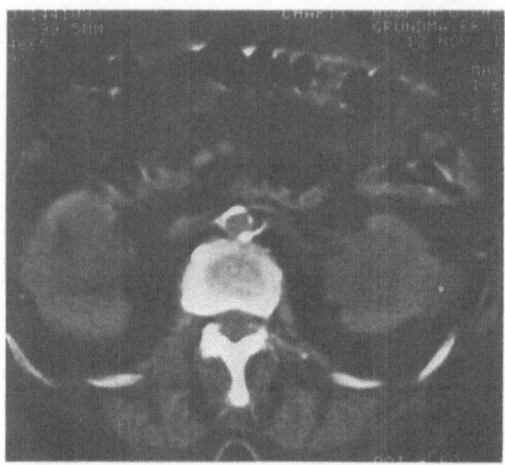

a

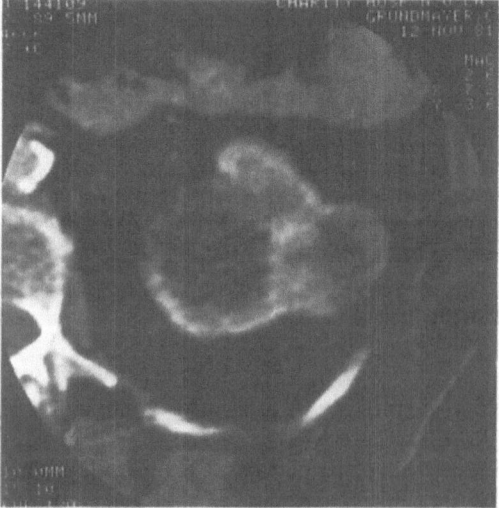

b

Fig. 9.19. a Computed tomogram suggesting a low density (0 IU) cystic lesion involving the lateral border of the lower pole of the right kidney. Irregularity of the inner contours raises the question of a necrotic and cystic renal carcinoma or an inflammatory or hemorrhagic cyst. **b** The dynamic CT recording the capillary phase of contrast medium transit demonstrates unequivocal enhancement of tumor nodules projecting into the lumen of the cystic lesion and establishes the diagnosis of a cystic necrotic renal carcinoma.

On unenhanced computed tomograms, most tumors feature a poorly marginated mass, with attenuation coefficients similar to those of normal renal tissues. However, necrosis, hemorrhage, or calcifications may occasion significant variability in attenuation coefficient readings obtained over the lesion [7]. After administration of intravenous contrast medium, renal tumors show less enhancement than normal renal parenchyma. Destruction of tubular elements and lack of opacification of tubular elements within the tumor are responsible for this phenomenon. On dynamic computed tomograms, a characteristic transient enhancement of viable tumor components is documented during the phase of capillary transit of contrast medium [24, 25]. Even in predominantly necrotic and cystic tumors, some areas may enhance [7, 25] (Fig. 9.19). Demonstration of a central stellate scar on ultrasonograms or computed tomograms, a spokewheel enhancement pattern on late phase dynamic computed tomograms, and sharp demarcation against adjacent normal parenchyma should suggest the histologic diagnosis of an oncocytoma rather than a renal cell carcinoma [29]. Computed tomography has largely obviated the use of arteriograms [32, 49].

Angiomyolipoma

Angiomyolipomas are hamartomatous malformations that contain fat, blood vessels, and smooth muscles.

On ultrasonograms, these tumors are characteristically hyperechoic. The presence of multiple interfaces between fat globules separated by septa occasions the marked echogenicity. However, if associated with a hematoma, hypechoic areas may be present [40, 45, 48].

Most angiomyolipomas are readily diagnosed on computed tomograms on the basis of the low attenuation coefficients (-30 to -100 units) characteristic for their fatty tissues. However, hemorrhage, necrosis, or calcifications may occasionally confuse the diagnosis [45, 48]. Dynamic computed tomograms add the criteria of opacified vessels with mulberry-like aneurysms demonstrable during the arterial phase of contrast medium transit [24] (Fig. 9.20). Dynamic CT is also best capable of differentiating areas of hemorrhage from vascular tumor elements, the latter showing enhancement [13, 25].

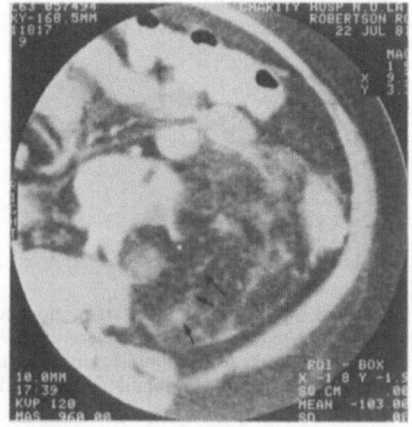

Fig. 9.20. Dynamic computed tomogram demonstrating a multilobulated mass replacing portions of the lower pole of the left kidney. The lesion is sharply demarcated against normal renal parenchyma. Attenuation coefficients obtained over most areas of the lesions indicate fat content. There are, however, serpiginous structures that light up and demonstrate contrast medium accumulation (arterial phase) (*arrows*). These are characteristic of the mulberry-like aneurysms seen in angiomyolipomas.

Lymphomas and Metastatic Lesions

Although metastatic tumors to the kidney are the most common malignant renal neoplasm, their premortem diagnosis is rare.

The ultrasonic appearance is related to the cellular organization and vascularity of such metastases. Vascularized tumors feature echo-producing interfaces and therefore present as relatively echogenic tumors. Hypovascular metastases with necroses and hemorrhage may present as relatively hyperechoic lesions.

The appearance of metastatic lesions on computed tomogram also varies with tissue characteristics and particularly its vascularity. Although a definitive diagnosis may not be possible, dynamic computed tomograms have been found helpful in identifying hypervascular metastases.

Transitional Cell Carcinoma

Infiltrative transitional cell carcinoma may present as a renal mass lesion. The appearance on ultrasonograms is variable, though most often it presents as a relatively hyperechoic mass.

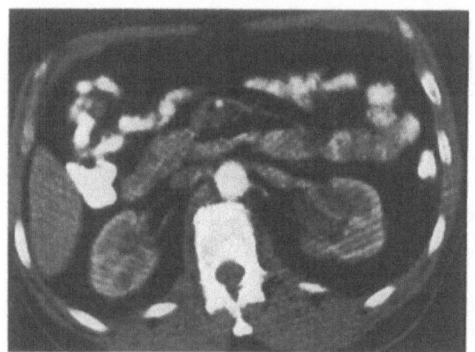

a

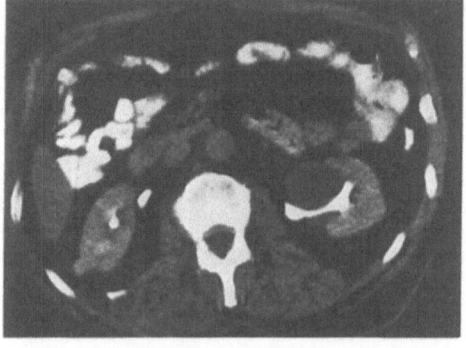

b

Fig. 9.21. a Dynamic computed tomogram demonstrating a low density spherical mass in a parapelvic position. Attenuation coefficients measured over the mass are low on the pre-enhancement study and remain unchanged after administration of intravenous contrast medium. **b** Postenhancement CT demonstrates splaying of infundibula around the mass. The appearance is considered characteristic for a parapelvic cyst.

Computed tomograms are particularly useful in differentiating pelvocalyceal filling defects on the basis of the attenuation coefficient [35, 39]. This criterion permits differentiation of uric acid or cystine calculi, blood clots, or transitional cell carcinoma presenting as filling defects in the pelvis and parapelvic cysts (Fig. 9.21). Dynamic computed tomograms are useful in identifying infiltrative transitional cell carcinoma. Despite the relative avascularity of this lesion, a distinct enhancement is documentable during the early capillary phase of contrast medium transit [24] (Fig. 9.22). This feature is particularly useful if infiltrative transitional cell carcinoma is associated with hyperdense cystic lesions, i.e., obstructed calyces with protein-rich urine.

Renal Pseudotumors

Invaginated cortical tissues (column of Bertin) may present as a renal pseudomass. Scintiscanograms with technetium glucoheptonate demonstrate normal uptake of the radionuclide in the suspected mass and thus definitively establish the diagnosis of a column of Bertin or invaginated renal cortex [24, 36] (Fig. 9.23).

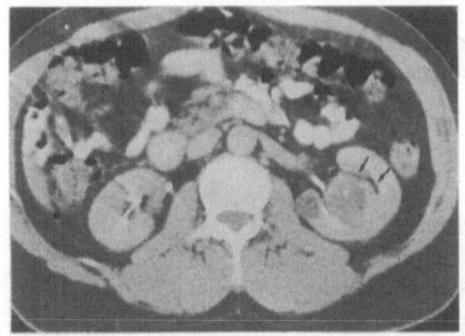

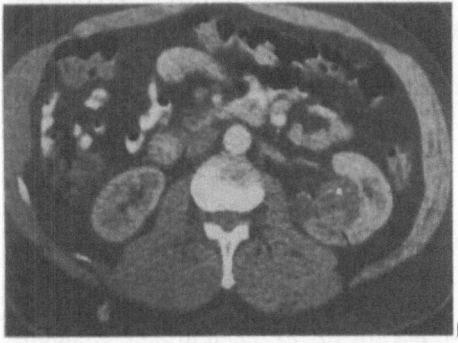

Fig. 9.22. a Computed tomogram demonstrating a space-occupying lesion in the parapelvic area. Note splaying of the pelvic fat by the mass. In contradistinction to a parapelvic cyst, the attenuation coefficients obtained over the mass are in the range of 20–30 on pre-enhancement studies. **b** However, during the phase of capillary transit of contrast medium recorded on dynamic CT, a sharp step-up is observed. This identifies the mass as a solid neoplasm, probably a transitional cell carcinoma extending from the pelvis into the parapelvic space and renal parenchyma. As an incidental finding, a typical benign cortical renal cyst, is demonstrated.

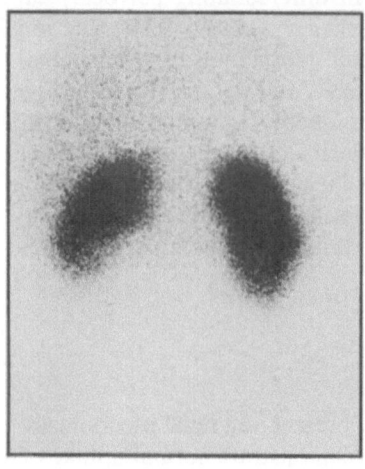

Fig. 9.23. Ascintiscanogram performed after administration of technetium glucoheptonate, demonstrating normal and even uptake of the radionuclide throughout the kidney and in the area of the suspected mass. This establishes the diagnosis of a pseudotumor attributable to a column of Bertin.

Generalized Cystic Mass Lesions of the Kidney

Adult and infantile type polycystic disease are the two principal representatives of cystic disease causing generalized enlargement of the kidney.

Polycystic Disease, Adult Type

Ultrasonograms demonstrate the presence of numerous cysts. Many of the cysts are too small to be resolved individually, but cast abnormal small echo complexes. The central echo complex tends to be distorted. Because of disparing size of the cyst, a typical cyst pattern may be obtained only from a few areas.

On computed tomograms, innumerable renal masses are documented, most with an attenuation value of about water. After administration of intravenous contrast medium, there is no enhancement of the cysts; however, study of tissue attenuation coefficients is subject to error due to partial volume effect, integrating interposed renal parenchyma and cyst into the evaluated pixel [38].

Polycystic Disease, Infantile Type

Infantile and juvenile polycystic disease may present with a spectrum of clinical manifestations. Dependent on the age of onset of clinical presentations, manifestations of renal or hepatic pathology may predominate. In older children, periportal fibrosis and the complications of hepatic involvement are the predominant feature. In younger children, renal disease is responsible for the clinical manifestations [4].

The radiologic diagnosis is usually made on intravenous urograms featuring large kidneys with a mottled nephrogram and characteristic medullary striation.

Innumerable cysts, particularly in the medulla, occasion many interfaces which on ultrasound produce a highly echogenic pattern.

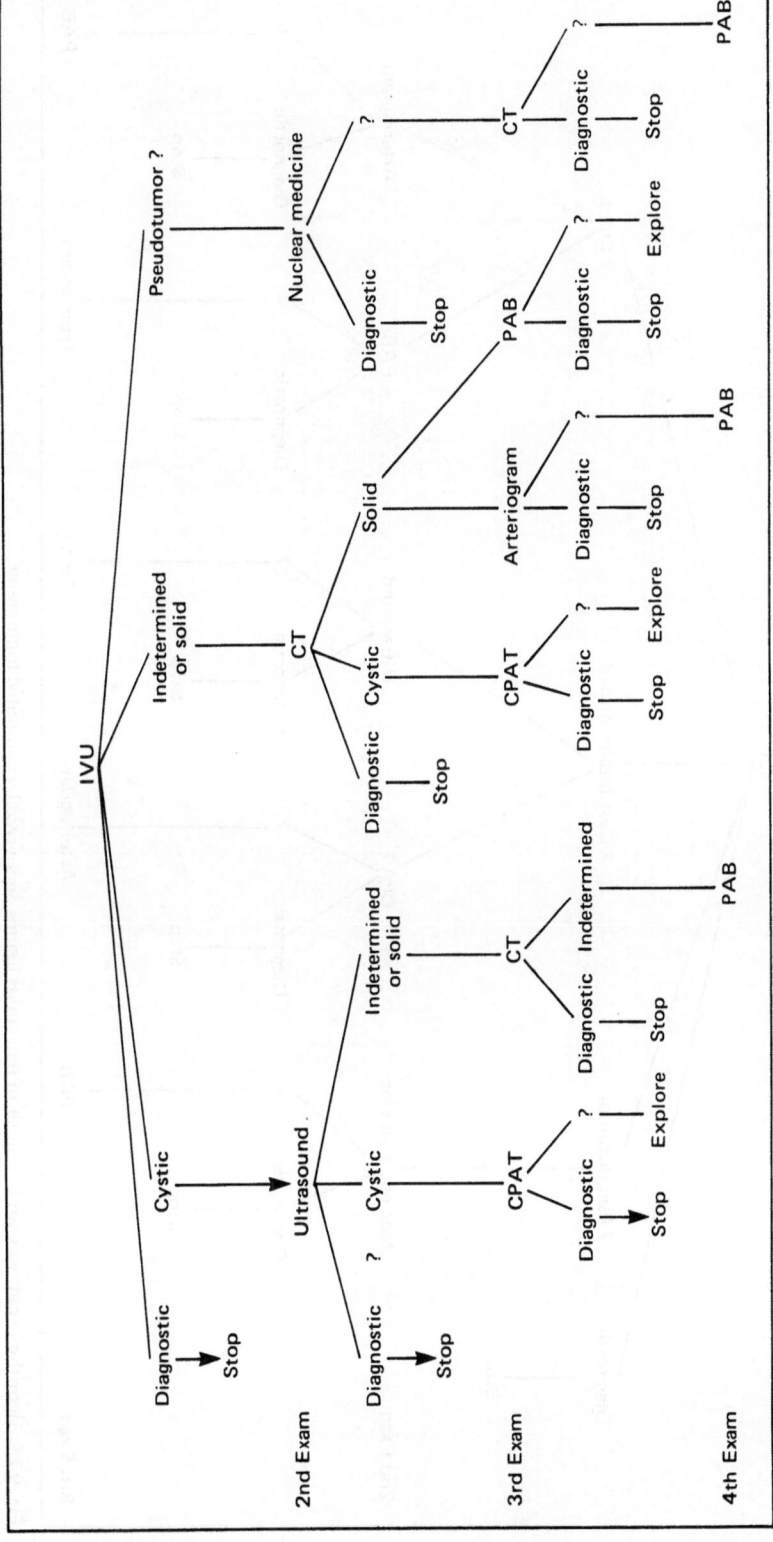

Fig. 9.24. Algorithmic pathway for diagnosis of renal mass lesions discovered by intravenous urography (IVU).

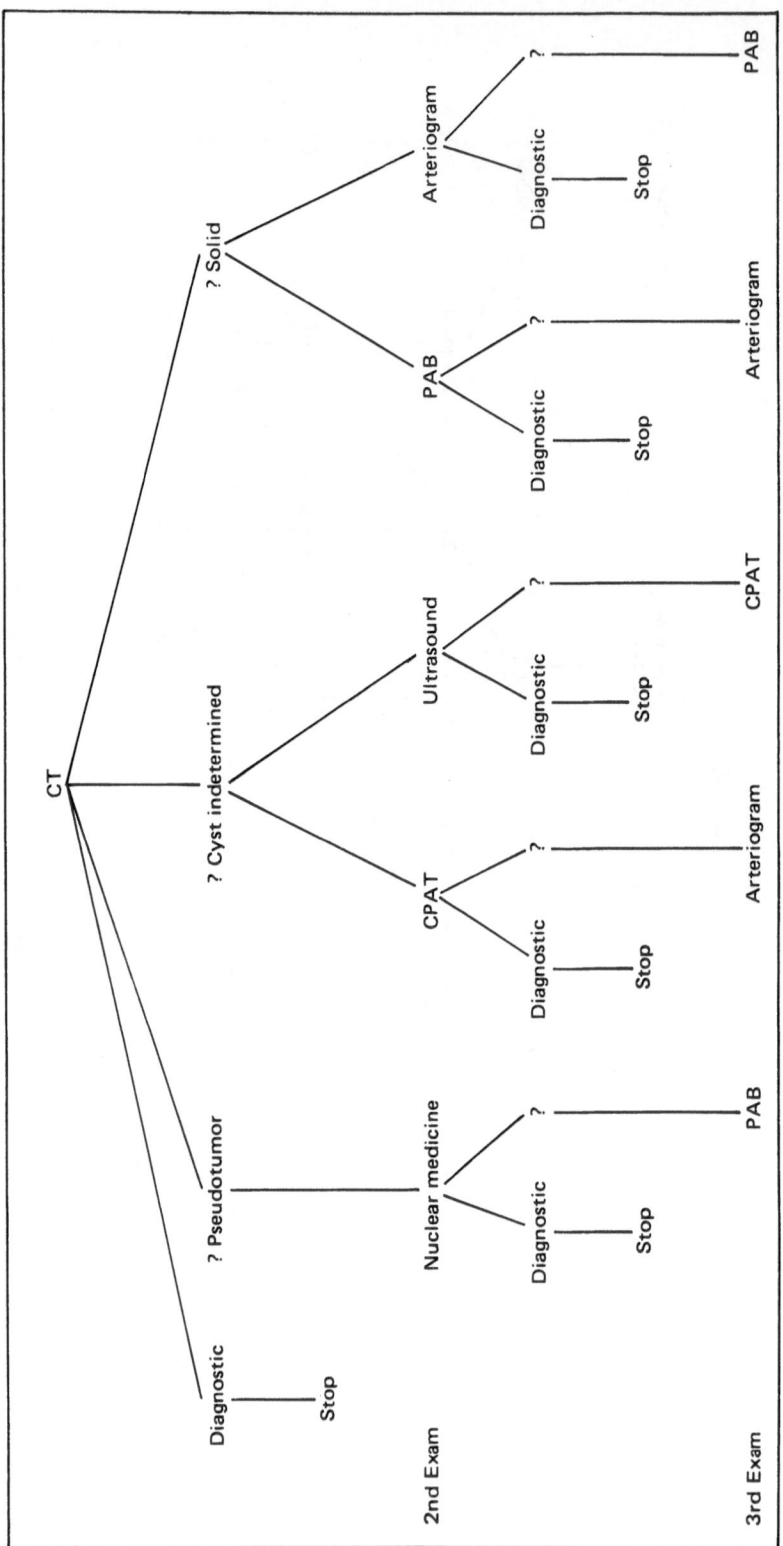

Fig. 9.25. Algorithmic pathway for diagnosis of renal mass lesions discovered by computed tomograms.

Economic Implications of Renal Cysts

The ubiquitous nature of renal cysts emphasizes the need for a cost-effective diagnostic approach. However, the very similar presentation of some renal cysts, asymptomatic neoplastic renal masses, and arteriovenous fistulas mandates their investigation to such a degree as will establish the diagnosis with acceptable confidence.

Despite some projections to the contrary, improved technology in the last decade has in fact reduced the cost for the workup of such lesions [51]. The reason for this lies in increased speed of diagnosis, increased use of noninvasive tests, and improved accuracy, sensitivity, and specificity of tests. Specifically, the fact that 45% of all lesions are diagnosed by the discovering examination (the computed tomogram) has significantly decreased the cost of diagnosis. Moreover, another 28% of all lesions are diagnosed by the relatively inexpensive ultrasonogram used as second examination.

The composition of asymptomatic space-occupying lesions of the kidney, with 70% due to benign renal cysts, obviously lowers the cost of diagnosis since this most common lesion is definitively diagnosed either by the discovering examination, the computed tomogram, or by the second examination, the ultrasonogram. Even the small group (about 27% of the patients) that remain undiagnosed after the initial studies can usually be definitively assessed by other relatively noninvasive techniques. Many of those lesions initially discovered on intravenous urograms and thought to be solid lesions on subsequent ultrasonograms can be diagnosed by computed tomograms (Fig. 9.24). Those refractory to diagnosis by both computed tomography and ultrasonography are usually diagnoseable by guided cyst puncture, aspiration, and/or biopsy (Figs. 9.24, 9.25).

Replacement of the costly and highly invasive arteriogram by CT and guided puncture, aspiration, and biopsy is the third factor that has greatly curtailed costs.

Thus, despite the introduction of more costly examinations (CT), the increased speed with which diagnosis can be rendered and particularly the attendant reduction in hospitalization cost has more than offset the procedural cost. Consequently, despite a further increase in the recognition of asymptomatic space-occupying lesions of the kidney, particularly in older patients, the cost of establishing a definitive diagnosis has declined substantially. The number of patients refractory to diagnosis by the proposed imaging algorithms (Figs. 9.24, 9.25) has also declined and the need for surgical exploration for diagnostic purposes has been reduced to about 1% of the patients.

References

1. Ambrose SS, Lewis EL, O'Brien EP, et al. (1977) Unsuspected renal tumors associated with renal cysts. J Urol 117:704
2. Balfe DM, McClennan BL, Stanley RJ, Weyman PJ, Sagel SS (1982) Evaluation of renal masses considered indeterminate on computed tomography. Radiology 142:421–428
3. Banner MP, Pollack HM, Chatten J, Witzleben C (1981) Multilocular renal cysts: Radiologic-pathologic correlation. AJR 136:239–247

4. Blyth H, Ockendon B (1971) Polycystic disease of kidneys and liver presenting in childhood. J Med Genet 8:257–284
5. Burnstein J, Woodside JR (1977) Malignant hemorrhagic renal cyst with occult neoplasm. Radiology 123:599
6. Carlson DH, Carlson D, Simon H (1978) Benign multilocular cystic nephroma. AJR 131:621–625
7. Clouse ME, Lee RG, Evans DD (1983) Multicystic renal cell carcinoma. CT 7:195–198
8. Coleman BG, Arger PH, Mintz MC, Pollack HM, Banner MP (1984) Hyperdense renal masses: A computed tomographic dilemma. AJR 143:291–294
9. Federle MP, Kaiser JA, McAninch JW, Jeffrey BR Jr, Mall JC (1981) The role of computed tomography in renal trauma. Radiology 141:455
10. Fishman MC, Pollack HM, Arger PH, Banner MP (1983) High protein content: Another case of CT hyperdense benign renal cyst. J Comput Assist Tomogr 7:1103–1106
11. Glazer GM, London SS (1981) CT appearance of global renal infarction. J Comput Assist Tomogr 5:847–850
12. Griscom ND, Vawter GF, Fellers RX (1975) Pelvo infundibular atresia: the usual form of multicystic kidney: 44 unilateral and 2 bilateral cases. Semin Roentgenol 10(2):125–132
13. Hilton S, Bosniak MA, Megibow AJ, Ambos MA (1981) Computed tomographic demonstration of a spontaneous subcapsular hematoma due to a small renal cell carcinoma. Radiology 141:743–744
14. Hricak H, Williams RD, Moon KL, Moss AA, Alper C, Crooks L, Kaufman L (1983) Nuclear magnetic resonance imaging of the kidney: renal masses. Radiology 147:765
15. Jackman RJ, Stevens GM (1974) Benign hemorrhagic renal cyst. Radiology 110:7–13
16. Kim WS, Goldman SM, Gatewood OMB, Marshall FF, Siegelman SS (1981) Computed tomography in calcified renal masses. J Comput Assist Tomogr 5:855–860
17. Kressel HY, Filly RA (1978) Ultrasonic appearance of gas containing abscesses in the abdomen. AJR 130:71–74
18. Lang EK (1971) Coexistence of cyst and tumor in the same kidney. Radiology 101:7–16
19. Lang EK (1973) Roentgenographic assessment of asymptomatic renal lesions. Radiology 109:257
20. Lang EK (1975) Roentgenologic assessment of medullary cysts. Seminar Roentgenol 10(2):145–154
21. Lang EK (1977) Asymptomatic space-occupying lesions of the kidney, a programmed sequential approach and its quality and cost of health care. South Med J 70:77
22. Lang EK (1980) Asymptomatic space-occupying lesions of the kidney. Minn Med 89:733
23. Lang EK (1980) Roentgenologic approach to the diagnosis and management of cystic lesions of the kidney: Is cyst exploration mandatory? Urol Clin North Am 7:677–688
24. Lang EK (1984) Evaluation of renal mass lesions by imaging examinations. In: Libertino JA (ed) Current concepts of uroradiology—Interventional perspectives in urology. Williams & Wilkins, Baltimore, pp 86–101
25. Lang EK (1984) Angiocomputed tomography and dynamic tomography in staging of renal cell carcinoma. Radiology 151:149–155
26. Lang EK (to be published) Assessment of asymptomatic space-occupying lesions of the kidney. J Urol
27. Lee JKT, McClennan BL, Melson GL, Stanley RJ (1980) Acute focal bacterial nephritis: Emphasis on grey scale sonography and computed tomography. AJR 135:87–92
28. Leopold GR, Talner LB, Asher WM, et al. (1973) Renal ultrasonography: an updated approach to the diagnosis of renal cysts. Radiology 109:671
29. Levine E, Hunrakoon M (1983) Computed tomography of renal oncocytoma. AJR 141:741
30. Madewell JE, Hartman DS, Lichtenstein JE (1979) Radiologic pathologic correlation in cystic disease of the kidney. Radiol Clin North Am 17:261–279
31. Madewell JE, Goldman SM, Davis CJ, Hartman DS, Feigin BS, Lichtenstein JE (1983) Multilocular cystic nephroma: A radiologic pathologic correlation of 58 patients. Radiology 146:309–322
32. Mauro MA, Wadsworth DE, Stanely RJ, McClennan BL (1982) Renal cell carcinoma: Angiography in the CT era. AJR 139:1135–1138
33. McClennan BL, Stanley RJ, Melson GL, Levitt RG, Sagel SS (1979) CT of renal cyst: Is cyst puncture and aspiration necessary? AJR 133:671–675
34. Parienty RA, Pradel J, Imbert M, Picard JD, Savert P (1981) Computed tomography of multilocular cystic nephroma. Radiology 140:135–139
35. Parienty RA, Ducellier R, Pradel J, Lubrano JM, Coquill EF, Richard F (1982) Diagnostic value of CT numbers in pelvocalyceal filling defects. Radiology 145:743–747
36. Pollack HM, Edell S, Morales JO (1974) Radionuclide imaging in renal pseudo tumors. Radiology 111:639

37. Pollack HM, Goldberg BB, Morales JO, Bogash MA (1974) A systemized approach to the differential diagnosis of renal masses. Radiology 113:653–659

38. Pollack HM, Banner MP, Arger TH, Goldberg BB, Mulhern CB Jr (1979) Comparison of computed tomography in ultrasound and diagnosis of renal masses. Clin Diagn Ultrasound 2:25–72

39. Pollack HM, Arger BH, Banner MP, Mulhern CT, Coleman BJ (1981) Computed tomography of renal pelvic filling defects. Radiology 138:645–651

40. Ragahavendra BN, Bosniak MA, Megibow AJ (1983) Small angiomyolipoma of the kidney: sonographic evaluation. AJR 141:575–578

41. Richie JP, Jarnick MB, Seltzer S, Bettmann MA (1983) Computerized tomography scan for diagnosis and the staging of renal cell carcinoma. J Urol 129:1114–1116.

42. Sagel SS, Siegel MJ, Stanley RJ, Jost RG (1977) Detection of retroperitoneal hemorrhage by computed tomography. AJR 129:403–407

43. Saxton HM, Golding SJ, Chantler C, Haycock JD (1981) Diagnostic puncture in renal cyst dysplasia (multicystic kidney): evidence on the etiology of the cysts. Br J Radiol 54:555–561

44. Shanser JD, Hedgcock MW, Korobkin M (1978) Transit of contrast material into renal cyst following urography and arteriography. AJR 130:584

45. Sherman JL, Hartman DS, Friedman AC, Madewell JC, Davis CJ, Goldman SM (1981) Angiomyolipoma: Computed tomographic-pathologic correlation of 17 cases. AJR 137:1221–1226

46. Sussman S, Cochran ST, Pagani JJ, McArdle C, Wong W, Austin R, Curry N, Kelly KM (1984) Hyperdense renal masses: A CT manifestation of hemorrhagic renal cysts. Radiology 150:207–211

47. Sussman S, Cochran ST, Pahani JJ, McArdle C et al. (1984) Hyperdense renal masses: A CT manifestation of hemorrhagic renal cysts. Radiology 150:207–211

48. Totty WG, McClennan BL, Melson GL, Patel R (1981) Relative value of computed tomography and ultrasonography in the assessment of renal angiomyolipoma. J Comput Assist Tomogr 5:173–178

49. Weyman PJ, McClennan BL, Stanley RJ, Levitt RJ, Sagel SS (1980) Comparison of computed tomography and angiography in the evaluation of renal cell carcinoma. Radiology 137:417–424

50. Weyman PJ, McClennan BL, Lee JKT, et al. (1982) Computed tomography of calcified renal masses. Am J Roentgenol 138:1095

51. Zimmer WD, Williamson B Jr, Hartman GW, Hattery RR, O'Brien TC (1984) Changing patterns in the evaluation of renal masses: Economic implications. AJR 143:285–289

Transcatheter Embolization in the Management of Neoplastic and Benign Disease of the Kidney

Leif Ekelund

Introduction

Transcatheter occlusion of the renal artery and its branches has been used for a wide variety of indications. These include tumors, either in combination with subsequent nephrectomy or for palliation in poor surgical candidates, gross hematuria secondary to trauma, arteriovenous fistulas or other types of vascular malformations, and aneurysms. "Percutaneous transcatheter nephrectomy" may be an alternative to surgery in end-stage renal disease and the technique has also been utilized in patients with intractable symptoms from various types of fistula formation between the urinary tract and other organs such as the vagina or colon.

Several embolic agents have been used, including autologous clot, muscle tissue, Gelfoam, cyanoacrylate, Ivalon (polyvinyl foam), stainless steel coils, detachable balloons, radioactive seeds, and absolute ethanol. It is important to realize that some of these will provide only temporary occlusion. Examples of such materials are autologous clot, oxycel, Gelfoam, Spongostan, and occasionally cyanoacrylate. They are therefore not well suited if permanent vascular occlusion is desired. The interventional radiologist must have a thorough knowledge of the characteristics of the various embolic materials available so that the right agent can be selected for the proper indication.

Renal Tumor Infarction

Considerable experience has been gathered over the last decade since the technique was first suggested by Lalli et al. in 1969 [15]. Encouraging results were reported by Lang [16] using radioactive infarct particles, and by Almgård et al. [1] using autologous muscle tissue as an embolic agent. This pioneering work has been followed by a multitude of reports describing the results with various embolic materials, often in limited study groups. Also, no controlled studies seem to have been undertaken and therefore the indications for transarterial renal tumor ablation are still not well settled. The largest case material has been collected at the M. D. Anderson Hospital and their results will be briefly summarized [22]. One hundred patients were embolized with a combination of Gelfoam particles for the peripheral arterial bed and stainless steel coils for the central renal vessels. The material was divided into three groups based on the extent of the disease and the type of management. The *first* group consisted of 25 patients with large localized tumors without metastases. Embolization was followed 1–6 days later by nephrectomy. Fifteen of these 25 patients were still alive 11–61 months following treatment. Forty-nine patients in the *second* group had metastases to the lung or bone and were treated by embolization, nephrectomy, and hormonal therapy with progesterone. Eighteen (36%) responded to therapy, seven showing a complete response, i.e., total disappearance of metastases for 7–44 months. In the *third* group of 26 patients, four had inoperable tumors and 22 had diffuse metastatic disease, usually involving the liver and brain. They were treated with palliative embolization without subsequent nephrectomy and were also given hormonal and/ or chemotherapy. Of these, only two were alive at the time of follow-up.

Reviewing these figures it is obvious that the group of patients with metastases to the lung or bone, who were treated by embolization, nephrectomy, and hormonal therapy, showed the best results. However, the value of renal tumor embolization has been questioned in two recent papers. MacErlean et al. [18] reported their experience with 16 patients, which seemed to indicate that routine preoperative embolization is of limited value and that surgery is facilitated only in patients with large, hypervascular tumors. Teasdale et al. [20] reported on 26 patients who had preoperative and two who had palliative embolization of renal carcinoma. Histologic examination in 24 of the embolized kidneys failed to demonstrate complete infarction of either the tumor or the kidney, and eight tumors showed no evidence of infarction at all. An explanation for these poor results may be that Gelfoam was used as the sole embolic agent in the majority of these patients, and it is well known that this material provides only temporary vascular occlusion.

Our own experience is based upon some 40 patients, who can be divided into two groups according to the technique of embolization. The first group consists of 19 patients who had palliative embolization for renal carcinoma (without subsequent nephrectomy) [10]. Seventeen of the patients had metastatic disease at the time of embolization. Early in the series bucrylate (isobutyl-2-cyanoacrylate) was used for occlusion of the renal artery in six patients, while the majority were embolized with a combination of Spongostan (similar to Gelfoam) and metallic coils. Adjuvant hormonal therapy was given in ten patients. Temporary remission of pulmonary metastases was seen in two patients (Fig. 10.1). The survival data in this series are given in Fig. 10.2. Today, however, only one patient from this group is still alive. It was concluded that transcatheter embolization alone is not curative; however, local tumor symptoms like hematuria and pain may be palliated, as shown in ten of the patients.

Owing to inherent risks of complication with most of the previously used particulate embolic agents (reflux into the aorta with peripheral nontarget embolization), continuous research has been going on to find safer materials. After initial testing in the experimental laboratory [9, 13], absolute ethanol has recently been advocated as a safe and reliable agent for transarterial infarction of renal

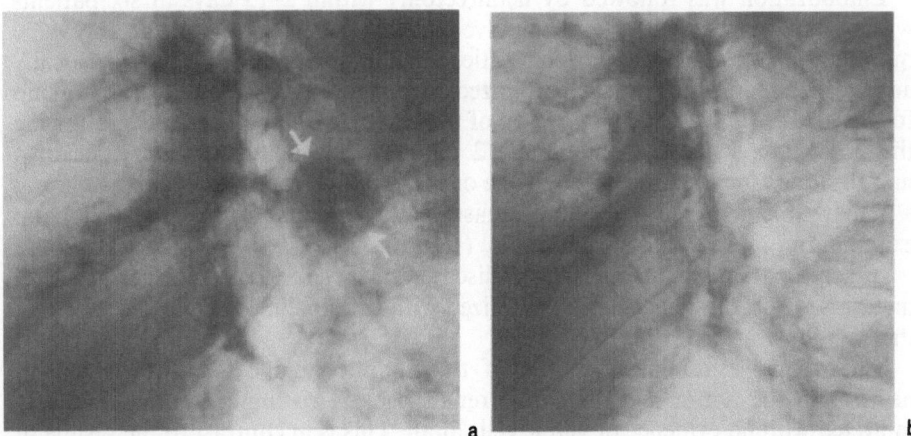

a   b

Fig. 10.1a,b. 48-year-old man with a large carcinoma of the left kidney. **a** Lateral chest film at admission. A right hilar mass was interpreted as a metastasis (*arrows*); however, biopsy was not performed. **b** Lateral chest film 10 months following transcatheter ablation of the renal carcinoma with Spongostan and coils. The hilar mass has disappeared. (From Ekelund et al. [10])

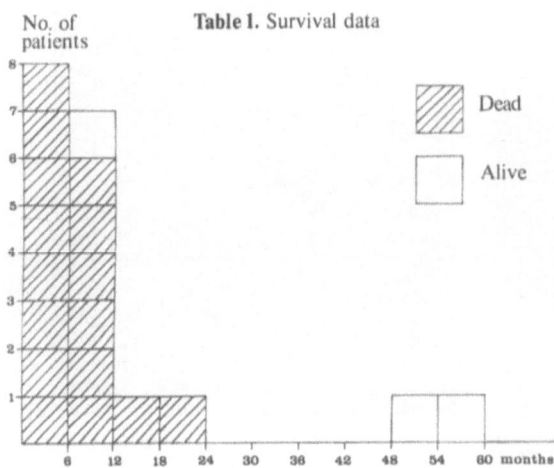

Fig. 10.2. Survival data in 19 patients with palliative embolization of renal carcinoma, presented in Ekelund et al. [10].

carcinoma [14, 19, 23]. We have used this technique in 20 patients so far [12]. Similar to Rabe et al., we have injected the ethanol through balloon occlusion catheters for the following purposes: (1) to prevent reflux of ethanol into the aorta; (2) to interrupt the renal circulation in order to prolong the contact time of ethanol with the vascular endothelium; and (3) to accomplish effective infarction by injection of the main renal artery without the necessity of segmental artery catheterization. The balloon occlusion technique is simple to use and also shortens the procedure.

Embolization was followed by nephrectomy within 2–13 days in six patients without metastases, all of whom are alive and without evidence of recurrence 4–20 months after treatment. Fourteen patients with generalized (eleven) or locally advanced disease (three) were embolized to palliate pain or hematuria, and no further treatment was given. Only two of these are alive 4 and 18 months following the procedure, while the remaining 12 patients died within a mean time of 4 months following the procedure. In one of the two survivors in the palliative group a remarkable reduction of tumor mass could be demonstrated at follow-up examination by computed tomography (Fig. 10.3).

In some patients with generalized disease and severe local pain from skeletal metastases, these lesions may be embolized with good palliative effect, as shown in the case illustrated in Fig. 10.4.

Microscopic examination in ten of the infarcted kidneys showed extensive necrosis of the tumor and remaining renal tissue. Two tumors were completely infarcted with no evidence of viable cells at all. This is in contrast to the results of Teasdale et al. [20], who, when using Gelfoam embolization, were unable to find histologic evidence of complete tumor infarction in any of 24 embolized kidneys. This fact would seem to indicate that absolute ethanol is more efficient in producing tumor necrosis than Gelfoam alone.

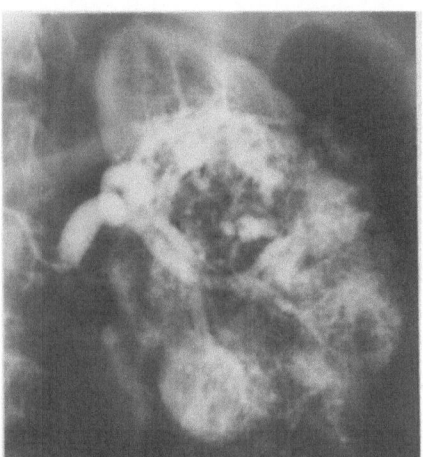

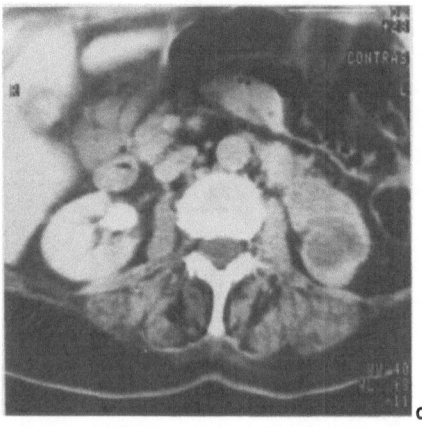

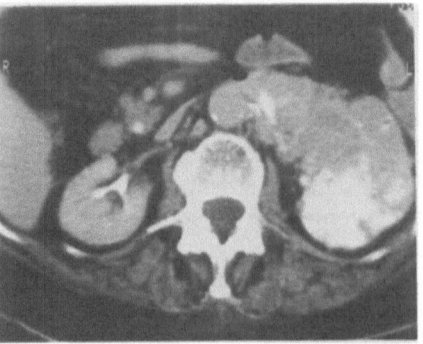

Fig. 10.3. a Preembolization angiogram in an 81-year-old woman with a large hypervascular carcinoma of the left kidney. The patient's general condition was too poor for surgery. b CT scan 1 h following ethanol embolization shows persistent contrast stain within parts of the large tumor, indicating arrested perfusion of the kidney. c Repeat CT scan 9 months later shows a remarkable decrease in tumor bulk. The patient was in good general condition at this time.

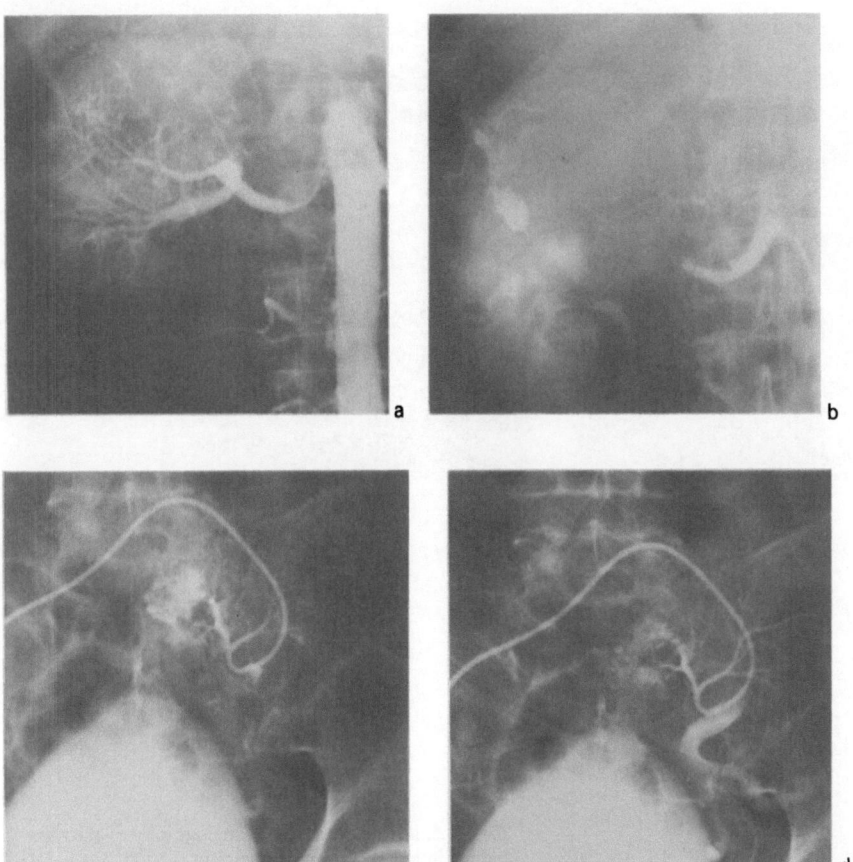

Fig. 10.4a–d. 65-year-old man with a large carcinoma of the right kidney and severe back pain from a metastasis to the sacrum. **a** Preembolization arteriogram. **b** Fifteen minutes following ethanol embolization the main renal artery is occluded. A superior capsular artery is still patent. **c** Selective angiography of the left iliolumbar artery shows hypervascularization of the sacral metastasis. **d** Following superselective embolization with small Gelfoam pieces there is a marked decrease in vascularity of metastatic lesion. Note that the muscular branch of the iliolumbar artery is still patent. The patient had temporary palliation from this additional procedure.

The occluding balloon catheter allows effective renal infarction by the injection of ethanol into the main renal artery, as mentioned previously. In some instances, however, segmental ablation of the kidney may be preferred, as, for example, in a case of localized tumor in a solitary kidney or with a nonfunctioning contralateral kidney. As we have shown in animal experiments, under such circumstances slow injection of ethanol into the superselectively catheterized segmental renal artery may produce a nice subtotal nephrectomy with preservation of normally functioning remaining parenchyma (Fig. 10.5) [11].

Another approach to the percutaneous treatment of advanced renal cell carcinoma was developed by Lang [16] (Fig. 10.6). The results from transcatheter embolization with radioactive infarct particles in 24 patients over a decade were analyzed recently [17]. The effectiveness of this treatment modality was shown by improved cumulative survival rates (59% for patients with metastases and at risk

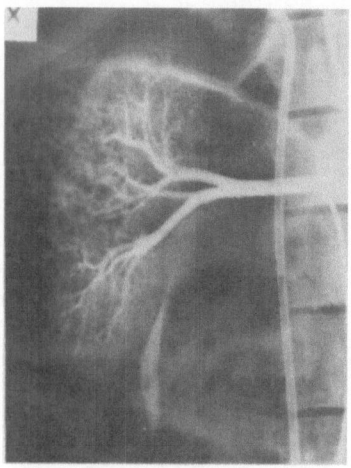
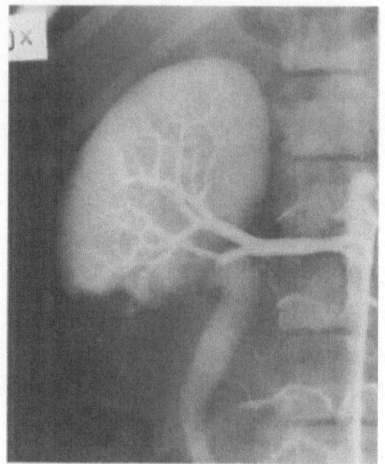
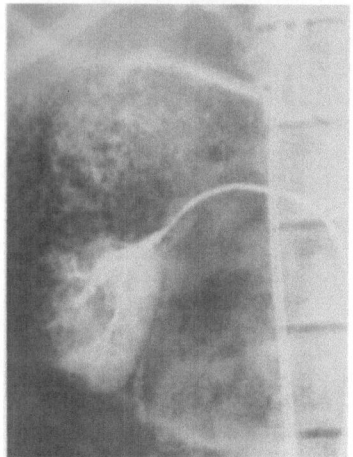

Fig. 10.5. a Baseline selective angiography of the right kidney in a pig. (Second catheter in the IVC for sampling purposes.) **b** Superselective segmental catheter position before injection of absolute ethanol. **c** Repeat arteriogram 10 days later shows ablation of the lower pole with preservation of remaining renal parenchyma and good function. (From Ekelund et al. [11])

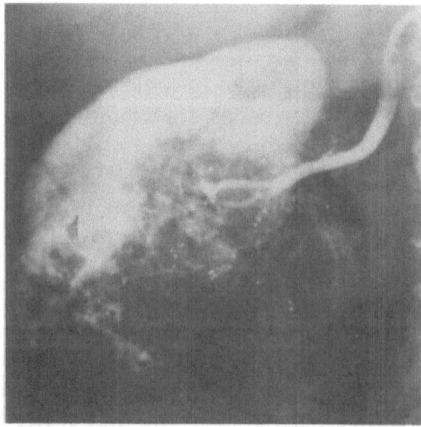

Fig. 10.6. A portion of a large renal cell carcinoma has been seeded with I-125 infarct particles introduced by a transcatheter approach. The infarct implant is delivered in three separate increments to take advantage of the changing flow characteristics within an irradiated tumor, facilitating distribution of infarct particles into hitherto underirradiated components of the neoplasm.

at 2 years, and 50% for those at risk at 5 years). The best results were obtained in patients with skeletal metastases.

Immunologic Aspects

Renal tumor infarction has been suggested to induce a release of tumor antigens into the circulation, possibly triggering an antitumor response. Wallace et al. [22] studied the general immunocompetence and immunodeficiency in 18 patients before and approximately 2 weeks after infarction and nephrectomy. Eleven patients demonstrated increased general immunocompetence as manifested by an increase in the skin test reaction.

Bakke et al. [2] investigated natural killer (NK) cell activity in peripheral blood before and at different time intervals after occlusion of the renal artery by coils in 13 patients with renal carcinoma. A slight increase in NK activity could be observed 24 h postembolization, while a marked augmentation was seen after 48 h in most of the patients. It was suggested that interferon produced by macrophages activated by the necrotizing tumor might be responsible for the increase in NK activity. Using the same technique we determined the level of NK activity before and 48 h after ethanol occlusion of the renal artery in seven patients with renal carcinoma [12]. Four of the patients displayed increased NK activity after renal artery occlusion, two reductions, and one unaltered values (Fig. 10.7). The mean cytotoxicity increased from 10% to 17%, this increase being statistically nonsignificant in this small patient sample.

In conclusion it seems reasonable to assume that an immunologic response is induced by tumor infarction. However, it is important to realize that increased NK activity will probably affect prognosis only in the early stages of renal carcinoma and not in advanced cases in which macrometastases are already established.

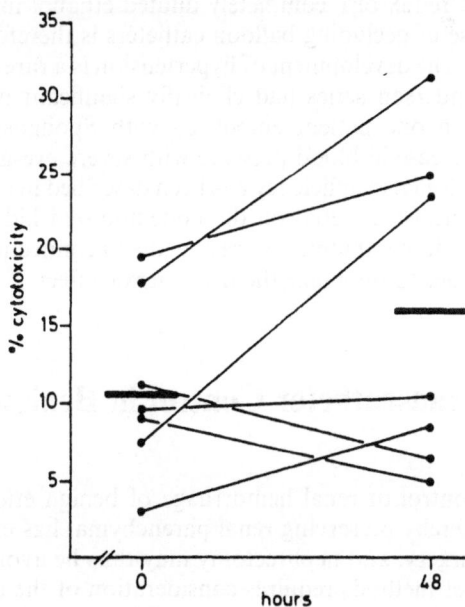

Fig. 10.7. Pre- and postocclusion NK activities in seven patients with ethanol embolization of renal carcinoma. (From Ekelund et al. [12])

Postembolization Syndrome

This is seen in most patients and consists of local pain, fever, nausea, vomiting, and a moderate paralytic ileus lasting for 1–5 days. The severity of the syndrome seems to be related to the bulk of tumor mass infarcted.

Using absolute ethanol as the embolic agent, Ellman et al. [14] reported milder postembolization symptoms than in patients previously treated with embolization using other techniques. The same experience was recently reported by Wells et al. [23] in ten patients. This is in agreement with our results, as the 20 patients in the ethanol embolization group developed milder side-effects as compared with those in 19 previous patients who had palliative embolization of renal tumors with other occlusive agents [10]. The reason for this difference is not clear.

Complications

Unintentional nontarget embolization due to reflux of embolic material is a serious complication. Escape of coils from the intended vessel occurred in two patients from the M. D. Anderson series [22]. Successful nonoperative retrieval with a Dormia basket was accomplished in one of these cases [5]. A few further cases with this type of complication have been reported and we have also experienced one case in which the coil was dislodged into the left femoral artery so that it had to be removed surgically. Peripheral embolization complicating bilateral renal infarction with Gelfoam has been described [24], and it has to be emphasized that the delivery of emboli should be performed under careful fluoroscopic control with frequent small test injections of contrast medium.

No complications were encountered in our series of 20 patients with ethanol occlusion of the renal artery. However, there is one recent report of two cases of large bowel infarction complicating ethanol ablation of renal tumors [7]. No occluding balloon catheter was used and the underlying mechanism was thought to be reflux of incompletely diluted ethanol into the inferior mesenteric artery. The use of occluding balloon catheters is therefore strongly recommended.

The development of hypertension is a rare complication. No patient in the M. D. Anderson series had clinically significant persistent hypertension [22]. We have seen one patient embolized with Spongostan and coils who had a significant increase in blood pressure with severe eye-ground changes.

Renal insufficiency has been described in a few cases, being due to an overload of contrast material on the nonembolized kidney [22]. Our present policy is to use modern nonionic contrast media in connection with the embolization procedure in order to minimize the nephrotoxic effect.

Transcatheter Control in Benign Disease of the Kidney

Control of renal hemorrhage of benign etiology by superselective embolization, thereby preserving renal parenchyma, has emerged as an attractive alternative to surgery, and nephrectomy may thus be avoided. Proper application of transcatheter methods requires consideration of the etiology and location of bleeding, the

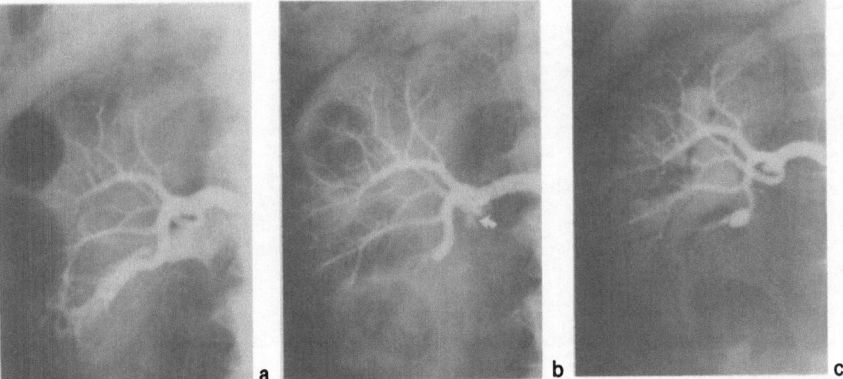

Fig. 10.8. a Selective angiography of the right kidney in a patient with gross hematuria following renal biopsy. A large arteriovenous fistula is seen in the lower pole of the kidney with early opacification of the renal vein. **b** The arteriovenous fistula has been occluded with small Gelfoam pieces following subsegmental catheterization of the feeding artery. Note slight extravasation of contrast medium at the renal hilum due to iatrogenic damage from the catheterization procedure (*arrow*). Preserved perfusion of remaining renal parenchyma. Hematuria stopped almost immediately following this procedure. **c** Follow-up arteriogram 2 months later when the patient was in excellent condition and normotensive. An aneurysm has developed at the site of the previously occluded artery and there is reduced perfusion of the lower pole. Also note a small aneurysm in renal hilum in the region of the previous extravasation. However, the arteriovenous fistula is closed and there is preserved perfusion of the remaining renal parenchyma.

suitability of the vascular anatomy for embolic occlusion, and the general condition of the patient.

Successful transcatheter management of traumatic bleeding renal arteriovenous fistulas has been described in several reports [3, 6, 21]. Most of these fistulas are secondary to renal biopsy and it should be stressed that the majority of these are nonsymptomatic, will ultimately heal spontaneously, and do not require interventional techniques [8]. If symptomatic (gross hematuria), these fistulas can be readily controlled by embolization of the feeding artery close to the fistula, thus preserving functioning renal parenchyma (Fig. 10.8). Most of these fistulas can be managed by embolization with autologous clot, Gelfoam, or Spongostan, while for large shunts a detachable balloon or a large coil may be necessary to prevent flow into the general circulation.

Arteriovenous fistulas have also been occluded from the venous side. Wallace et al. [21] placed two coils in the renal vein to obliterate successfully an intrarenal arteriovenous fistula in a patient with renal artery stenosis which made the arterial approach difficult.

Chang et al. [4] used Gelfoam for the embolization of post-traumatic bleeding pseudoaneurysms, and we have used coils for control of hemorrhage from an aneurysm secondary to percutaneous nephrostomy (Fig. 10.9).

Hypertension rarely develops following embolization, even if a segmental renal artery is occluded. This is confirmed in the literature and from our own experience.

We have also successfully applied "percutaneous transcatheter nephrectomy" in three females with intractable symptoms from ureterovaginal and/or ureteroenteric fistulas secondary to widespread pelvic malignancies, who were not considered for surgery because of the extent of the disease. Good palliative effect was achieved and the urinary leakage stopped soon after the procedure.

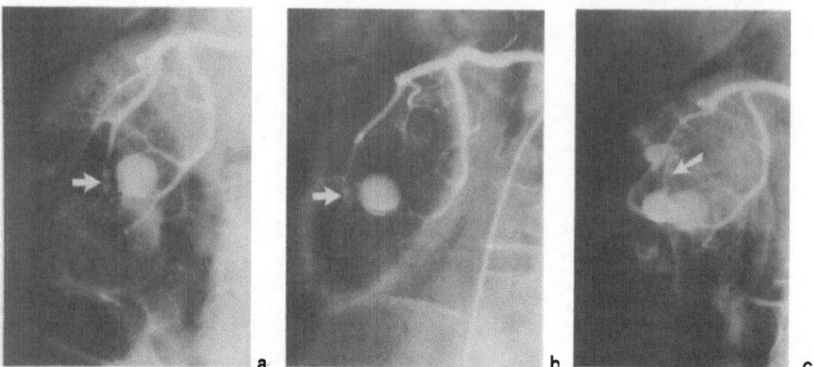

a   b   c

Fig. 10.9a–c. Elderly woman who developed gross hematuria and right flank pain following percutaneous nephrostomy. **a** AP and **b** oblique selective arteriograms of the right kidney demonstrate a pseudoaneurysm emanating from the ventral branch of the renal artery (*arrow*). The contrast-filled balloon of the Foley nephrostomy catheter is also seen in the renal pelvis. **c** After superselective catheterization the major branch of the ventral artery was occluded with two coils (*arrow*). The dorsal artery as well as a smaller branch of the ventral artery are still patent. There is contrast medium in the collecting system which contains blood clots. Bleeding promptly stopped following the procedure.

Conclusion

Transcatheter embolization of a main or segmental renal artery can be used for a wide variety of indications. Most rewarding is perhaps the control of renal hemorrhage of benign etiology, where the bleeding can be stopped and at the same time functioning renal parenchyma preserved. It is also clear that good palliation can be achieved in nonoperable patients with generalized renal carcinoma, and occasionally remission of pulmonary metastases may be seen. There is also some evidence that embolization in combination with subsequent nephrectomy may improve the prognosis in patients with renal carcinoma and limited metastatic spread.

References

1. Almgård LE, Fernström I, Haverling M et al. (1973) Treatment of renal adenocarcinoma by embolic occlusion of the renal circulation. Br J Urol 45:474–479
2. Bakke A, Göthlin JH, Haukaas SA et al. (1982) Augmentation of natural killer cell activity after arterial embolization of renal carcinomas. Cancer Res 42:3880–3883
3. Barry JW, Bookstein JJ (1981) Transcatheter hemostasis in the genitourinary tract. Urol Radiol 2:211–221
4. Chang J, Katzen BT, Sullivan KP (1978) Transcatheter Gelfoam embolization of posttraumatic bleeding pseudoaneurysms. AJR 131:645–650
5. Chuang VP (1979) Nonoperative retrieval of Gianturco coils from abdominal aorta. AJR 132: 996–997

6. Clark RA, Gallant TE, Alexander ES (1983) Angiographic management of traumatic arterio-venous fistulas: clinical results. Radiology 147:9–13
7. Cox GG, Rak Lee K, Price HJ (1982) Colonic infarction following ethanol embolization of renal cell carcinoma. Radiology 145:343–345
8. Ekelund L, Lindholm T (1971) Arteriovenous fistulae following percutaneous renal biopsy. Acta Radiol Diagn 11:38–48
9. Ekelund L, Jonsson N, Treugut H (1981) Transcatheter obliteration of the renal artery by ethanol injection: experimental results. Cardiovasc Intervent Radiol 4:1–7
10. Ekelund L, Karp W, Månsson W et al. (1981) Palliative embolization of renal tumors: follow-up of 19 cases. Urol Radiol 3:13–18
11. Ekelund L, Lin G, Jonsson N et al. (1983) Partial ablation of the kidney by intraarterial ethanol in domestic swine. Urol Radiol 5: 233–241
12. Ekelund L, Ek A, Forsberg L et al. (1984) Occlusion of renal arterial tumor supply with absolute ethanol: experience with 20 cases. Acta Radiol Diagn 25:195–201
13. Ellman BA, Green CE, Eigenbrodt E et al. (1980) Renal infarction with absolute ethanol. Invest Radiol 15:318–322
14. Ellman BA, Parkhill BJ, Curry TS et al. (1981) Ablation of renal tumors with absolute ethanol: a new technique. Radiology 141:619–626
15. Lalli AF, Peterson N, Bookstein JJ (1969) Roentgen-guided infarctions of kidneys and lungs. A potential therapeutic technique. Radiology 93:434–435
16. Lang EK (1971) Superselective arterial catheterization as a vehicle for delivering radioactive infarct particles to tumors. Radiology 98:391–399
17. Lang EK, Sullivan J, De Kernion JB (1983) Work in progress: Transcatheter embolization of renal cell carcinoma with radioactive infarct particles. Radiology 147:413–418
18. MacErlean DP, Owens AP, Bryan PJ (1980) Hypernephroma embolization—is it worthwhile? Clin Radiol 31:297–300
19. Rabe FE, Yune HY, Richmond BD et al. (1982) Renal tumor infarction with absolute ethanol. AJR 139: 1139–1144
20. Teasdale C, Kirk D, Jeans WD et al. (1982) Arterial embolisation in renal carcinoma: a useful procedure? Br J Urol 54:616–619
21. Wallace S, Schwarten DE, Smith DL et al. (1978) Intrarenal arteriovenous fistulas: transcatheter steel coil occlusion. J Urol 120:282–286
22. Wallace S, Chuang VP, Swanson D et al. (1981) Embolization of renal carcinoma. Experience with 100 patients. Radiology 138:563–570
23. Wells IP, Hammonds JC, Franklin K (1983) Embolisation of hypernephromas: a simple technique using ethanol. Clin Radiol 34:689–692
24. Woodside J, Schwartz H, Bergreen P (1976) Peripheral embolization complicating bilateral renal infarction with Gelfoam. AJR 126:1033–1034

Chapter 11

Transcatheter Embolization of Renal Cell Carcinoma with Radioactive Infarct Particles

Erich K. Lang

Introduction

Radical nephrectomy has proven reasonably effective in the management of renal cell carcinoma contained within the kidney. However, more than 30% of all patients with renal cell carcinoma have either distant metastases or invasion of surrounding organs at the time of diagnosis [12]. Although there have been significant advances in immunotherapy and combinations of chemotherapy and immunotherapy, these methods must still be considered experimental and await judgment based on 5-year survival statistics [2, 3, 15].

Radiation therapy by interstitial implant has been advocated to reduce the tumor burden and perhaps downstage the tumor and to render an inoperable neoplasm operable [6–8]. Transcatheter embolization of the neoplasm with radioactive infarct particles is a convenient technique to seat the implant [4, 5]. Although external radiation therapy has been found ineffective for downstaging of primary lesions, the much higher dose range achieved by an interstitial implant can effectively reduce the tumor burden of the primary lesion [6–8].

Disappearance of pulmonary metastases has been reported in patients treated by transcatheter embolization of the primary tumor with inert embolic material, subsequent nephrectomy, and hormone therapy with Provera [14]. Reduction of the tumor burden and stimulation of the host immune mechanism by antigens released from the necrotic tumor have been credited with this beneficial response. The gradual reduction of tumor burden by interstitial radiation therapy and the continued stimulation of the host immune mechanism by release of antigens should therefore theoretically generate an even better host immune response [7, 8].

Recent advances make possible a more accurate estimation of the host immune status. Assays of tumor-produced hormones, monoclonal antibodies, T-lymphocyte activity, and killer cell indices should yield a more accurate picture of the host immune status versus the tumor burden [1, 4, 11, 13].

Interstitial radiation therapy is also effective in ameliorating symptoms of pain and hemorrhage [7, 8]. For these reasons, transcatheter embolization with radioactive infarct particles has been advocated in the management of advanced stage renal cell carcinoma either as the exclusive treatment modality or to render operable an initially inoperable neoplasm and also to ameliorate symptomatology, particularly pain attendant upon bone metastases [7, 8].

Technique

The goal of transcatheter embolization with radioactive infarct particles is the creation of an interstitial implant capable of delivering a dose of about 16 000 rads (160 Gy) to the tumor.

Rate of delivery and rapidity of dose falloff in adjacent tissues is determined by the physical characteristics of the radionuclide used. I-125 has a relatively long half-life of 60 days and a low keV [7, 8]. Radiation is, therefore, delivered over a prolonged period and there is a rapid falloff of dose rate in adjacent tissues. This permits delivery of a high tumor dose while maintaining a low integral dose to the host. The prolonged exposure to radiation theoretically increases the probability of irradiating tumor cells during the mitotic phase, at which time they are most sensitive to radiation damage.

However, if subsequent surgery is contemplated, a radionuclide with a short half-life must be chosen. Radon, with a half-life of 3.83 days, is considered ideal for this purpose. After eight or nine half-lives (about 5 weeks) have elapsed, the specimen implanted with the radioactive material can be handled safely by the surgical team without risk of undue exposure to radiation.

To achieve homogeneous irradiation of the entire tumor volume, the sources should be distributed evenly throughout the tumor. Superselective catheterization of as many tumor branch vessels as possible and the use of the greatest number of infarct particles possible will optimize an even spacing of radioactive particles throughout the tumor. The number of infarct particles that can be deployed, however, is governed to some degree by the vascularity of the neoplasm. Seating of an infarct particle results in occlusion of an end-branch vessel. The tumor volume supplied by this vessel depends then on collateral supply from adjacent vessels. In highly hypervascular renal cell carcinomas occasional occlusion of terminal end-branches by radioactive infarct particles poses no threat to the vascular supply of the tumor. Adequate oxygenation of the neoplasm is important to ensure effectiveness of radiation therapy. In hypovascular tumors, the number of infarct particles needs to be curtailed to avoid creation of a hypoxic milieu in the infarcted tumor and thereby render radiation therapy ineffective.

Even though it may not be feasible to engage each tumor branch vessel selectively, the propensity toward temporary spasm of vessels recently embolized tends to alter flow characteristics within the tumor and thereby channels subsequently released infarct particles into different regions of the neoplasm (Fig. 11.1) [7, 8]. The distribution of infarct particles depends largely on flow characteristics existing within the tumor. For this reason, actively growing and well vascularized tumor components tend to receive more of the infarct particles released in the midstream of the tumor supply vessel than necrotic tumor areas or components undergoing regression.

Fractional dispensation of the radioactive infarct implant by three transcatheter

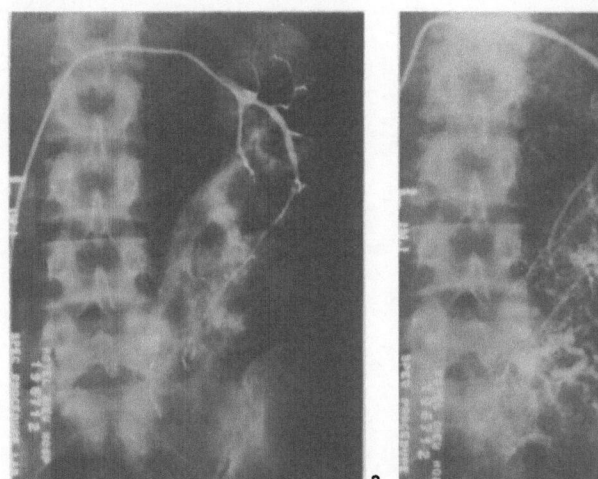

a   b

Fig. 11.1. a Arteriogram delineating the volume of tissues supplied by a branch artery. **b** Radioactive infarct particles released into this tumor branch vessel are seated in the smaller radicals. The presence ol extensive collaterals in this hypervascular tumor assures continued adequate vascular supply and oxygenation of tissues.

embolization procedures spread over 3 months takes advantage of the change in perfusion characteristics within the tumor that accompany irradiation. Following heavy irradiation of a section of tumor, fibrosis ensues and the perfusion to this segment decreases. Release of radioactive infarct particles into the midstream of the tumor supply vessel at this point in time will therefore tend to channel infarct particles into regions of the tumor featuring a high flow, which are segments that have been undertreated by the initially seated infarct implant. Thus, fractional placement of the infarct implant will improve uniformity of distribution of infarct particles throughout the entire tumor volume, capitalizing on the changing preferential vascular flow.

Dose Calculation

The precise location of each radioactive infarct particle can be determined on computed tomograms (Fig. 11.2). The dose delivered to the tumor and adjacent tissues is readily calculable by computers [9]. The shrinkage of tumor attendant upon interstitial radiation therapy and the resultant change of geometry of sources mandate recomputation of the dose rate at appropriate intervals. The final tumor dose is established as the sum of the fractional doses.

The low gamma energy of I-125 (27.3 and 35.4 keV) results in almost complete absorption of the radiant energy in the tumor itself and minimizes exposure of adjacent tissues and, hence, integral dose to the patient.

Once the I-125 particles are seated in the tumor, there is no significant emission of radiation to the outside, and nursing personnel and attendants are not subject to radiation exposure.

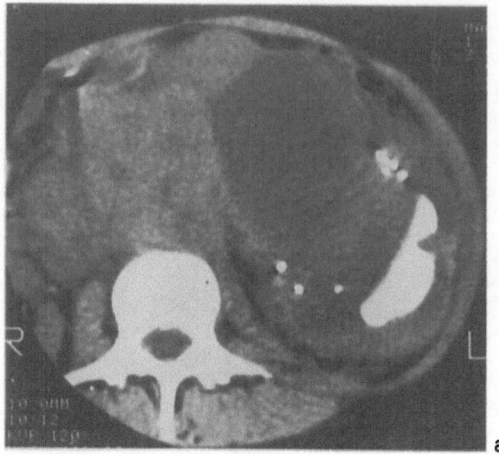

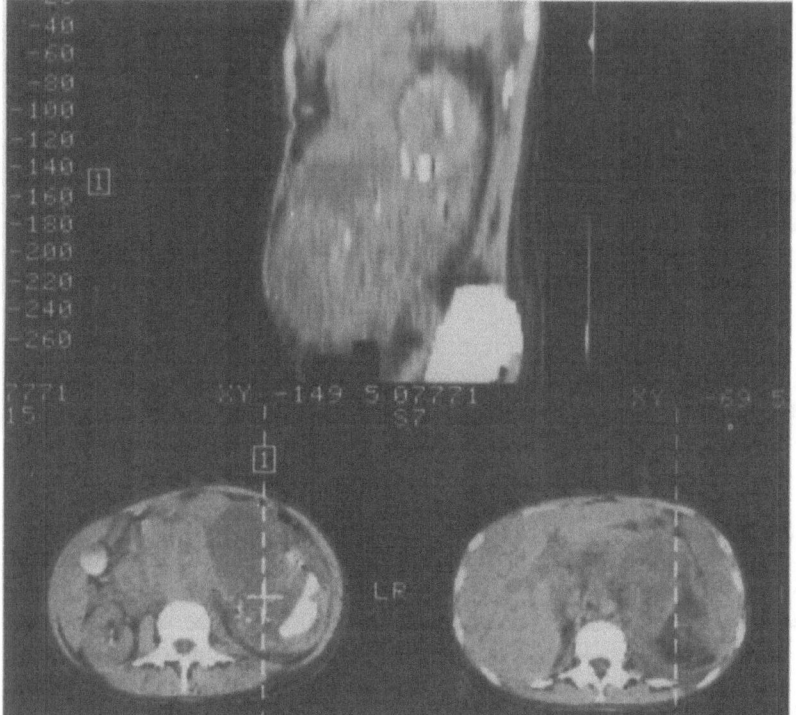

Fig. 11.2. a The precise location of each radioactive infarct particle is established on axial tomograms. The dose rate delivered to the tumor is calculated based on the location and strength of each infarct particle and its geometric relation to the entire tumor volume. **b, c** Reconstruction in sagittal and coronal planes facilitates understanding of the location of the first fractional infarct implant and selection of suitable vessel groups for seating subsequent infarct particles. In this patient, most of the infarct particles are seated in the posterior circumference of the neoplasm. The infarct implant had been delivered into a branch vessel supplying the posterior third of the tumor. **d** A computer printout demonstrates the dose delivered to a section of the tumor. Note the rapid falloff of dose rate in adjacent normal structures.

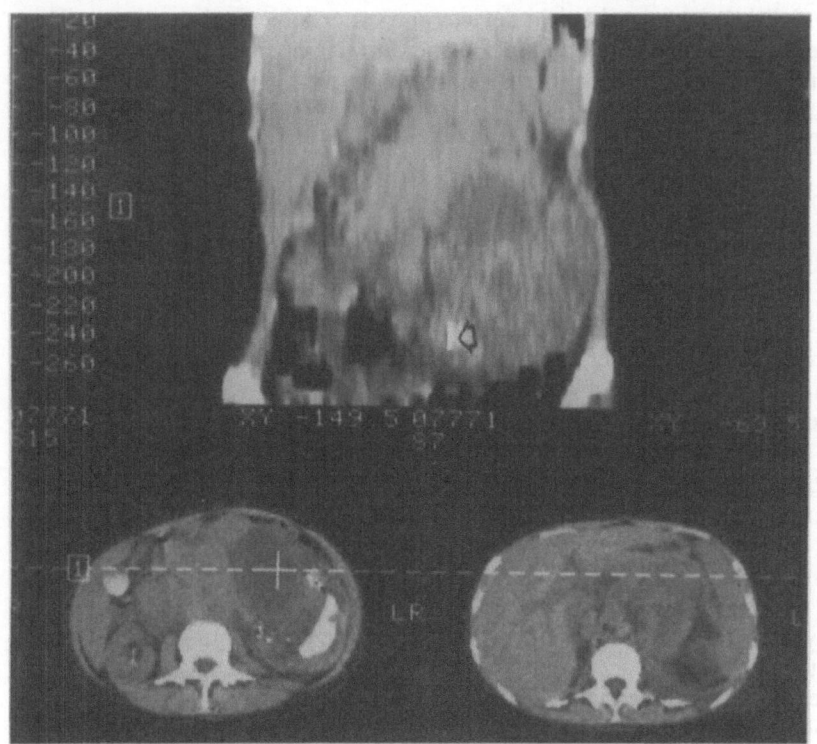

▲ Fig. 11.2c

▼ Fig. 11.2d

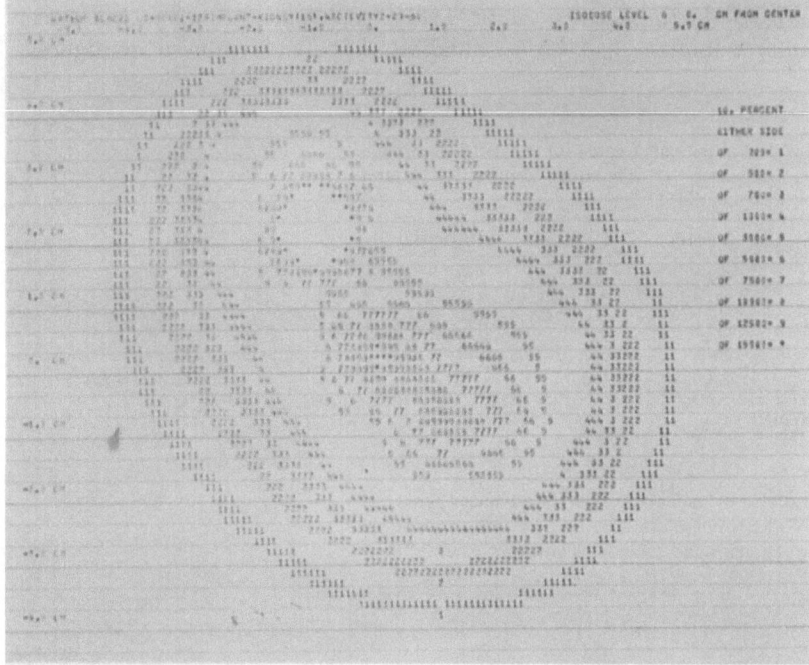

Most recently, propelling and expulsion of the sources through the catheter have been accomplished by a mechanical device (gun) attachable to the catheter. This device shields and protects the hand of the operator against radiation exposure. In the past, the sources had to be loaded individually with a long forceps into the catheter and driven through it and expelled from it by means of a guide wire [4, 6–8].

Results

The effectiveness of treatment of renal cell carcinoma by interstitial radioactive infarct implant is best judged on the basis of patient survival, amelioration of symptoms, and ability of patients to pursue a normal life.

Of our patients treated for advanced primary lesions and known metastatic disease, 16 of 33 at risk were alive after 2 years, 7 of 18 after 5 years, and none of seven after 10 years (Table 11.1). The survival statistics for a group of patients treated by interstitial radiation therapy and multiple courses of arterial chemotherapy to first downstage advanced renal cell carcinoma and then resect the primary neoplasm were even more favorable; 55% of those at risk were alive at 2 years, 33% at 5 years, and 11% at 10 years (Table 11.2). The combination of interstitial radiation therapy, arterial chemotherapy, and surgery in the management of early renal cell carcinoma resulted in a 72% 2-year survival rate, a 57% 5-year rate, and a 33% 10-year rate (Table 11.3).

Reduction of tumor mass appeared to be a consistent response to interstitial radiation therapy. Only in 4 of 88 patients in our series could we not document a decrease in size of the thus treated tumor. Two of these patients died within weeks after the infarct implant had been seated. Both patients showed contiguous

Table 11.1. Survival of patients treated for renal cell carcinoma with known metastases by interstitial radioactive infarct implant

Stage	2 years	5 years	10 years
$T_4(N_{4-3})M_1$	4/2[a]	4/2	3/0
$T_4N_xM_1$	9/3	4/1	1/0
$T_3(N_{3-0})M_1$	3/3	3/2	1/0
$T_3N_xM_1$	16/7	6/2	2/0
$T_2N_2M_1$	1/1	1/0	–

[a] At risk/surviving

Table 11.2. Survival of patients treated for advanced renal cell carcinoma by interstitial radioactive infarct implant, arterial chemotherapy, surgery, and sometimes adjuvant external therapy

Stage	2 years	5 years	10 years
$T_{3-2}N_{2-x}M_{1-0}$	9/5	9/3	9/1

[a] At risk/surviving

Table 11.3. Survival of patients treated for early renal cell carcinoma by interstitial radioactive infarct implant, arterial chemotherapy, and surgery

Stage	2 years	5 years	10 years
$T_{2-1}N_{1-0}M_0$	7/5	7/4	6/2

[a]At risk/surviving

extension of the neoplasm into the spleen. Two other patients were lost for follow-up and reassessment of the lesion was therefore not possible.

Hematuria also responded favorably to treatment by interstitial infarct implant. In 18 of 22 patients, hematuria ceased completely within 3 weeks after seating of the infarct implant.

Pain was controlled in 18 of 21 patients by the infarct implant. Most impressively, pain was controlled in all 16 of our patients in whom causative skeletal metastases were treated by a radioactive infarct implant (Fig. 11.3) [7, 8].

A significant weight gain occurred within 6 weeks after seating of the interstitial infarct implant in 30 of 33 patients, paralleling what appeared to be clinical remission. All but one of these patients showed normalization of the erythrocyte sedimentation rate [7, 8]. There was also a drop in tumor markers such as prostaglandin A and E, renin, and erythropoietin in all but one of the patients in whom such markers were initially present [7, 8]. Killer cell indices improved in 14 of 15 patients who appeared to be in clinical remission.

Fourteen patients disabled by metastatic disease to bones or generalized cachexia were able to resume a normal lifestyle, including gainful employment, after the interstitial radioactive infarct implant had initiated a remission of tumor activity, improved metabolic rate, and stabilized disabling osseous metastases by redeposition of calcium and restitution of weight-bearing bone matrix.

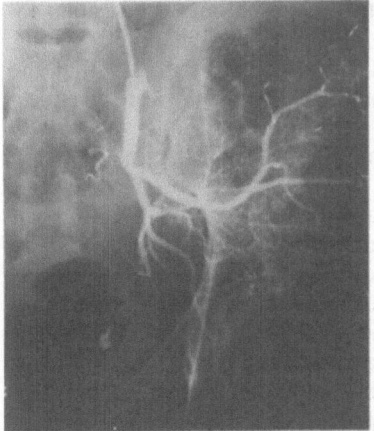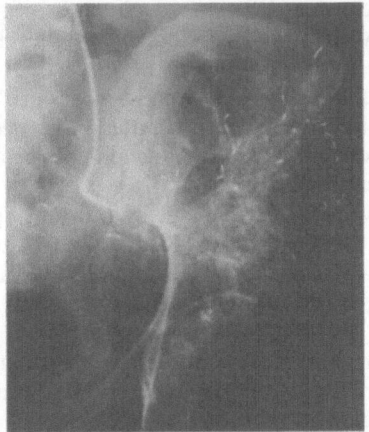

a   b

Fig. 11.3. a A selective arteriogram of the posterior division of the left hypogastric artery demonstrates extensive tumor neovascularity in the region of the gluteal muscles and destroying the left iliac wing. **b** A radioactive infarct implant has been seated into the metastasis. Good reduction in the size of the tumor, cessation of pain, and deposition of calcium occurred promptly in response to the radioactive infarct implant.

Table 11.4. Relationship between location of metastases and survival in 33 patients

Metastatic site	At risk at/alive at		
	2 years	5 years	10 years
Skeletal	5/3	2/1	1/0
Pulmonary	5/1	1/0	2/0
Liver	3/1	1/0	–
Spleen	2/0	1/0	–
CNS	1/0	1/0	–
Pulmonary and skeletal	8/6	5/3	2/0
Pulmonary and other	3/1	2/0	–
Skeletal and other	3/3	2/2	–
Other locations	3/1	2/1	2/0

Survival of patients differed vastly depending on the location of metastases. Irregardless of the size of the primary lesion and/or the coexistence of other metastases, patients with skeletal metastases fared better than those with metastases to other sites. After seating of an interstitial radioactive infarct implant into skeletal metastases, 75% of those at risk were alive at 2 years and 66% at 5 years (Table 11.4). Conversely, of patients with metastases to the liver, spleen, or central nervous system, only two of nine at risk survived for 2 years and one of five for 5 years. Patients with pulmonary metastases showed a similarly low survival rate unless skeletal metastases were also present.

The Place of the Interstitial Radioactive Infarct Implant in the Management of Renal Cell Carcinoma

The impressive treatment results of interstitial radioactive infarct implant in patients with advanced stage renal cell carcinoma raises the question of modus operandi. The survival statistics approach those of radical nephrectomy in early renal cell carcinoma [10]. The effectiveness of radical nephrectomy in the management of early renal cell carcinoma is generally attributed to the ability of this procedure to totally eradicate the disease. It is because of this ability that the cumulative survival rates at 3 and 5 years are similar: 73% and 66% respectively [10]. Similar favorable survival rates have been reported by Skinner for locally advanced lesions managed by radical nephrectomy. The success is again attributed to eradication of all neoplastic disease.

The effectiveness of treatment by infarct implant with radioactive material can be explained in two ways. Reduction of tumor burden might substantially *downstage the lesion* and prove capable of converting initially inoperable lesions into operables ones (Fig. 11.4) [4]. Conceivably, a subsequent radical nephrectomy can eradicate the neoplastic process. However, the survival rate of patients treated solely by interstitial radiation therapy is similar to that of the group with followup radical nephrectomy. Yet autopsies in a number of patients treated only by interstitial radiation therapy revealed residual tumor. One must therefore assume that a substantial reduction in tumor burden, accompanied by stimulation of the host immune system by continuously released antigens, initiated a clinical re-

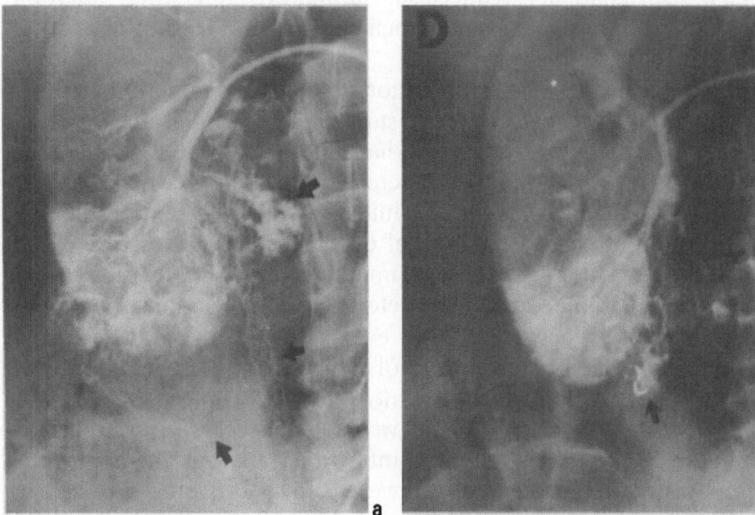

Fig. 11.4. a A selective injection of a lower polar artery demonstrates a huge tumor extending into the perirenal space as well as tumor neovascularity in metastases to regional nodes. (By courtesy of the Journal of Urology). **b** A control arteriogram obtained 8 weeks after an infarct implant with radon gold seeds had been seated shows marked regression in the extracapsular tumor extension as well as in the neovascularity of nodal metastases. Despite a relatively low dose delivered to the tumor-bearing area, this lesion proved resectable at the second attempt.

mission. Thus the improved survival of the patients appears to be based on improved host immune competence and reduction of tumor burden [7, 8]. This supposition is supported by a number of observations. Demonstrable reduction of the tumor mass, weight gain of the patient, normalization of erythrocyte sedimentation rate, disappearance of tumor markers, and improvement of killer cell indices are factors supporting the presence of such a mechanism.

Remission of tumor activity tends to be only temporary and appears to be related to such measurable host immune responses as erythrocyte sedimentation rate, level of tumor markers, killer cell indices, and sensitivity to recall antigens (dermatophytin).

Although *eradication and sterilization of a tumor* by interstitial radiation therapy is theoretically possible, existing inhomogeneity in distribution of radionuclide sources and resultant low isodose areas throughout the tumor make this difficult to achieve. In all but one of our 11 patients who came to autopsy, residual viable tumor was identified, though it was often encased by areas of fibrosis. Similarly, viable tumor cells surrounded by areas of a fibrotic capsule have been identified in all biopsy specimens obtained from patients thought to be in clinical remission.

The prolonged interstitial radiation at a relatively low dose rate may be one other key factor in control of the neoplasm. As stated above, this technique increases the probability of irradiating cells in a state of mitosis at which time the cells are most sensitive to radiation damage.

The unusually salutary response of patients with known skeletal metastases to interstitial radioactive infarct implant also suggests an altered host immune response. The ability of such patients to have survived extensive primary and metastatic tumors implies some balance mechanism between host and neoplasm. If the tumor burden in such a patient is reduced substantially (by interstitial radiation therapy), the host immune mechanisms may then control or at least retard future tumor growth for a prolonged period.

Our best results were achieved by a combination of interstitial radiation therapy, intraarterial chemotherapy, and subsequent surgical resection of the primary lesion. Even though the neoplasm may not have been eradicated totally, the additional debulking of the tumor must be credited for the success rate. The combination of downstaging of the tumor by initial interstitial radiation therapy and subsequent resection of at least the bulk of the tumor undoubtedly exceeded the control of the primary tumor achievable by interstitial radiation therapy alone.

Eventually, however, immunocompetence deteriorated and tumor growth and dissemination of metastases occurred. This event was heralded by a rising erythrocyte sedimentation rate, deterioration of killer cell indices, recurrence of elevated tumor markers, and clinical deterioration, such as weight loss.

Unlike the experience reported by Wallace, we have not seen disappearance or regression of pulmonary metastases following interstitial radiation therapy to the primary tumor or other metastases [14]. However, since Provera was used in Wallace's patients, an apparent decrease in the size of pulmonary metastases could be mimicked by the disappearance of edema surrounding such metastases in response to the hormone.

Our experience suggests that the technique of creating an interstitial radioactive infarct implant by transcatheter embolization is useful in the management of renal cell carcinoma (a) for the treatment of extensive primary lesions and metastases which are not amenable to surgical intervention and (b) for reducing the size of the primary neoplasm, effectively downgrading the lesion and rendering the neoplasm amenable to surgical resection. As outlined in the text, short half-life radionuclides are utilized for the latter purpose whereas I-125 is favored if interstitial radiation therapy is pursued as the exclusive treatment modality.

References

1. Bander NH, Cordon-Cardo C, Finstad CL, et al. (1984) Results of the study of human renal cancer with monoclonal antibodies. 79th meeting of the American Urologic Association, 6–10 May 1984, paper #297
2. DeKernion JB, Katsuoka Y, Ramming KP (1980) Immunology of human renal adenocarcinoma. In: Sufrin G, Beckley SA (eds) Renal adenocarcinoma, a series of workshops on the biology of human cancer. International Union Against Cancer, Geneva (Report #10) 49:96–113
3. Droller MJ, Levy HJ (1984) Immunotherapy of metastatic renal cell carcinoma with poly IC-LC. 79th meeting of the American Urologic Association, 6–10 May 1984, paper #301
4. Lang EK (1971) Superselective arterial catheterization as vehicle for delivering radioactive infarct particles to tumors. Radiology 98:391–399
5. Lang EK (1982) Advanced renal cell carcinoma treated by transcatheter embolization with inert material and radioactive particles. In: Ariel IM (ed) Progress in clinical cancer, vol 8. Grune and Stratton, New York, pp 299–310
6. Lang EK (1984) Transcatheter embolization of renal cell carcinoma. In: Lang EK (ed) Current concepts of uroradiology. Williams and Wilkins, Baltimore, pp 224–236
7. Lang EK, DeKernion JB (1981) Transcatheter embolization of advanced renal cell carcinoma with radioactive seeds. J Urol 126:581–586
8. Lang EK, Sullivan J, DeKernion JB (1983) Work in progress: transcatheter embolization of renal cell carcinoma with radioactive infarct particles. Radiology 147:413–418

 9. Ling CC, Yorke ED, Spiro IG, et al. (1978) Physical dosimetry of I-125 seeds of a new design for interstitial implant. N.C.R.P. Publications, C.A. 30378 and C.A. 07020, N.C.I.
10. Robson CJ, Churchill BM, Anderson W (1969) The results of radical nephrectomy for renal cell carcinoma. J Urol 101:297–301
11. Scharfe T, Becht E, Kaltwasser R, et al. (1984) Monoclonal antibodies tumors specific for renal cell carcinoma. 79th meeting of the American Urologic Association, 6–10 May 1984, paper #103
12. Skinner DJ, DeKernion JB (1978) Clinical manifestations and treatment of renal parenchymal tumors. In: Skinner DJ, DeKernion JB (eds) Genitourinary cancer. W. B. Saunders, Philadelphia, pp 107–133
13. Sufrin G, Mirand EA, Moore RH et al. (1977) Hormones in renal cancer. J Urol 117:433–438
14. Wallace S, Chuang VP, Swanson D, et al. (1981) Embolization of renal carcinoma: Experience with 100 patients. Radiology 138:563–570
15. Williams RD, Jensen B, Higgins M, et al. (1984) Alpha 2 interferon therapy of disseminated renal cell carcinoma, 79th meeting of the American Urologic Association, 6–10 May 1984, paper #298

Chapter 12

Transcatheter Embolization in the Management of Intractable Hemorrhage from Pelvic Organs

Erich K. Lang

Transcatheter embolization of pelvic vessels has been advocated as both a temporary and a definitive measure to control intractable hemorrhage from pelvic organs. While the technique is identical, there are notable differences in the materials used for embolization, depending on the therapeutic intent [10].

In patients presenting with life-threatening hemorrhage caused by traumatic injury, puerperal hemorrhage, or hemorrhage complicating transurethral resection of the prostate and such orthopedic procedures as hip replacement surgery, the aim of transcatheter embolization is to control bleeding and stabilize the patient's condition but without total or permanent disruption of the vascular channels [5, 7, 14]. For this reason embolic material prone to lysis, facilitating later restitution of flow, is used.

Conversely, intractable hemorrhage from pelvic vessels in patients with extensive pelvic neoplasms and often after radiation therapy requires permanent disruption of the blood supply to reduce effectively the pulse pressure [10–12]. Inert embolic material prone to cause semipermanent occlusion of muscular size arteries is deployed for this purpose.

Concepts Governing Management of Intractable Hemorrhage from Pelvic Organs by Transcatheter Embolization

Acute hemorrhage attendant upon trauma or iatrogenic injury calls for occlusion of the responsible vessels at the earliest possible time to avoid further blood loss and to stabilize the patient's condition [1]. Diagnostic arteriography is charged with identifying the offending vessel or vessel groups (10, Fig. 12.1).

Transcatheter embolization should be limited to the offending vessel or vessels only. In general the embolic material is seated in vessels of the muscular type. Occlusion at this level fosters maintenance of some perfusion via the precapillary

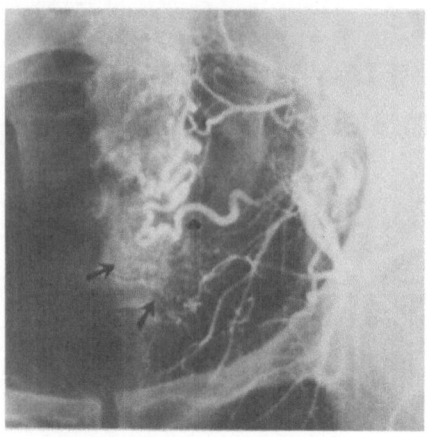

Fig. 12.1. A selective left hypogastric arteriogram demonstrates a prominent marginal segment uterine artery (*short arrow*) and extensive neovascularity in the region of the uterine cervix (*long arrows*) supplied from the cervicovaginal branch vessels. Early puddling suggests this as a source of the hemorrhage.

collateral network and thus prevents occurrence of an ischemic milieu [2, 10].

At times, however, injury may afflict a larger size vessel and occlusion of this larger vessel proximal to the site of severance and bleeding must be accomplished. This is easiest done with Gianturco coils of appropriate size.

The physiology of pelvic blood flow calls for a relatively peripheral site for effective occlusion with embolic material. Only peripheral obstruction will cause a substantial reduction in the blood flow and a drop in pulse pressure.

As demonstrated by Burchell, unilateral ligation of the hypogastric artery has but little effect on pulse pressure (ipsilateral 77% of preligation pressure) and blood flow (ipsilateral 49% of preligation value) [3]. An extensive intercommunicating network ensures substantial collateral flow via some major vessels unless the occlusion is set so far peripherally as to eliminate this component of the collateral network. However, once the pulse pressure is reduced adequately, intra-arterial thrombus formation will occlude the bleeding vessels. The propensity of fibroblasts to permeate a clot within 8–24 h means that occlusion of the vessel need be for that length of time only. Thereafter, fibroblastic activity will seal the bleeding site effectively. For this reason material prone to dissolution, such as autologous blood clot, is favored. Thereby reconstitution of flow to nearly all of the affected area is assured, which reduces the risk of tissue necrosis [10].

At times the precise bleeding site or bleeding vessels may not be identifiable. This occurs not infrequently in patients with intractable hemorrhage after transurethral resection of the prostate or puerperal bleeding. Under these circumstances embolic material is seated in the major branches of the anterior division of the hypogastric arteries [5, 7]. It is hoped that the resulting reduction in pulse pressure and blood flow will be of a magnitude to permit formation of clots at the often multiple bleeding sites and later sealing by fibroblastic activity.

Embolization of major branches of the anterior division of both hypogastric arteries is tolerated if the occlusion is set at a proximal site, permitting collateral flow from other sources such as the posterior hypogastric branches and presacral, epigastric, and circumflex femoral vessels [2, 3, 8].

Management of intractable hemorrhage from pelvic organs as a complication of neoplasms and/or radiation therapy calls for yet another approach [6, 10–13]. A precise bleeding site is hardly ever identifiable (9, Fig. 12.2a). Usually a large tumor mass with areas of necrosis and suspect as a source of the bleeding is identified on

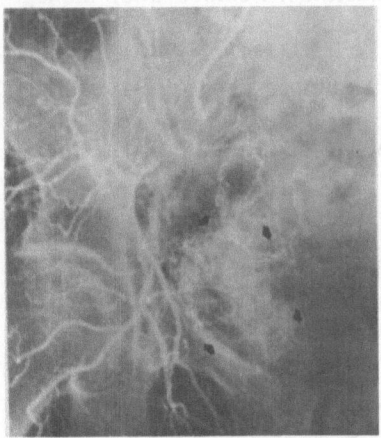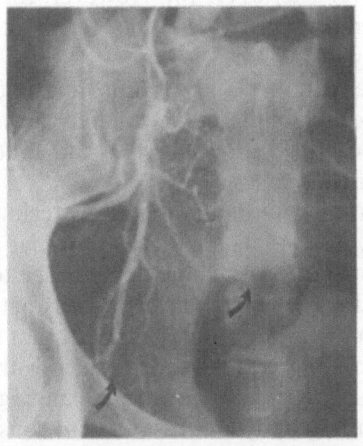

a   b

Fig. 12.2. a A selective hypogastric arteriogram demonstrates dense staining of a tumor mass invading the right half of the bladder (*arrows*). A precise bleeding site is not identifiable. **b** Following transcatheter embolization of the superior and inferior vesical and internal pudendal branches of the anterior division of the hypogastric artery there is appropriate cessation of flow to the tumor. The infarct particles are lodged in the muscular size arteries (*curved arrows*), which permits collateral perfusion via the precapillary plexus. Note unimpeded flow to the branches of the posterior division of the hypogastric artery. (From Lang [10], with permission)

the diagnostic arteriogram (Fig. 12.2a). Embolization must be directed to the vessels supplying the neoplasm. Frequently its vascular supply is derived from multiple branches of both the right and the left anterior divisions of the hypogastric arteries [9].

Embolic material is seated at such locations in major branch vessels as to eliminate the more proximal collateral supply but maintain flow via the distal and particularly the precapillary collateral network (10–12, Fig. 12.2b). This is to safeguard against further tissue necrosis and resultant sloughs brought on by ischemic conditions and causing renewed hemorrhage. In patients bleeding from neoplasms a more permanent occlusion of the vessels is needed to ensure a long-term reduction in pulse pressure and blood flow. For this reason material not prone to lysis or dissolution is favored. Moreover, material not prone to fragmentation and hence antegrade migration of the embolic fragments into more distal branches is preferred, as peripheral occlusion increases the chance for further ischemic slough and thereby sets the stage for a vicious circle with repeat hemorrhage after only a short reprieve.

Methods

Catheterization of the hypogastric arteries is possible via a femoral or axillary artery approach. The axillary artery approach is favored in patients with traumatic injury to the pelvis since massive hematomas in the groin usually preclude entry into the femoral arteries [1, 10]. However, for transcatheter embolization managing pelvic hemorrhage attributable to all other causes, catheterization via the femoral artery is favored.

For catheterization via an axillary approach a number 5.8- to 6.3-F catheter featuring a renal double curve configuration is favored. RC 1 or RMI Cook catheters appear to conform best to the anatomy to be negotiated if a femoral approach is used.

In combination with digital recording techniques a 4-F catheter will provide an adequate flow rate [4]. The latter method has the advantage of reducing substantially the amount of contrast medium needed to demonstrate the vascular network but it limits the size of embolic particles that can be delivered (a 6.3-F catheter allows transmission of particles almost 1 mm in diameter).

Survey arteriograms are first performed with injections of contrast medium into the hypogastric arteries [9]. For routine angiography a bolus of 12 ml is necessary; for digital arteriography a bolus of 10 ml consisting of 3 ml contrast medium and 7 ml saline will offer identical detail. Thereafter, superselective engagement of the branch or branches incriminated on the preceding study is carried out. For digital arteriography 2 ml contrast medium mixed with 2 ml saline suffices.

Superselective engagement of the bleeding branch vessel or vessels should be attempted for embolization of traumatic injury sites. Conversely, in patients bleeding from other conditions the catheter may be placed into the main or a major branch of the anterior division of the hypogastric artery.

Pharmacologic manipulation of blood flow may be used to identify the bleeding site and to channel infarct particles selectively into such bleeding vessels. The propensity of normal arterioles to constrict in response to intra-arterial administration of adrenaline hydrochloride and the notable lack of this response by injured vessels makes possible the creation of almost selective flow into the injured vessel group [10]. Elimination of flow to adjacent normal vessels seemingly accentuates the bleeding on the diagnostic study and subsequently siphons infarct particles released into the main branch selectively into the vessels responsible for the bleeding. The pathophysiologic explanation for this phenomenon lies in the increase in the peripheral resistance in normal vessels attendant upon intra-arterial injection of adrenaline hydrochloride versus the lowered peripheral resistance in actively bleeding vessels.

Embolic Material

Autologous blood clot is the material of choice for embolization of traumatic bleeding sites. The propensity for fragmentation to a particle size prone to lodge in muscular type arteries results in occlusion at a level which causes a substantial reduction in the pulse pressure while retaining collateral perfusion via the precapillary plexus, thus safeguarding against avascular tissue necrosis.

The propensity for lysis within 8–24 h ensures reconstitution of flow in the initially occluded vessel group (Table 12.1).

At times massive use of blood transfusions may result in an abnormal clotting mechanism. If an autologous blood clot does not form readily, addition of Amicar (ε-aminocaproic acid) will encourage clot formation (10, Table 12.1).

Table 12.1. Characteristics of materials used for transcatheter embolization

Material	Usual embolization site (vessel size)	Longevity of occlusion	Potential for restoration of vascular continuity
Autologous blood clot	Muscular branch arteries	8–24 h	Excellent
Amicar (ε-aminocaproic acid) reinforced clot	Muscular branch arteries	24–96 h	Excellent
Gelfoam particles	Muscular branch arteries	2–3 weeks	Good
Ivalon (polyvinyl alcohol) 1 × 1 × 1 mm cubes	Muscular branch arteries	Semipermanent	Limited
Ivalon shavings suspended	Arterioles	Semipermanent	Limited
6-Cyanoacrylate	Branch arteries to arterioles (dependent on admixture of contrast medium)	Permanent	None
Detachable balloons	Larger arteries	Permanent	None
Gianturco coils	Larger arteries	Permanent	None

Gelfoam is the most readily available material for semipermanent occlusion of a vessel. Small cubes of approximately 1 × 1 × 1 mm are prepared. These cubes can be soaked in contrast medium prior to their deployment, which facilitates identification and localization on high-detail radiographs and particularly digital radiographs [4]. Although administered as a 1-mm^3 cube, these particles tend to fragment during the process of ejaculation and therefore may be seated in somewhat smaller caliber vessels.

Ivalon (dehydrated polyvinyl alcohol) can be administered in similar size cubes or in the form of a suspension of large shavings. This material, however, is dehydrated, compressed, and less prone to fragmentation. Moreover, once seated in a vessel it tends to enlarge due to absorption of water and therefore causes a particularly solid occlusion. Ivalon particles are favored whenever seating in a particular size vessel is of critical importance.

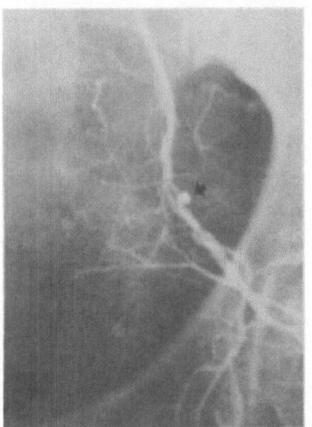 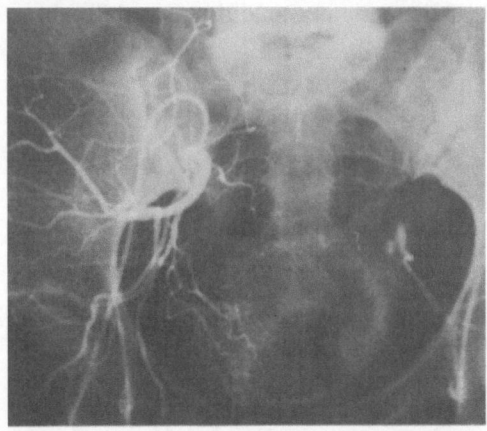

Fig. 12.3. a A branch of the anterior division of the left hypogastric artery is engaged superselectively. A mycotic aneurysm is demonstrated. This is presumed to be the source of the hemorrhage. **b** The offending vessel has been cast with 6-cyanoacrylate. Contrast medium added to the compound to modify the speed of setting causes opacification of the cast.

6-Cyanoacrylate is reserved for occlusion of vessels weakened by neoplasms and undergoing formation of myotic aneurysms (Fig. 12.3). The ability to modify the speed of setting of the compound by admixing contrast medium makes it possible to float the forming embolus to the desired location before it hardens and attaches to the wall (Fig. 12.3b).

With the notable exception of arteriovenous malformations, embolization of capillary beds with material such as Gelfoam powder is not indicated since it creates a totally ischemic field and may provoke extensive tissue necrosis (Table 12.1).

Therapeutic Results

Transcatheter embolization has been particularly successful in the management of intractable hemorrhage as a consequence of pelvic trauma. It is the procedure of choice to control temporarily hemorrhage from medium or small size arteries [1, 10].

Particularly when associated with venous bleeding, surgical intervention is contraindicated since it destroys the fascial barriers which contain venous hemorrhage (Fig. 12.4). Therefore, control of concomitant arterial bleeding rests upon transcatheter embolization. Venous bleeding eventually stops attendant upon the tamponading effect of the hematoma; arterial bleeding will stop as a result of lowered pulse pressure, which sets the stage for intra-arterial clot formation.

With all pelvic embolization procedures care must be exercised so as not to compromise the vascular supply to skin areas. Concomitant use of "M.A.S.T." pants carries the risk of compromising perfusion of skin areas if, at the same time, the deep circulation is repressed by transcatheter embolization. All adjunctive therapies such as M.A.S.T. pants are therefore discontinued once the patient's condition is clinically stabilized and arterial bleeding controlled by transcatheter embolization. Orthopedic and all other surgical reconstructions are deferred until such time as the patient's condition is stabilized.

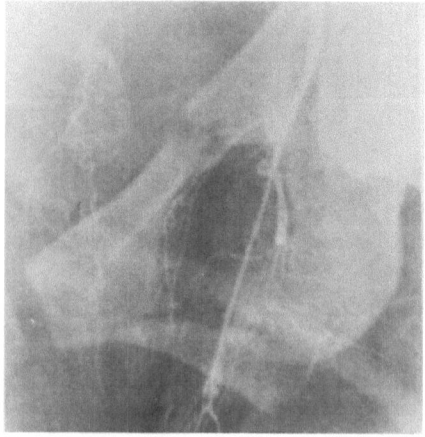

Fig. 12.4. Although there are fractures of the left pubic and ischial ramus and spasm of the obturator artery, there is no evidence of arterial injury. The associated hematoma is due to venous bleeding.

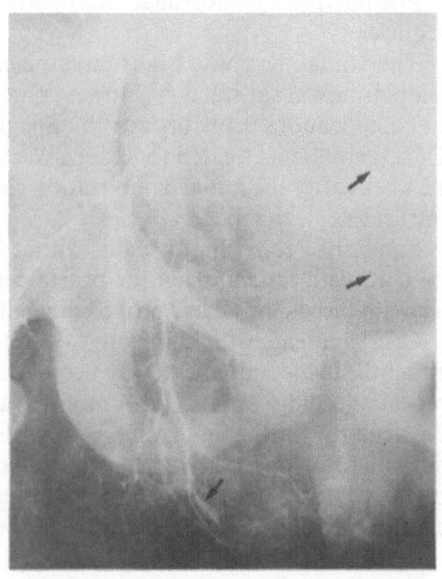

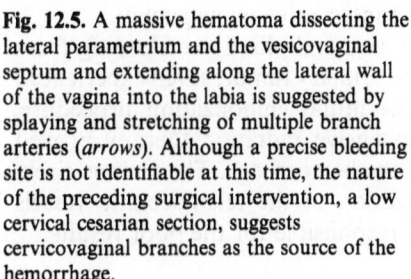

Fig. 12.5. A massive hematoma dissecting the lateral parametrium and the vesicovaginal septum and extending along the lateral wall of the vagina into the labia is suggested by splaying and stretching of multiple branch arteries (*arrows*). Although a precise bleeding site is not identifiable at this time, the nature of the preceding surgical intervention, a low cervical cesarian section, suggests cervicovaginal branches as the source of the hemorrhage.

Transcatheter embolization of bleeding sites in the prostate bed after transurethral resection is resorted to only after such conservative attempts as tamponade by a Foley balloon catheter, fulguration, packing, and surface coagulation with silver nitrate have failed [5]. The diffuse nature of this type of hemorrhage usually requires embolization of the inferior vesical, obturator, and pudendal arteries of both sides. In general, bleeding is controlled promptly; however, repeat bleeding episodes may occur after clot lysis and/or slough of further tissue.

Patients with puerperal hemorrhage likewise respond satisfactorily to transcatheter embolization. If the source of bleeding can be defined on the diagnostic arteriogram, superselective embolization with Ivalon shavings has proven successful as a means of control [9]. This is particularly true in patients with low cervical cesarean section, often subject to complicating, intractable hemorrhage from small cervical branch arteries that were not ligated (Fig. 12.5).

Transcatheter embolization for intractable hemorrhage from pelvic organs involved by neoplasms and often after radiation therapy may yield only temporary success. The usually marginal vascular supply of neoplastic tissues sets the stage for continued tissue necrosis and hence reactivation of bleeding [9, 10]. Particularly tissues compromised by extensive radiation therapy are prone to complicating late hemorrhage.

In our institution transcatheter embolization successfully stabilized 18 of 19 patients presenting with intractable hemorrhage as a consequence of pelvic trauma. In one patient multiple bleeding sites were identified and despite multiple superselective transcatheter embolizations the patient succumbed to irreversible shock.

The initial bleeding was controlled in our five patients embolized for hemorrhage from the prostate bed following transurethral resection. However, in two of these patients a delayed hemorrhage occurred on the 7th and 10th post embolization days respectively. These cases were controlled by conservative measures.

Postpuerperal hemorrhage was controlled in all of our five patients without late sequelae.

The initial response to transcatheter embolization of hemorrhaging pelvic neoplasms was satisfactory. However, in many instances late hemorrhage occurred or complications probably attributable to the embolization procedures developed. Of seven patients treated for extensive carcinoma of the bladder, two rebled 2 and 12 weeks after the initial embolization respectively, and one of them succumbed to intractable hemorrhage.

Similarly, rebleeding, usually within 2 weeks, was observed in three of eight patients with carcinoma of the prostate and treated by external radiation therapy. These rebleeds, however, proved amenable to conservative management.

Of 21 patients with carcinoma of the cervix and embolized for bleeding from either the bladder permeated by neoplasm or the primary tumor, seven experienced repeat bleeding 7 days to 3 months after the initial embolization procedure. Particularly the patients who had received extensive radiation therapy proved refractory to conservative measures to control the hemorrhage. The vicious circle of further tissue necrosis induced by embolization of the telangiectatic vessels caused by prior radiation therapy can be held responsible for the poor results.

Complications of Transcatheter Embolization

Overzealous embolization may result in deprivation of the vascular supply of large tissue elements. This is particularly so when attempting bilateral embolization of all branches of the anterior division of the hypogastric arteries by seating emboli at the periphery of branch vessels. Avascular necrosis of the bladder can result [2, 8]. In our experience three patients suffered a reduced bladder capacity as a result of compromised blood supply to the bladder.

Overzealous embolization of tissues, particularly muscle, in patients who have sustained traumatic injuries increases the risk of acute tubular necrosis. Traumatic injury of muscle has set the stage for this by the release of myoglobin. Unnecessary embolization of additional muscle masses (such as the gluteal muscle supplied by the posterior division of the hypogastric arteries) may lead to irreversible acute tubular necrosis. We noted episodes of transient renal failure in at least four of our patients. However, myoglobinuria and transient elevation of serum creatinine levels were present in all of our patients who sustained extensive pelvic trauma.

Transcatheter embolization of pelvic vessels must be considered a temporary intervention intended as a life-saving procedure in patients with intractable hemorrhage. Properly performed, this procedure can stop intractable hemorrhage. Overextended use of this technique, however, may cause complications that outweigh the temporary benefits and ultimately hasten the demise of the patient.

Injudicious embolization of the vascular supply to a hemorrhaging tumor that also serves as the sole collateral supply to other organ systems may produce severe complications. The sole vascular supply to such organs is then derived from collaterals from pelvic vessels, such as the uterine artery, which in turn may also be the major supply vessel to a hemorrhaging tumor (Fig. 12.6). Occlusion of this vessel, however, would cause avascular necrosis of the rectum and rectosigmoid and thus ultimately worsen rather than improve the patient's condition.

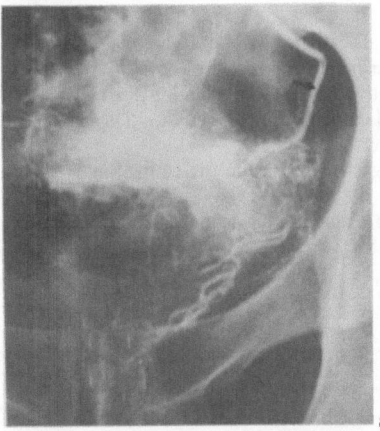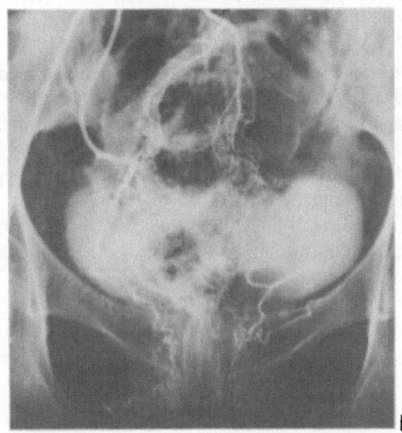

a b

Fig. 12.6. a A superselective arteriogram demonstrates a huge, densely staining tumor mass in the vesicovaginal septum supplied predominantly by the superior and inferior vesical arteries. **b** A superselective injection of the right cervicovaginal branch demonstrates extensive tumor neovascularity in the vaginal fornix. However, there is retrograde filling of the inferior mesenteric artery via collaterals from the vaginal branches to the external hemorrhoidals, mid-hemorrhoidals, superior hemorrhoidals, and inferior mesenteric artery. This finding indicates the dependency of the rectum and rectosigmoid on this source of vascular supply and militates against embolization of the vessel (From Lang [10], with permission)

Despite the caveats that must be observed, the often life-saving contributions of the transcatheter embolization justify its consideration in patients with intractable pelvic hemorrhage.

References

1. Ayella RJ, DuPriest RW, Khaneja SC, et al. (1978) Transcatheter embolization of autologous clot in the management of bleeding associated with fractures of the pelvis. Surg Gynecol Obstet 147:849–852
2. Braf ZF, Koontz WW Jr (1977) Gangrene of bladder. Complication of hypogastric artery embolization. Urology 9:670–671
3. Burchell RC (1968) Physiology of internal iliac artery ligation. J Obstet Gynaecol Br Comm 75:642–651
4. Crummy AB, Stieghorst MF, Turski PA, Strother CM, Lieberman RP, Sackett JF, Turnipseed WD, Detmer DE, Mistretta CA (1982) Digital subtraction angiography: current status and use of intra-arterial injection. Radiology 145:303–308
5. Fysal M (1979) Angiographic management of post-prostatectomy bleeding. J Urol 122:129–131
6. Goldstein HM, Medellin H, Ben-Menachem Y, et al. (1975) Transcatheter arterial embolization in the management of bleeding in the cancer patient. Radiology 115:603–608
7. Heaston DK, Mineau DE, Brown BJ, et al. (1979) Transcatheter arterial embolization for control of persistent massive puerperal hemorrhage after bilateral surgical hypogastric artery ligation. Am J Roentgenol 133:152–154
8. Hietala SO (1978) Urinary bladder necrosis following selective embolization of the internal iliac artery. Acta Radiol (Diagn) 19:316–320
9. Lang EK (1980) Angiography in the diagnosis and staging of pelvic neoplasms. Radiology 134:353–358

10. Lang EK (1981) Transcatheter embolization of pelvic vessels for control of intractable hemorrhage. Radiology 140:331–339
11. Lang EK, Deutsch JS, Goodman JR, et al. (1979) Transcatheter embolization of hypogastric branch arteries in the management of intractable bladder hemorrhage. J Urol 121:30–36
12. Miller FJ Jr, Mortel R, Mann WJ, et al. (1976) Selective arterial embolization for control of hemorrhage in pelvic malignancy: femoral and brachial catheter approaches. Am J Roentgenol 126:1028–1032
13. Smith DC, Wyatt JF (1977) Embolization of the hypogastric arteries in the control of massive vaginal hemorrhage. Obstet Gynecol 49:317–322
14. Smith JC Jr, Kerr WS, Athanasoulis CA, et al. (1975) Angiographic management of bleeding secondary to genitourinary tract surgery. J Urol 133:89–92

Chapter 13

Balloon Embolization for the Treatment of Primary Varicocele

Klemens H. Barth

Introduction

Varicocele represents a dilatation of the pampiniform plexus and the cremasteric veins associated with retrograde blood flow through the internal spermatic vein (ISV) [8, 16]. The mechanism is analogous to lower extremity varicosity with insufficiency of the venous valves. Insufficiency of the ISV can be documented on retrograde venography in the reverse Trendelenburg or upright position [2, 13, 16]. The great majority of varicoceles are left-sided; however, as bilateral ISV venography indicates, left-sided varicocele is not infrequently associated with right ISV insufficiency despite absence of a palpable right varicocele [2, 7]. Varicocele is mostly idiopathic and referred to as primary varicocele, whereas secondary varicocele develops on the basis of obstruction, usually by tumor, and is not considered in this context.

Apart from the infrequent incidence of a large varicocele causing pain and discomfort [8], the clinical significance of varicocele is mainly related to its well established association with male infertility [2–4, 8, 14, 15]. Oligospermia, abnormal morphology, and decreased sperm motility are found with varicocele [4, 8, 14, 15].

Varicoceles apparently develop during adolescence, sometimes earlier, and are rather common. Records from military draftees shows an incidence of 15%–17% [11, 20]. According to Shirren and Klosterhalfen [11], 40%–50% of patients with varicocele are subfertile. It is also known that about 40% of infertile men have a varicocele [6].

The pathogenetic mechanism leading to impairment of spermatogenesis secondary to varicocele is not completely clear. Increased testicular temperature induced by retrograde venous blood flow is one, if not the, key factor [11].

Surgical treatment of varicocele consists of "high" retroperitoneal or suprainguinal ligation of the ISV or direct ligation of the cremasteric plexus [2, 3, 8, 15]. Improvement in sperm count and semen quality has been reported in up to 80% after treatment. Reported persistence or recurrence of varicocele after surgical ligation averages around 10% [2, 3, 11]. Bypass collaterals are the most frequent reason for recurrence [2, 3, 5, 10, 11, 15, 16]. Improvement of spermatogenesis does not equally relate to the generation of offspring. Such has been reported in as many as 50%, but a more reasonable figure averages around 30%–35% [4, 8, 14, 16].

Whether early treatment of varicocele will improve the chances for normal fertility is not established; however, it appears likely. Interestingly, there is no correlation between the size of the varicocele and the outcome of treatment.

Surgical ligation, as well as the herein described alternative, embolotherapy, aim at eliminating retrograde blood flow in the ISV.

Anatomy of the Internal Spermatic Veins

The left ISV enters the left renal vein in all instances. In duplicated renal veins, the spermatic vein may enter either distal to the branch point or into the lower, retroaortic branch [8, 19]. Duplication of the ISV at various levels is frequent [2, 15]. Anastomoses to renal capsular veins, lumbar veins, and other retroperitoneal veins are practically always present. The intrapelvic portion of the ISV has the lowest likelihood of branch veins; however bi- or trifurcation of the ISV above the inguinal canal is the rule rather than the exception [2, 13, 15]. On the right, the ISV most frequently enters the anterior–lateral portion of the inferior vena cava just caudad to the right renal vein [2, 19]. The relatively rare junction of the right ISV with the right renal vein appears to be found disproportionately more frequently in patients with right-sided varicocele [2]. The diameter of the ISV needs to be determined prior to balloon embolotherapy and ranges between 4 and 11 mm in patients with varicocele [15, 19].

Balloon Embolization Technique

Details of the technique have been described elsewhere [19]. Our present, slightly modified procedure is summarized as follows: Under local anesthesia, a 9-F self-sealing, thin wall sheath is placed into the femoral vein, mostly in the right. The sheath is rinsed continuously through a side arm with heparinized saline. Through this sheath, a 6- or 7-F pre-curved catheter, usually a "cobra" shape for the left ISV and a "shepherd's crook" catheter for the right, is placed into the ISV orifice. With this catheter, a retrograde spermatic venogram under the Valsalva maneuver is obtained. Contrast should fill the distal spermatic vein to the level of the inguinal canal. A 1 to 2 film venogram is obtained (Fig. 13.1). There is no need to visualize the pampiniform plexus. The testicles are covered with an appropriate radiation shield both anteriorly and posteriorly throughout the procedure. In this fashion, the mean testicular dose was measured at 26 mrad [19]. The venogram serves as a guide to determine the exact level of balloon occlusion, usually the intrapelvic portion of the vein for the reasons indicated above (Fig. 13.2).

Two balloons are available; the smaller 1-mm balloon can inflate up to 4 mm diameter, while the larger balloon with an uninflated diameter of 2 mm can inflate

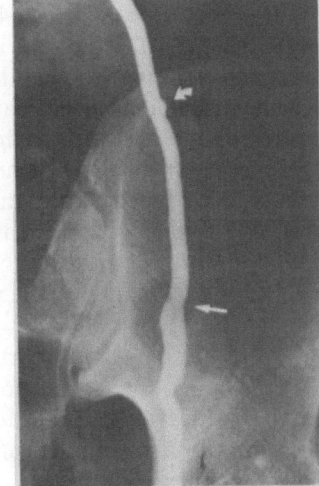

Fig 13.1. Single film pre-embolization left internal spermatic venogram, showing retrograde contrast filling of a valveless vein to the level of the inguinal canal. There is bifurcation of the vein at the midpelvic level (*arrow*). Protrusion of vein just below the iliac crest indicates branch vein entry (*curved arrow*). The level of spermatic vein occlusion is to be chosen above the bifurcation and below the branch vein entry.

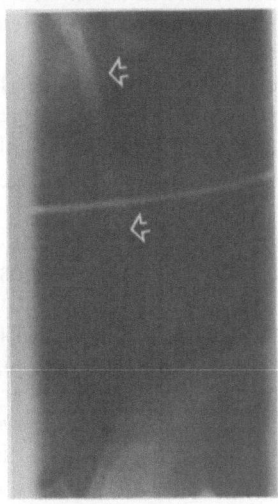

Fig. 13.2. 7-mm diameter balloon occluding left internal spermatic vein above its bifurcation and below the level of the branch vein. Contrast stasis in the proximal spermatic vein (*arrows*) indicates occlusion of the vein by the balloon.

up to 9 mm. Inflation medium is isomolar contrast (Becton Dickinson & Co., Rutherford, NJ 07070.

Following venography and selection of the most appropriate occlusion site, the diagnostic catheter is exchanged over guide wire for the nontapered balloon-introducing catheter. For the 1-mm balloon, a 5-F thin wall catheter is adequate, while for the 2-mm balloon an 8.8-F catheter needs to be used. It is important that the guide wire be introduced as gently as possible and advanced as deeply into the spermatic vein as possible, particularly when exchange for the larger caliber catheter is needed. Venous spasm does occur frequently during the exchange maneuver and needs to resolve prior to balloon embolization. If spasm occurs, the procedure is interrupted while the catheter is slowly rinsed with normal saline. Within 5–15 min, the venous spasm is expected to resolve. The introducer catheter only needs to be placed well into the orifice of the spermatic vein. The balloon is injected through the introducer catheter and should be propelled into the vicinity of the inguinal canal. The balloon will need to be adjusted to the occlusion position. Then the balloon is inflated, a test injection determines adequacy of occlusion, and, if adequate, the balloon is detached (Fig. 13.2). The exact inflation volumes specified by the manufacturer need to be observed. Sometimes one or several collateral veins not discovered on initial venography will become evident after occlusion of the primary venous channel. These collaterals, even if small, should be occluded during the same procedure to prevent continued reflux.

Bilateral varicocele is usually treated in one session. Embolization of the right ISV is carried out similarly to the left-sided embolization. Since the left varicocele frequently predominates, the venous caliber on the right is expected to be generally smaller.

Except for some discomfort during venous spasm and the need to anesthetize the puncture site, the procedure is painless. Patients are frequently given some sedation during the procedure and are kept supine for 2–3 h following the procedure to allow sealing of the venous puncture site. Normal physical activity can be resumed within 24 h.

Potential complications of the procedure include premature balloon detachment and subsequent balloon dislodgement into the lung. This complication occurred once in our early experience, when detachment was made into a spastic vein [19]. Premature detachment is otherwise possible by improper handling of the balloon inside the vein, particularly if backfolding of the balloon is not recognized and the balloon is retracted forcibly into the introducer catheter. Extravasation by direct trauma to the venous wall rarely prevents successful completion of the procedure. Allergy to contrast material needs to be assessed before any embolization is considered as routine for every angiographic procedure. The incidence of severe contrast reaction is not expected to be higher than for intravenous contrast injection for other purposes [17].

Persistent or recurrent varicocele after balloon embolization was found in 11% of our first 70 patients [10]. Analysis of these cases, most of them successfully treated by repeat embolization, showed that unoccluded bypass collaterals or untreated right-sided varicoceles were the most frequent cause of recurrence. Presently, we occlude anywhere in the intrapelvic portion of the ISV proximal to the inguinal canal and distal to collaterals. We do not routinely investigate for right ISV insufficiency but instead follow the same regimen the surgeon would follow when performing suprainguinal ligation. There are, however, convincing arguments on the basis of the rather frequent right-sided ISV insufficiency [2] that the insufficient right ISV should be occluded concomitantly to improve treatment results and prevent recurrences.

Alternative Embolization Techniques

Sclerotherapy of the ISV was the first reported nonsurgical treatment for varicocele [9, 15, 20]. This method is relatively simple, can be administered quite quickly by occluding the ISV orifice with a balloon catheter and, according to reported experience, is quite effective [9, 17, 20]. Theoretical limitations are the lack of total control over the extent of the venous occlusion with the potential for penetration of the sclerosing agent into the varicocele proper, causing painful inflammation [9, 17, 20]. Paravenous sclerosis affecting the adjacent ureter has not been reported. Steel coils and other metallic implants have been used for ISV occlusion and require distal venous catheterization in order to ensure proper placement of the device [1, 7, 18]. Distal ISV catheterization with its associated venospasm can easily lead to improper placement of the occlusion device, whose position is not correctable. Tissue adhesive (IBC) has been used successfully [12]. This treatment may be quite appropriate for occlusion of smaller veins, particularly collateral channels, since it can employ small catheters which are less prone to induce spasm. The embolization technique is rather delicate because of the need for the fast setting material to clear the catheter completely (if it fails to do so, the catheter tip may become embedded in the acrylic cast) [12].

Embolotherapy Versus Surgical Treatment

To a large extent embolotherapy is as effective as surgical ligation, and it has the advantage of guidance by venography, delineating the variable anatomy. It also affords treatment of bilateral varicoceles at the same session with a single venous puncture. Balloon embolization is performed with minimal discomfort and no post-treatment disability. Using the present balloon embolization technique, recurrences should not exceed 5% [10].

On the other hand, in experienced hands surgical ligation of the ISV is a quite simple and quick procedure and less time consuming than most embolization procedures. Ligation can be performed under local anesthesia as an outpatient procedure. Postoperative disability for a week is expected during the healing process.

In our opinion, the clinician examining the patient and making the indication for treatment should be open-minded to available treatment modalities. The real choice lies between embolotherapy and outpatient surgery. Pros and cons should be explained to the patient. Bilateral varicocele and postoperative recurrences should definitely be investigated by ISV venography and embolized if technically feasible.

References

1. Berkman WA, Price RB, Wheatley JK, Fajman WA, Sones PJ, Casarella WJ (1984) Varicoceles: a coaxial coil occlusion system. Radiology 151(1):73–77
2. Comhaire F, Kunnen M, Nahoum C (1981) Radiological anatomy of the internal spermatic vein(s) in 200 retrograde venograms. Int J Androl 4:379–387
3. Coolsaet BLRA (1980) The varicocele syndrome: venography determining the optimal level for surgical management. J Urol 124:883–839
4. Davidson HA (1954) Varicocele and male sterility. Br Med J I:1378
5. Dubin L, Amelar RD (1970) Varicocele size and results of varicocelectomy in selected subfertile men with varicocele. Fertil Steril 21:606–609
6. Dubin L, Amelar RD (1971) Etiologic factors in 1924 consecutive cases of male infertility. Fertil Steril 22:469–474

7. Formanek A, Rusnak B, Zollikofer C, Castaneda-Zuniga WR, Narayan P, Gonzalez R, Amplatz K (1981) Embolization of the spermatic vein for treatment of infertility: a new approach. Radiology 139:315–321
8. Hanley HG, Harrison RG (1962) The nature and surgical treatment of varicocele. Br J Surg 50:64–67
9. Iaccarino V (1979) A non-surgical treatment of varicocele: trans-catheter sclerotherapy of gonadal veins. Eur Soc Cardiovasc Radiol 369–370, May 1979
10. Kaufman SL, Kadir S, Barth KH, Smyth JW, Walsh PC, White RI (1983) Mechanisms of recurrent varicocele after balloon occlusion or surgical ligation of the internal spermatic vein. Radiology 147:435–440
11. Klosterhalfen H, Schirren C, Wagenknecht LV (1979) Pathogenese und Therapie der Varicocele. Urologe [Ausg A] 18:187–192
12. Kunnen VM (1980) Neue Technik zur Embolisation der Vena Spermatica Interna: Intravenöser Gewebekleber. Fortschr Röntgenstr 133:625–629
13. Lien HH, Kolbenstvedt A (1977) Phlebographic appearances of the left renal and left testicular veins. Acta Radiol [Diagn] 18:321–332
14. MacLeod J (1969) Further observations on the role of varicocele in human male infertility. Fertil Steril 20:545–563
15. Riedl P (1979) Selektive Phlebographie und Katheterthrombosierung der Vena testicularis bei primärer Varikocele. Eine angiographisch-anatomische und klinische Studie. Wien Klin Wochenschr 91 Jahrgang, Supplementum 99
16. Sayfan J, Adam YG (1978) Intraoperative internal spermatic vein phlebography in the subfertile male with varicocele. Fertil Steril 29: 669–675
17. Seyferth W, Jecht E, Zeitler E (1981) Percutaneous sclerotherapy of varicocele. Radiology 139:335–340
18. Weissbach L, Thelen M, Adolphs H-D (1980) Treatment of idiopathic varicoceles by transfemoral testicular vein occlusion. J Urol 126:354–356
19. White RI, Kaufman SL, Barth KH, Kadir S, Smyth JW, Walsh PC (1981) Occlusion of varicoceles with detachable balloons. Radiology 139:327–334
20. Zeitler VE, Jecht E, Richter E-I, Seyferth W (1980) Perkutane Behandlung männlicher Infertilität im Rahmen der selektiven Spermatikaphlebographie mit Katheter. Fortschr Röntgenstr 132:294–300

Chapter 14

Urologic Applications of Regional Chemotherapy

John D. Maldazys and Jean B. deKernion

Introduction

Since its beginnings, the goal of cancer chemotherapy has been the selective destruction of cancer cells without systemic toxicity. The narrow margin between therapeutic and toxic doses with the presently available drugs has prevented this. The report by Klopp and co-workers in 1950 [20] of the injection of nitrogen mustard directly into the arterial supply of tumors raised hope that this goal would soon be realized. In the 1950s and 1960s enthusiasm for regional chemotherapy led clinicians to investigate its use against neoplasms of many cell types and organ sites. Ingenious methods were devised for drug administration in attempts to gain the maximum benefit.

The perspectives of time and experience have pointed out the limitations of regional chemotherapy, and we now have a better understanding of its place in the management of cancer patients. At present, regional chemotherapy has two roles. First, it can provide palliation for symptomatic, locally extensive tumors that are not satisfactorily treated by other means; and second, it can be used as an adjunct to surgery or radiation in the treatment of potentially curable localized tumors. Regional chemotherapy is of known benefit in the management of a number of human tumors (Table 14.1).

The following discussion will consider the use of regional chemotherapy for urologic tumors and include methods, drug and dose selection, and vascular access.

Table 14.1. Regional chemotherapy—present role

Head and neck	Squamous carcinoma
Extremity	Melanoma
	Soft tissue sarcomas
	1° bone tumors
Liver	Metastases from breast, colon

General Considerations

Regional chemotherapy can be defined as the administration of cytotoxic drugs to a limited anatomic area in an attempt to obtain greater antitumor effect with less general toxicity. High drug concentrations are introduced into a tumor's arterial supply by one of two methods: regional perfusion or intra-arterial infusion.

Regional Perfusion

In regional perfusion the arterial and venous supplies of a tumor-containing region are isolated from the general circulation after systemic heparinization. Following placement of vascular cannulae, the isolated region is perfused for 30–60 min with heparinized whole blood containing the cancericidal drug by means of an extracorporeal pump. At the end of this time the regional circuit is flushed with fresh blood or solution *not* containing the drug to minimize the release of the drug to the systemic circulation. Finally, the cannulae are removed, vessels repaired, and circulatory continuity restored.

Theoretically, regional perfusion allows drug concentrations to be used in the perfused area that are many times higher than those seen with intravenous chemotherapy, but with little escape of the drug to the rest of the body. In addition, regional hyperthermia or hyperoxygenation can be employed by placing an oxygenator and a heat exchange unit into the circuit. In the case of limb perfusion the theoretical goals are met because the single vessels supplying the limb can easily be controlled, and collateral vessels can be occluded by placing a tourniquet at the junction of the limb with the trunk. However, perfusion of pelvic tumors poses a greater problem.

Since bilateral arterial supply from many branches of the iliac system is the rule for pelvic tumors, cannulation of single vessels is not appropriate. Therefore, to perfuse the entire tumor, temporary occlusion of the aorta and vena cava is required. The aorta must be occluded below the inferior mesenteric artery so that intestine is not perfused. Input and return catheters are usually introduced via the superficial femoral vessels through a small groin incision. They are then directed upward to the region of the aortic bifurcation. Control of the aorta and vena cava can be "open," with vascular exposure and occlusion during laparotomy, or "closed," using balloon catheters threaded upwards from the femoral vessels as described by Watkins et al. [43]. In either case, general anesthesia and two incisions are needed. To exclude the chemotherapeutic agent from the legs, pneumatic tourniquets are placed high on the thighs before beginning pelvic perfusion.

Another problem is the extensive collateral flow between the upper and lower halves of the body through vessels in the vertebral area and body wall despite occlusion of the vena cava and aorta. This has two consequences: the drug leaks into the general circulation, allowing systemic toxicity, and the concentration of the drug in the perfused area is continuously diluted. Measurements of leakage using chromium-tagged red blood cells, radioactive iodinated albumin, or the dye T-1824 showed rates of 0.5%–1.5%/min of perfusion [3, 8, 16]. In large tumors with many collateral vessels, the leakage rate can exceed 3%/min, soon obviating any advantage in drug concentration gained by the perfusion technique [3].

Intra-arterial Infusion

Infusion of cytotoxic drugs into the vessels feeding a tumor is considerably simpler than perfusion. Although the drug may be given by bolus injection, infusions lasting from several hours to several months are more commonly used. The basic equipment required is a catheter placed in the appropriate artery, connecting tubing, and an infusion pump capable of delivering the solution at higher than systemic arterial pressure. As with perfusion, the goal of intra-arterial infusion is to obtain higher drug concentration in the tumor vascular bed without increasing systemic toxicity. During infusion no attempt is made to restrict the egress of drug from the tumor, so any concentration differential depends on achieving a high concentration within the limited volume of the tumor, which falls substantially after distribution into the larger fluid volume of the remainder of the body.

Eckman et al. [11] developed a mathematical model for the pharmacokinetics of intra-arterial infusions to identify the parameters that affected response and toxicity. Their analysis showed that local drug concentration increased compared with systemic concentration as the infused artery received a smaller percentage of cardiac output (effect and flow inversely related). This suggests that infusion catheters should be positioned as distally and selectively as possible. In addition, they determined that the higher the total body elimination of the drug, the greater the difference between local and systemic drug concentration. However, a reduction in systemic toxicity only occurred if the infused site metabolized or excreted the drug; the greater the ability of the infused region to eliminate the drug, the greater the reduction in toxicity. Therefore, regional infusion does not reduce systemic effects unless the target area eliminates the drug.

Few reports of actual drug levels during intra-arterial infusion have been published. Stewart et al. measured serum platinum concentration at the infused artery, regional vein, and distant veins during cisplatin infusion [36]. They found that the intra-arterial infusion indeed produced higher concentration at the infusion site, while platinum concentration at a distant site was similar to that produced by intravenous cisplatin. Clarkson and Lawrence found local concentrations of methotrexate to be 3–4 times higher than systemic concentrations during carotid artery infusion [8].

Technical Considerations

Vascular Access

Catheter placement for infusion chemotherapy may be gained either surgically or percutaneously. With the refinement of percutaneous catheter techniques over the last 10 years, operative placement is seldom necessary for technical reasons. But under some circumstances open placement remains proper: (a) insertion of a catheter intended for prolonged infusion and (b) catheter placement at the time of exploratory surgery when a mass is found to be unresectable and infusion chemotherapy is planned.

Surgical Insertion

During open placement, the target vessel should be dissected for a distance of several centimeters and positively identified. If infusion of nearby branches is not desired (i.e., superior gluteal artery during hypogastric artery perfusion), then that vessel should either be ligated, or the catheter tip positioned distal to it. The catheter can be inserted by several methods: through the lumen of a needle passed into the desired vessel, through a small stab wound in the vessel wall made by a pointed scalpel blade or an 18-gauge needle, or through a ligated small branch artery not supplying the tumor [38]. Regardless of method, attention should be paid that the catheter tip lies within the artery's lumen and not intramurally, and that the position of the tip is correct. A nonabsorbable purse string suture is used to secure the catheter at the arterial entrance point. Nevin et al. also recommended that a small loop be formed and the catheter anchored again to prevent dislodgement by arterial pulsations [27]. The catheter is directed to a convenient area and brought through the body wall via the lumen of a needle. Care must be taken to avoid kinking or obstruction by shear effect in the body wall. The catheter is trimmed to a convenient length, the end flared, a stopcock attached, and the catheter flushed with heparinized saline. It is then secured to the skin.

Percutaneous Insertion

Percutaneous catheter placement is performed through an accessible artery using standard needle/guide wire/catheter technique [35]. The femoral vessels are suitable for short infusions (up to several days), but the brachial or axillary arteries allow greater patient mobility during lengthier infusions. Puncture opposite the dominant hand allows the greatest freedom of movement. A catheter no larger than 5-F should be used in the brachial artery because of its small size. If two arteries need to be infused (i.e., bilateral hypogastric), infusion can be simultaneous using two catheters or asynchronous by infusing each side in turn.

The infusion catheter should have several side holes near the tip, besides an end hole. This helps prevent obstruction from impingement against the vessel wall or an endothelial flap. A trade-off exists regarding catheter size. Although a larger catheter is less likely to become occluded, the larger size increases the risk of arterial thrombosis.

Catheter Maintenance

The infusion catheter should be secured to the skin with suture and tape to prevent inadvertent dislodgement. Scrupulous cleanliness of the entry site is desired to avoid infection. The site should be washed with a bactericidal detergent such as povidine-iodine every other day. Then bactericidal ointment is applied, followed by an occlusive dressing. Skin care is particularly important for percutaneously inserted catheters because of the proximity of the arterial wall to the skin. During lengthy infusions, the position of the catheter tip should be checked periodically with a plain film or injection of a small amount of contrast. Comparison with films from the time of catheter insertion allows any change in position to be detected.

To prevent catheter thrombosis the lumen should always be filled with fluid. At times when infusion is not in progress, the catheter should be flushed with 5–10 ml of heparinized saline twice a day. If a catheter becomes obstructed, thrombus might be cleared by forceful injection or passage of a guide wire. Thomson and Goldin discuss methods for percutaneous replacement of an occluded catheter [39]. Some authors advocate systemic heparinization during infusion [42], while others mix small amounts of heparin with the infusate [6] or use no anticoagulants [21, 27, 38]. Heparin should never be mixed with infusions containing doxorubicin because precipitation results.

Discontinuation of percutaneously placed catheters is accomplished by simple withdrawal. Simultaneous aspiration with a syringe may help recover any thrombus adherent to the outside of the catheter and minimize distal embolization. After withdrawal, moderate pressure is placed on the puncture site for 30 min, and motion of the limb avoided for 6 h. When a surgically implanted catheter is no longer needed, it can be allowed to thrombose. It is then cut short, cold sterilized, and ducked into the subcutaneous tissue at the entrance point [37].

Determination of Area Infused

The effectiveness of intra-arterial chemotherapy will be compromised if a sizeable portion of the tumor is fed by arteries not being perfused. Several methods help ascertain that the catheter will distribute drug to the entire tumor. At the time of surgical placement, injection of methylene blue or fluorescein followed by observation of the area stained is a useful adjunct to careful vessel identification and manual positioning. During percutaneous placement, standard arteriography helps define the extent of the tumor, but the high injection rates tend to opacify an area larger than that actually fed by the infusion artery. Arteriography at a rate similar to that of the infusion gives a truer picture, but visualization is limited because of the small amount of contrast delivered. Scanning with a gamma camera after injection of radiolabeled colloids at infusion rate is reported to give an accurate depiction of the tumor's vascular bed. This is because the larger particles are temporarily trapped in tumor capillaries. Both ^{99m}Tc sulfur colloid and ^{99m}Tc macro-aggregated albumin have been used [18, 42]. The information gained may be helpful in adjusting the dose proportions in a two catheter system as is used in bladder cancer.

Infusion Pumps

Any system capable of delivering fluid at higher than arterial pressure can be used for regional chemotherapy. Standard intravenous administration sets can be used as long as care is taken to make connections securely. Pressure is generated either by raising the fluid container (gravity) or by using a blood pump. The infusion rate is then controlled with any of the available IV regulation devices. The infusate container should not be allowed to empty completely; if this happens, air embolism is a hazard when glass containers are used. With plastic containers, fluid flow will stop and the arterial catheter may thrombose.

Several portable, self-contained infusion pumps are now available. Their differences and performance were recently reviewed [31].

In the last decade a totally implantable catheter/pump system powered by the vapor pressure of a volatile liquid has been developed [4]. Catheter insertion via laparotomy, cutdown, and percutaneous routes has been described [9, 13].

Complications

Related to Vascular Access

There is a small but definite risk attached to percutaneous arterial catheterization. The most devastating complication, arterial thrombosis at the site of introduction, is fortunately rare, although in one report it occurred in 5 of 30 patients [14]. Loss of radial pulse is seen in 10%–20% of brachial artery catheterizations, but arm viability is rarely in jeopardy because of collateral flow [45]. Embolization of thrombus attached to the catheter may occur upon withdrawal. As the catheter is usually coated with a thin fibrin layer after a period in situ, subclinical emboli are probably more common than recognized, but gross embolization and tissue infarction are virtually unheard of. However, transient cerebral ischemic symptoms during transbrachial artery infusion have been reported, probably being the result of small fibrin emboli [45]. Risk of this may be reduced by using only the left brachial artery [15]. Infection at the puncture site can progress to septic endarteritis with associated bacteremia and septic embolization. Signs of this are local inflammation, purulent discharge, and bleeding from the puncture site. If these are noted, the catheter should be removed, cultures of blood and the catheter tip obtained, and antibiotics started. *Staphylococcus aureus* is the organism most commonly implicated [24]. In this setting, surgical intervention for abscess drainage or vascular repair may be necessary. Other problems such as hematoma at the puncture site, connector leak, or catheter cracking and leakage can be avoided by attention to detail.

Related to Cytotoxic Drugs

Because the techniques of regional chemotherapy release varying amounts of cytotoxic drugs into the systemic circulation, the physician administering such treatment must be familiar with the management of the toxicities of these drugs. Nausea and vomiting, fatal myelosuppression, stomatitis, and alopecia have all been reported, as well as renal dysfunction related to cisplatin infusion. The incidence and severity of these depend on the drug and dose given, the duration of infusion, and the patient's overall condition. Appropriate dose reduction should be made for patients with prior radiation, or hepatic or renal impairment. The high drug concentration in the area of infusion can produce local complications such as skin erythema or necrosis, edema, and neuritis. Regional chemotherapy has been reported to cause intestinal perforation and formation of vesicovaginal and rectovaginal fistulas [16]. The cause was rapid necrosis of a bulky tumor that formed part of the wall of the organ involved.

Drug Selection and Schedule

The most important factor in drug selection is efficacy against the tumor being treated. Knowledge of this may be empiric or based on previous response to intravenous chemotherapy in a given patient. In the future, in vitro chemosensitivity assays may be useful. Auersperg and Us-Krašovec described a rapid sensitivity test based on cell morphology [2]. They performed thin needle aspiration biopsy on tumors before, during, and after infusion chemotherapy and found a good correlation between cytologic changes during infusion and subsequent response.

When several choices are available, the drug with the highest elimination rate should be selected. Doxorubicin and 5-fluorouracil have clearances several times higher than that of endogenous creatinine, whereas clearance of methotrexate and cisplatin is much less [7, 10, 46]. Cyclophosphamide is not suitable for regional chemotherapy because it requires metabolic activation in the liver to become cytotoxic.

During perfusion the drug is only in contact with the target area for a short time. Therefore, alkylating agents or other non-cycle dependent drugs should be used. Doses used range from 1 to 3 times the recommended intravenous doses [8].

Antimetabolites are commonly used for intra-arterial infusion. Because their effectiveness depends on the tumor cell being in a sensitive phase of the cell cycle, longer infusions are desirable. Sullivan has suggested that infusion duration should be the same as tumor doubling time [37]. Doses for intra-arterial infusion are generally similar to intravenous doses and are adjusted according to toxicity and the planned length of infusion. An exception is that the dose of 5-fluorouracil for intra-arterial infusion needs to be 2–3 times higher than the intravenous dose to produce equivalent toxicity. As the goal of regional infusion is to produce local toxicity with tolerable systemic toxicity, doses can be varied according to the length of infusion desired. When local toxicity develops, infusion is stopped until recovery. Therefore, with the same drug it is possible to use high dose, short infusions or lower dose, long infusions.

Another approach is that of using the combination of a drug regionally and its antagonist systemically. Sullivan [37] investigated this and found that methotrexate infused at 5 mg/day produced local toxicity in 5–6 days, while methotrexate 50 mg/day with simultaneous folinic acid (6 mg IM q 6 h) produced toxicity in 6–10 days. He felt that the high regional concentration would yield a therapeutic effect, but that the remainder of the body exposed to a lower concentration would be protected by the folinic acid. Further study of cisplatin and its antagonists, the thio compounds, seems in order. An advantage for intra-arterial cisplatin and systemic thiosulfate over cisplatin alone was demonstrated in a rat model with a transplanted bladder tumor [32].

Results in Urologic Tumors

No controlled studies have compared the relative effectiveness of intravenous and intra-arterial chemotherapy. For this reason, reported results of regional chemotherapy must be interpreted with caution, in particular because many of the responses recorded were subjective or involved unmeasurable masses.

Renal Carcinoma

Few patients have received regional chemotherapy for renal carcinoma. No response was found in four patients treated with intra-arterial methotrexate or 5-fluorouracil [5]. Kraybill and co-workers reported some effect in two of five patients who received doxorubicin, although their criteria for response were not clearly defined [21]. Concurrent intra-arterial actinomycin D and external beam radiation were used for two patients with unresectable tumors. One experienced some palliation, and in the other the tumor shrank by two-thirds and was resected, although differentiating the effect of drug from radiation is impossible [44].

In all, these findings reflect the poor results of intravenous chemotherapy for this disease. Improvement cannot be expected until a drug effective for renal carcinoma is developed.

One recent report described the combined use of arterial embolization and chemotherapy [19]. Large renal carcinomas were embolized with a mixture of pieces of absorbable gelatin sponge and ethylcellulose microcapsules which contained mitomycin C. Previous experimental work had shown that the micro-capsules had a sustained release effect with systemic drug levels about 40% less than those seen after comparable drug doses given by direct injection. Tumor shrinkage, vascular occlusion, and histologic necrosis were of much greater magnitude and duration in patients who received "chemoembolization" as compared with a previous group given intra-arterial injection of gelatin sponge and nonencapsulated mitomycin C. This approach deserves more study.

Prostate Cancer

Bilateral hypogastric infusion with 5-fluorouracil was performed in 22 patients with stages C and D prostate cancer by Nevin's group [25, 28]. First 15 mg/kg/day was given for 10 days, followed by 2500 mg every other week, alternating sides, for 3 months. In a group of six patients who had failed estrogen therapy and pelvic radiation, shrinkage of local tumor was observed in all, and ureteral obstruction improved in four of five patients. Sixteen other patients who were estrogen failures received the above infusion therapy followed by pelvic radiation. In this group eight patients were reported to have negative prostate biopsies after therapy, and five more had palpable shrinkage of tumor as determined by rectal examination. The authors felt survival was increased compared with historic controls from the literature, but their patients continued to die from disseminated tumor in spite of the local control achieved.

No patients had significant bone marrow depression, but 25% developed sciatic neuritis that required termination of infusion therapy. Toward the end of the 3 months of infusions, all patients had varying degrees of skin necrosis in the distribution of the superior gluteal arteries, and some required skin grafting.

Bladder Cancer

More experience with regional chemotherapy is available for bladder cancer. One of the first studies used mitomycin C at a dose of 5 mg/day for 3 days, then 2 mg/day for 3 weeks infused into one hypogastric artery [29]. Objective response in localized bladder tumors was seen in 9 of 16 T_1 tumors, 4 of 12 T_2 and T_3, and 4 of 5 T_4 lesions. Skin necrosis occurred in 27% and sciatic neuritis in 9%; two patients died of unstated causes as a result of therapy.

Nevin et al. gave 5-fluorouracil with the same protocol they used for prostate cancer [27] (see above). Of ten patients with recurrent bladder tumors after full course radiation, two were rendered free of disease and had prolonged survival. All patients in this group had radiation cystitis, which was worsened by the infusion. They also had 17 evaluable patients with stage C or D-1 tumors who were not surgical candidates whom they treated with 5-fluorouracil followed by radiation. Some of these were also given bleomycin or doxorubicin. Eight of ten stage C patients were made tumor-free, although follow-up was short. Six of seven patients with stage D-1 tumors had partial responses, and two were made tumor-free by radiation. The remainder progressed after shorter intervals. The authors noted that no patients with squamous carcinoma had a significant response.

In another report, doxorubicin at 0.4 mg/kg/day for 5 days gave some response in five of nine patients so treated [21]. One bladder was found to be tumor-free at later cystectomy.

Cisplatin was administered in doses of 80–120 mg/m^2 every 4 weeks in another series [42]. The dose was divided between two hypogastric artery catheters. The 15 patients included some with pelvic recurrence after cystectomy and the rest with extensive unresectable tumors. Complete response occurred in six (40%), partial response in three (20%), and the treatment failed in the rest. Hematuria was controlled in 8 of 10 patients, and 10 of 15 patients had improvement of pelvic pain.

Another study from the same group used a different drug protocol [23]. Hypogastric artery infusion with 5-fluorouracil (1 g/m^2/day) for 5 days was combined with intravenous doxorubicin (20 mg/m^2/day) and mitomycin C (5 mg/ m^2/day) for 2 days each. This cycle was repeated every 4 weeks. In 29 patients with locally advanced bladder tumors, 17 (58%) had some degree of objective response. Response was seen in transitional cell carcinoma and in adenocarcinoma, but not in squamous carcinoma. It is interesting that two of the four patients who had tumor-free bladders by cystoscopy after treatment later developed distant metastases while the bladder remained tumor-free. Complications were considerable. All patients had inflammatory skin changes, 38% had stomatitis, and 14% had sciatic neuropathy. More than 50% had leukopenic fever. One patient died of unsuspected mitomycin lung toxicity.

Doxorubicin was used as a surgical adjuvant for T$_3$ bladder tumors in 20 patients [34]. Patients received 80 mg divided between bilateral hypogastric artery catheters on two occasions a month apart. A complete or partial (> 50%) response was found in all evaluable bladders. Similar results were found after the same drug was given by infusion into the distal aorta [25]. In a phase I study, Jacobs and Lawson added intracavitary hyperthermia in patients with bulky stage C tumors prior to cystectomy [17]. They continuously irrigated the bladders with 39°–49°C saline during simultaneous hypogastric artery infusion of doxorubicin, 40–75 mg/ m^2 over 48 h. Tumor necrosis was found in all nine treated patients, with a gradient from severe necrosis at the mucosal surface to less necrosis and viable tumor on the serosal side. In spite of local control in seven of the nine patients, six died of metastases within a short time.

Progress has been made in the treatment of metastatic bladder cancer, and it might be argued that the responses listed above could be obtained with standard intravenous chemotherapy. Although no comparative studies are available, a review of the response to intravenous therapy by site of tumor yields some information. With methotrexate, an 18% objective response rate was found for local pelvic disease, compared with 48% for metastatic [40]. With cisplatin based combinations, responses of 29% and 33% were obtained for pelvic tumor in contrast to 62% and 67% for lung metastases [22, 33]. These figures suggest that intra-arterial infusion chemotherapy is more effective than intravenous for local bladder cancer, especially in light of the fact that many of the infusion patients had bulky tumors that had been previously radiated.

External Genitalia

There are no published series of intra-arterial chemotherapy for tumors of the penis, scrotum, or urethra. Recently a patient with squamous carcinoma of the penis who developed a large, biopsy-proven recurrence in the groin was treated by this method at UCLA (Fig. 14.1). Methotrexate (40 mg/m^2 on days 1 and 15), cis-platin (50 mg/m^2 on day 4), and bleomycin (30 units IM on days 1, 8, and 15) were given on a q 4 week schedule. The methotrexate and cisplatin were administered by infusion into the external iliac artery on the side of the mass. This protocol was chosen because of its effectiveness for squamous carcinoma of the head and neck [41]. After two courses, the mass had shrunk by more than 75%. Wide excision was performed, along with inguinal and ipsilateral pelvic node dissections. On patho-logic examination all resected nodes were free of tumor, and the mass contained only necrotic debris, scattered keratin pearls and foreign body giant cells, and a few microfoci of atypical squamous cells (Fig. 14.2).

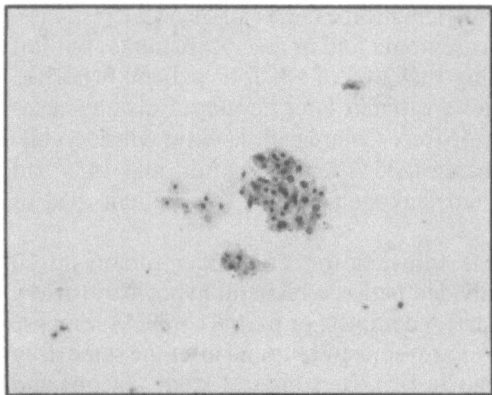

Fig. 14.1. Penile carcinoma: clusters of malignant squamous cells (fine needle aspiration of groin mass).

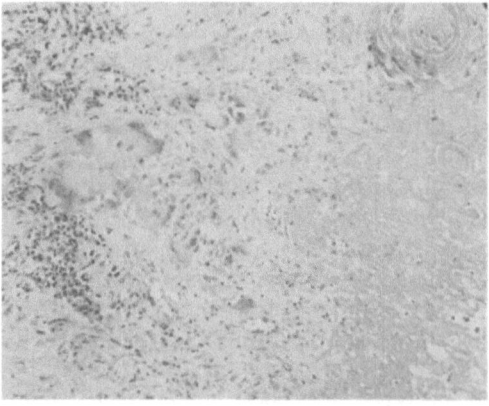

Fig. 14.2. Penile carcinoma after chemotherapy: necrotic debris, foreign body giant cells, inflammatory reaction.

Urogenital Sarcomas

Sarcomas in adults that arise from the kidney, bladder, prostate, retroperitoneum, or testicular adnexa have proven difficult to treat successfully. Doxorubicin has been effective in the treatment of soft tissue sarcomas in other locations, and administration by intra-arterial infusion has seemed to increase response [21, 30]. The extension of this to include planned regional chemotherapy, radiation, and surgery for limb sarcomas has yielded further improvement in response [12]. In view of the good results obtained in pediatric urogenital sarcomas with this approach, application of a similar plan to adults seems logical, although few patients so treated have been reported. In recent years, adults with nonmetastatic urogenital sarcomas at UCLA have been treated with the combination of intra-arterial doxorubicin (30 mg/day for 3 days), radiation, and excision of the primary tumor shortly after radiotherapy is completed. This regimen has resulted in tumor-free survival in four patients: one with poorly differentiated sarcoma of the kidney (Figs. 14.3–14.5), one with leiomyosarcoma of the bladder, and two with leiomyosarcoma of the prostate (Figs. 14.6, 14.7). The effect of this combination was demonstrated by the absence of recognizable residual tumor in the surgical specimen in the kidney and prostate patients (Figs. 14.8, 14.9).

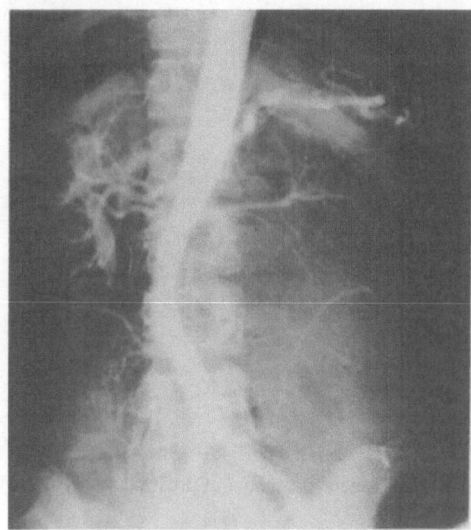

Fig. 14.3. Sarcoma of kidney: aortogram with deviation of aorta and hypovascular left renal mass.

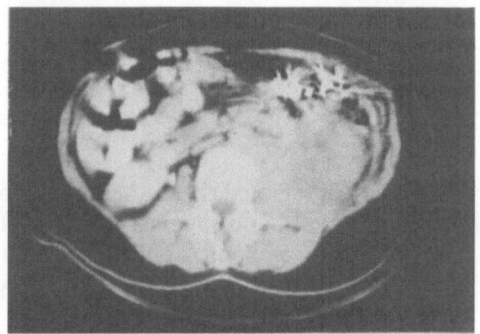

Fig. 14.4. Sarcoma of kidney: abdominal CT with large left renal mass.

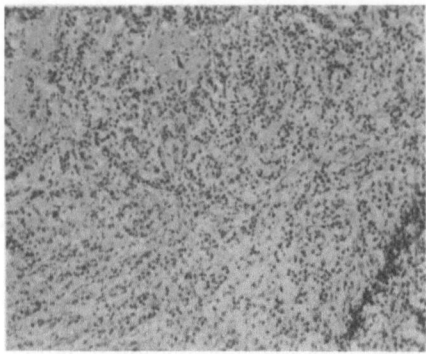

Fig. 14.5. Sarcoma of kidney: sheets of pleomorphic cells with scant cytoplasm.

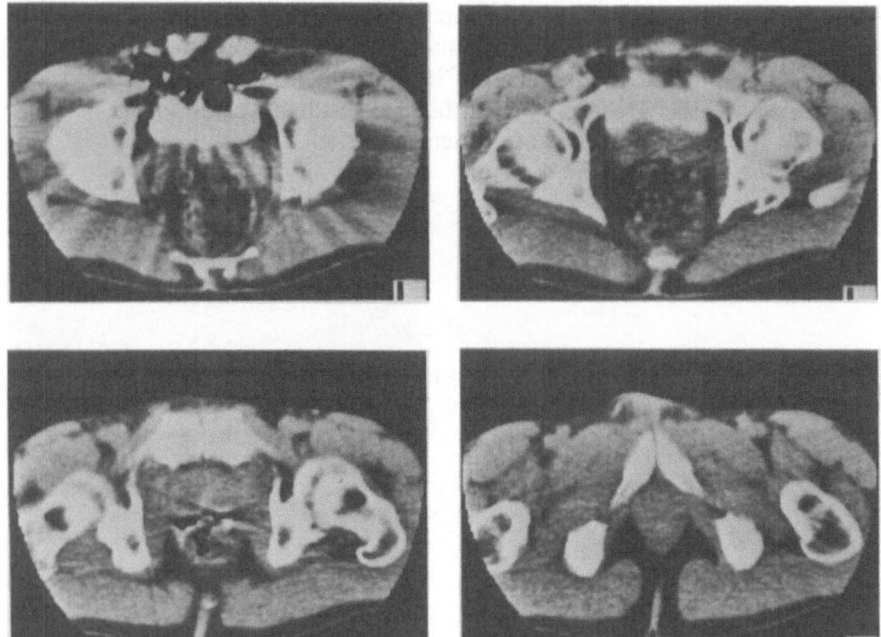

Fig. 14.6. Leiomyosarcoma of prostate: pelvic CT with enlarged prostate.

Summary

The history of regional chemotherapy has been typical of any new form of therapy, particularly that aimed against cancer. After an initial optimistic description, the new treatment is soon applied to many patients with little discrimination. Eventually, analysis of results and side-effects allows a realistic role, or lack of one, to be assigned.

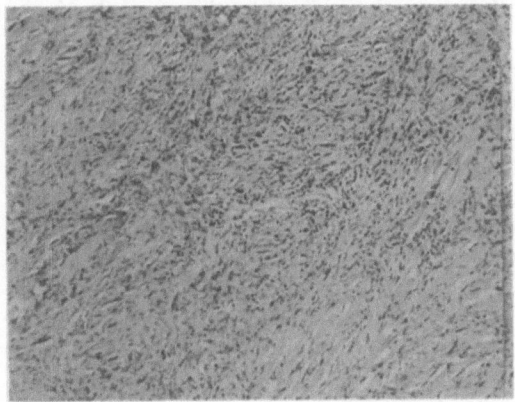

Fig. 14.7. Leiomyosarcoma of prostate: moderate sized spindle cells, rare mitotic figures.

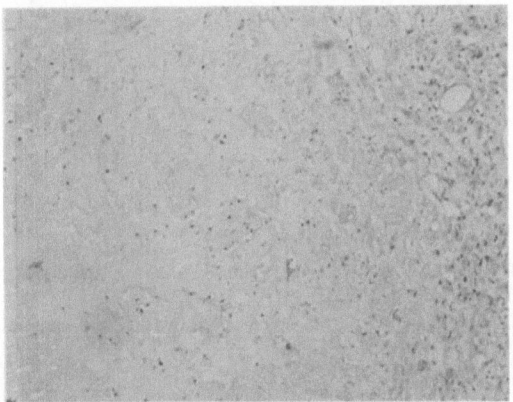

Fig. 14.8. Sarcoma of kidney after chemotherapy: necrotic debris, no viable tumor.

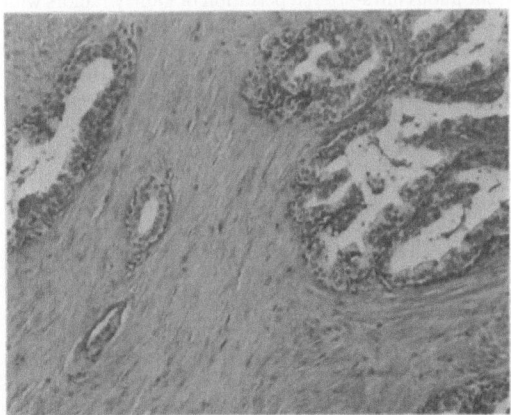

Fig. 14.9. Leiomyosarcoma of prostate after chemotherapy: inflammation, metaplasia of duct epithelium, no residual tumor.

Responsiveness to regional chemotherapy is determined by the tumor having a defined and limited arterial supply and by the availability of an effective drug, although response to intra-arterial infusion when intravenous therapy has failed is reported [1]. Maintaining acceptable toxicity requires the physician to be well versed in the use and complications of cytotoxic drugs. Because doses and schedules are not well defined, a certain amount of improvisation is necessary.

The situations in which regional chemotherapy is proper for the urologic cancer patient are few. The use of it for palliation of locally extensive pelvic tumors in patients with bladder or prostate cancer seems reasonable, especially when more conventional means have been exhausted. This would be true for patients with moderate life expectancy whether or not metastases were present. The use of regional chemotherapy as an adjunct to other measures in the attempt to cure nonmetastatic tumors deserves further study. Its use for urogenital sarcomas is justified by extrapolation of results attained with soft tissue sarcomas in other sites. Utility for other tumors, such as invasive bladder cancers, would best be established through the format of a planned clinical study. The small but impressive series employing intra-arterial doxorubicin in patients with bulky invasive bladder cancer may forecast a new dimension in preoperative adjuvant therapy.

References

1. Ansfield FJ, Ramirez G, Skibba JL, Bryan GT, Davis HL, Wirtanen GW (1971) Intrahepatic arterial infusion with 5-fluorouracil. Cancer 28:1147–1151
2. Auersperg M, Us-Krašovec M (1970) In vivo sensitivity test for guided chemotherapy of malignant tumors. Proc Sixth Int Congr Chemother 2:353–358
3. Austin WG, Monaco AP, Richardson GS, Baker WH, Shaw RS, Raker JW (1959) Treatment of malignant pelvic tumors by extracorporeal perfusion with chemotherapeutic agents. N Engl J Med 261:1037–1045
4. Blackshear PJ, Dorman FD, Blackshear PL, Varco RL, Buchwald H (1970) A permanently implantable self-recycling low flow constant rate multipurpose infusion pump of simple design. Surg Forum 21:136–137
5. Brendler H, Leiter E, Edelman S (1967) Continuous intra-arterial perfusion of kidney tumors with cytotoxic agents prior to nephrectomy. In: King JS (ed) Renal neoplasia. Little, Brown and Company, Boston
6. Calvo DB, Patt YZ, Wallace S, Chuang VP, Benjamin RS, Pritchard JD, Hersh EM, Bodey GP, Mavligit GM (1980) Phase I-II trial of percutaneous intra-arterial cis-diamminedichloroplatinum (II) for regionally confined malignancy. Cancer 45:1278–1283
7. Chabner BA (1982) Pyrimidine antagonists. In: Chabner BA (ed) Pharmacologic principles of cancer treatment. W. B. Saunders, Philadelphia, pp 183–212
8. Clarkson B, Lawrence W (1961) Perfusion and infusion techniques in cancer chemotherapy. Med Clin North Am 45:689–710
9. Cohen AM, Wood WC, Greenfield A, Waltman A, Dedrick C, Blackshear PJ (1980) Transbrachial hepatic artery chemotherapy using an implanted infusion pump. Dis Colon Rectum 23:223–227
10. Collins JM, Dedrick RL (1982) Pharmacokinetics of anticancer drugs. In: Chabner BA (ed) Pharmacologic principles of cancer treatment. W. B. Saunders, Philadelphia, pp 77–99
11. Eckman WW, Patlak CS, Fenstermacher JD (1974) A critical evaluation of the principles governing the advantages of intra-arterial perfusions. J Pharmacokinet Biopharm 2:257–285
12. Eilber FR, Mirra JJ, Grant TT, Weisenberger T, Morton DL (1980) Is amputation necessary for sarcomas? A seven-year experience with limb salvage. Ann Surg 192:431–438
13. Ensminger W, Niederhuber J, Dakhil S, Thrall J, Wheeler R (1981) Totally implanted drug delivery system for hepatic arterial chemotherapy. Cancer Treat Rep 65:393–400

14. Fortuny IE, Theologides A, Kennedy BJ (1975) Hepatic arterial infusion for liver metastases from lung cancer: comparison of mitomycin C (NSC-26980) and 5-fluorouracil (NSC-19893). Cancer Chemother Rep 59:401–404
15. Goldman ML, Bilbao MK, Rösch J, Dotter CT (1975) Complications of indwelling chemotherapy catheters. Cancer 36:1983–1990
16. Hurley JD, Wall T, Worman LW, Schulte WJ (1961) Experiences with pelvic perfusion for carcinoma. Arch Surg 83:127–137
17. Jacobs SC, Lawson RK (1982) Pathologic effects of pre-cystectomy therapy with combination intra-arterial doxorubicin and local bladder hyperthermia for bladder cancer. J Urol 127:43–47
18. Kaplan WD, D'Orsi CJ, Ensminger WD, Smith EH, Levin DC (1978) Intra-arterial radionuclide infusion: a new technique to assess chemotherapy perfusion patterns. Cancer Treat Rep 62:699–703
19. Kato T, Nemoto R, Mori H, Takahashi M, Tamakawa Y (1981) Transcatheter arterial chemoembolization of renal cell carcinoma with microencapsulated mitomycin C. J Urol 125:19–24
20. Klopp CT, Alford TC, Bateman J, Berry GN, Winship T (1950) Fractionated intra-arterial cancer chemotherapy with methyl bis amine hydrochloride: a preliminary report. Ann Surg 132:811–832
21. Kraybill WG, Harrison M, Sasaki T, Fletcher WS (1977) Regional intra-arterial infusion of adriamycin in the treatment of cancer. Surg Gynecol Obstet 144:335–338
22. Levi JA, Aroney RS, Dalley DN (1980) Combination chemotherapy with cyclophosphamide, doxorubicin and bleomycin for metastatic transitional cell carcinoma of the urinary bladder. Cancer Treat Rep 64:1011–1013
23. Logothetis CJ, Samuels ML, Wallace S, Chuang V, Trindade A, Grant C, Haynie TP, Johnson DE (1982) Management of pelvic complications of malignant urothelial tumors with combined intra-arterial and IV chemotherapy. Cancer Treat Rep 66:1501–1507
24. Maki DG, McCormick RD, Uman SJ, Wirtanen GW (1979) Septic endarteritis due to intra-arterial catheters for cancer chemotherapy. Cancer 44:1228–1240
25. Nakazono M, Iwata S (1981) Pre-operative intra-arterial chemotherapy for bladder cancer. Urol Res 9:289–295
26. Nevin JE, Hoffman AA (1975) Use of arterial infusion of 5-fluorouracil either alone or in combination with supervoltage radiation as a treatment for carcinoma of the prostate and bladder. Am J Surg 130:544–549
27. Nevin JE, Melnick I, Baggerly JT, Easley CA, Landes R (1974) Advanced carcinoma of bladder: treatment using hypogastric artery infusion with 5-fluorouracil, either as a single agent or in combination with bleomycin or adriamycin and supervoltage radiation. J Urol 112:752–758
28. Nevin JE, Melnick I, Baggerly JT, Esteves J, Landes R, Easley CA (1974) Arterial infusion of 5-fluorouracil as a treatment for carcinoma of the prostate. J Urol 112:114–119
29. Ogata J, Migita N, Nakamura T (1973) Treatment of carcinoma of the bladder by infusion of the anticancer agent (mitomycin C) via the internal iliac artery. J Urol 110:667–670
30. Pinedo HM, Kenis Y (1977) Chemotherapy of advanced soft tissue sarcoma in adults. Cancer Treat Rev 4:67–86
31. Plasse T. Ohnuma T, Bruckner H, Chamberlain K, Moss T, Holland JE (1982) Portable infusion pumps in ambulatory cancer therapy. Cancer 50:27–31
32. Sagiyama K, Uozumi J, Aoki K, Baba T (1983) Efficacy of "two-route chemotherapy" using intra-arterial cisplatin and IV sodium thiosulfate, its antidote, in rat bladder tumor. Cancer Treat Rep 67:567–572
33. Samuels ML, Moran ME, Johnson DE, Bracken RB (1979) CISCA combination chemotherapy for metastatic carcinoma of the bladder. In: Johnson DE, Samuels ML (eds) Cancer of the genitourinary tract. Raven Press, New York, pp 101–106
34. Schulman CC, Struyven J, Bredael JJ, Delcour A (1983) Intraarterial chemotherapy of infiltrative bladder tumors. Proc Am Urol Assoc, Abstr #348, p 178
35. Seldinger SI (1953) Catheter replacement of the needle in percutaneous arteriography. Acta Rad Stockh. 39:368–376, 1953
36. Stewart DJ, Benjamin RS, Zimmerman S, Caprioli RM, Wallace S, Chuang V, Calvo D, Samuels M, Bonura J, Loo TL (1983) Clinical pharmacology of intra-arterial cis-diamminedichloroplatinum (II). Cancer Res 43:917–920
37. Sullivan RD (1962) Continuous arterial infusion cancer chemotherapy. Surg Clin North Am 42:365–379
38. Sullivan RD, Watkins E, Oberfield RA, Khazei AM (1967) Current status of protracted arterial infusion cancer chemotherapy for the treatment of solid tumors. Surg Clin North Am 47:769–784
39. Thomson KR, Goldin AR (1979) Angiographic techniques in interventional radiology. Rad Clin North Am 17:375–391
40. Turner AG (1981) Methotrexate in advanced bladder cancer. Cancer Treat Rep 65 (Suppl 1):183–186

41. Vogl SE, Kaplan BH (1979) Chemotherapy of advanced head and neck cancer with methotrexate, bleomycin and *cis*-diamminedichloroplatinum II in an effective outpatient schedule. Cancer 44:26–31
42. Wallace S, Chuang VP, Samuels M, Johnson D (1982) Transcatheter intra-arterial infusion of chemotherapy in advanced bladder cancer. Cancer 49:640–645
43. Watkins E, Hering AC, Luna R, Adams HD (1960) The use of intravascular balloon catheters for isolation of the pelvic vascular bed during pump-oxygenator perfusion of cancer chemotherapeutic agents. Surg Gynecol Obstet 111:464–468
44. Wiley AL, Wirtanen GW, Joo P, Ansfield EJ, Ramirez G, Davis HL, Vermund H (1975) Clinical and theoretical aspects of the treatment of surgically unresectable retroperitoneal malignancy with combined intra-arterial actinomycin-D and radiotherapy. Cancer 36:107–122
45. Wirtanen GW (1973) Percutaneous transbrachial artery infusion catheter techniques. AJR 117:696–700
46. Zwelling LA, Kohn KW (1982) Platinum complexes. In: Chabner BA (ed) Pharmacologic principles of cancer treatment. W. B. Saunders, Philadelphia, pp 309–339

Chapter 15

Technique and Results of Percutaneous Renal Artery Dilatation (PTRD)

E. Zeitler

The suggestion that arterial stenosis could be permanently dilated with percutaneously introduced catheters was first made by Dotter and Judkins in 1964 [7]. We assessed this technique in the iliac and femoral arteries in more than 3000 patients and found clear indications for it.

In October 1970, we had our first opportunity to try the dilating technique in a patient with renal artery stenosis using a Teflon catheter in combination with a Fogarty balloon catheter after an unsuccessful thromboendarterectomy. The stenosis was very rigid and we had little success, but renin activity changed and the systolic peak pressure dropped from over 200 to 160 mmHg for more than 9 months. Two years later the patient died after a cerebral stroke. In 1974, Grüntzig and Hopff [12] refined the balloon dilatation concept by using a nonelastomeric balloon of fixed volume on a double-lumen catheter. Grüntzig, Kuhlmann, and Mahler [13, 20, 23, 24] were the first to employ such a coaxial balloon catheter for the dilatation of renal artery stenoses. Within a short time, early results were published by several working groups [3, 5, 10, 11, 15, 16–19, 21–25, 28, 31–39, 42–47]. The potential of dilating arterial stenoses of renal transplants was soon indicated by impressive examples [26, 37, 41, 46].

Diagnosis of Renal Artery Stenoses

Until a few years ago, in patients suffering from arterial hypertension, intravenous urograms, radionuclide nephrograms, and renin assays of the renal blood on both sides were used as screening and selective procedures prior to renal angiography and surgical treatment of renal artery stenoses [1, 9, 14, 48–51]. Recently, however, more effective and more economical diagnosis has become possible [15, 16].

The introduction of digital subtraction angiography (DSA) [2, 6, 27, 29, 40] improved the diagnostic accuracy of renal arteriography and opened the way for early diagnosis in outpatients.

The diagnosis of renovascular hypertension secondary to renal artery stenoses is of particular significance owing to the simple therapeutic technique of percutaneous dilatation.

Percutaneous treatment of renal artery stenoses aims at:

1. Normalizing the blood pressure of patients with arterial hypertension
2. Reducing the number and dose of antihypertensives and attaining a decrease in blood pressure
3. Improving creatinine clearance in patients with renal insufficiency

Medication Before PTRD

Due to the fact that an immediate reduction in blood pressure may occur after successful dilatation, antihypertensives are not given on the day of percutaneous dilatation of a stenosis. To avoid a thrombocyte thrombus at the site of the intimal lesion, a thrombocyte aggregation inhibitor (acetylsalicylic acid 0.5 g b.i.d. or t.i.d. or acetylsalicylic acid 330 mg and 75 mg dipyridamole b.i.d. or t.i.d.) is administered at least 1 day before the PTRD is performed. This treatment has to be continued for at least 3 months.

In addition, 5000 IU heparin are administered intra-arterially after sounding the renal artery stenosis in order to avoid deposition of hyalin thrombi at the surface of the catheter and at the intimal lesion in the area of the renal artery. Immediately prior to the dilatation the patient is given either nitroglycerin or nifedipine in order to avoid a spasm of the renal arteries.

Technique of PTRD

The selective catheterization of the renal artery is performed transfemorally. As recommended by Grüntzig [12, 13], a coaxial catheter system may be used together with a femororenal guiding catheter through which the balloon catheter is passed. Another possibility is to catheterize the renal artery stenosis with a sidewinder I or II [33, 39, 43, 45, 52].

A disadvantage of the sidewinder catheter technique is the necessity to advance the catheter within the aortic arch in order to turn it. At narrow aortic lumina, this approach may, in very rare cases, lead to shedding of plaque, a cerebral embolism, and a subintimal dissection at the stenosis by the catheter tip. Renal artery stenoses can, however, be passed easily. Thus it is not unnecessary to employ the coaxial technique with its larger diameter of guide wire, which may cause significant arterial wall defects. In occasional cases a sheath for the exchange of catheters may be required.

In evaluating hemodynamics the first steps are to measure the aortic blood pressure and record the poststenotic pressure when the stenosis has been passed. The position of the catheter may accentuate the gradient across a stenosis, but it generates a gradient of not more than 20 mmHg if the changes of the vessel walls do not cause hemodynamic effect. Regardless of the angiographic findings, we only dilate when a systolic gradient of more than 40 mmHg is encountered or a fibromuscular dysplasia is proven angiographically (Table 15.1).

Table 15.1. Results of pressure measurements and subsequent use of PTRD in 161 patients with 189 renal artery stenoses (RAST)

Not confirmed by pressure measurements	PTRD performed
↓	↓
11	178 RAST in 151 patients
(Radiological Center)	(Klinikum Nürnberg)

Dilatation

When a safe position of the catheter within the renal artery is attained poststenotically the sidewinder catheter is exchanged for a dilatation balloon catheter by means of a 2-m guide wire. The dilatation balloon catheter is then placed at the site of the stenosis which has previously been marked (Fig. 15.2).

Different balloon catheter types from various manufacturers are available:

1. Grüntzig-type double lumen balloon catheters made of polyvinyl chloride or special types of polyethylene with markers at both ends of the balloon. The length of the balloon varies between 2 and 4 cm and the diameter between 4 and 8 mm. When fully distended the pressure reaches 5 and 17 atm. We have not encountered any ruptures of these balloons.

2. Olbert-type double lumen balloon catheters made of a specially prepared latex, where the stretching is combined with a longitudinal displacement of the catheter. The deflation of this balloon catheter is more rapid [30].

3. Grüntzig-type coaxial balloon catheter with a diameter of only 5 F. The balloon is made of polyvinyl chloride or polyethylene. It is 2.5 cm long and shows a diameter of 3–8 mm. The guiding catheter has a diameter of 8–9 F.

The dilatation has to be performed under fluoroscopic control, since during dilatation the stenosis can easily cause the rather short balloon to slip to a distal or proximal position. The dilating force may thus be lost. The dilating procedure may be repeated up to five times for a period of 10–30 s. It is recommended that the guide wire be left peripherally in the renal artery while dilating, or, if the changes in poststenotic pressure ought to be controlled permanently, that a second guide wire be inserted by the contralateral femoral artery together with a further sidewinder catheter which will remain in the aorta [1]. Thus a sidewinder or balloon catheter may be introduced into the renal artery at any time. This approach may be required to block temporarily the site of an eventual perforation. Such a procedure makes possible safe measurements of the pressure after successful dilatation.

Immediate Control of the Success of the Treatment

After dilatation a pull back is generated. In the presence of a systolic gradient exceeding 40 mmHg, a balloon catheter with a larger balloon diameter may be inserted over the second guide wire. There is no risk of a dissection. If no second guide wire has been inserted into the renal artery, a repeat insertion of the balloon catheter across the dilatation site is not advisable because of the danger of a dissection.

Control angiography may be produced via a sidewinder catheter or a balloon catheter. It is best to utilize intra-aortic DSA (Fig. 15.3c).

After removal of the catheter using a guide wire, compression of the groin is necessary to control after-bleedings. A compression bandage has to be applied and the patient has to stay in bed for 24 h. During this period the blood pressure is measured every 2 h and subsequently three times a day so that appropriate additional drug treatment can be instituted if a sudden decrease in blood pressure occurs or if there is persisting hypertension. If no complications have been encountered the patient may be discharged from hospital on the third day after dilatation to be supervised on an outpatient basis.

Follow-up Controls

Follow-up controls are conducted in three ways:

1. Control of blood pressure values and dosage of antihypertensives.

2. A radionuclide scintigram [35] of the kidneys may be produced in order to compare it with a preliminary examination or an intravenous DSA 6–12 weeks following dilatation. This procedure is especially required when normalization of blood pressure values could not be achieved and there is a necessity to dilate a residual stenosis.

3. Transfemoral artery angiography or intra-arterial DSA may be performed in the presence of persistent hypertensive blood pressure values. During this angiographic procedure a repeat pressure measurement of the renal arteries on both sides as well as a repeat PTRD may be performed. In one patient we detected and dilated stenoses in as many as four renal arteries.

Example 1 (Figs. 15.1, 15.2)

A 45-year-old female received antihypertensive drugs over 9 years because of arterial hypertension. An increase in blood pressure values, varying between 170/110 and 220/135, had been noted for 1 year in spite of antihypertensive treatment. Determination of the renin values showed a clearly increased renin quotient on the right side. Abdominal aortography clearly showed fibromuscular dysplasia of the right renal artery as well as a ptotic right kidney and a left kidney enlarged by compensator hypertrophy. After drug pretreatment the right renal artery was investigated by a sidewinder II catheter and dilated using a polyethylene catheter with a balloon 4 cm long and 8 mm in diameter (Meditech). The systolic pressure gradient through an orthograde sidewinder catheter was 110 mmHg. No more pressure gradient was verified following dilatation. Control angiography still showed minimum wavy borderlines but no stenosis (Fig. 15.2b). Immediately after the dilatation a segmental spasm could be discerned. The patient was discharged from hospital on the third day following dilatation, showing normal blood pressure values and requiring no further drug treatment. The follow-up control 1 year later revealed normal blood pressure values. Scintigraphy and intravenous DSA were without pathologic findings.

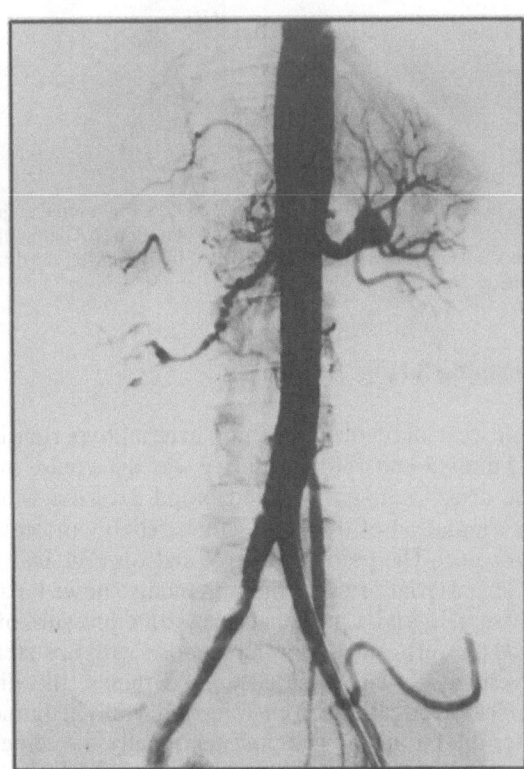

Fig. 15.1. Abdominal aortography showing fibromuscular dysplasia of the right renal artery.

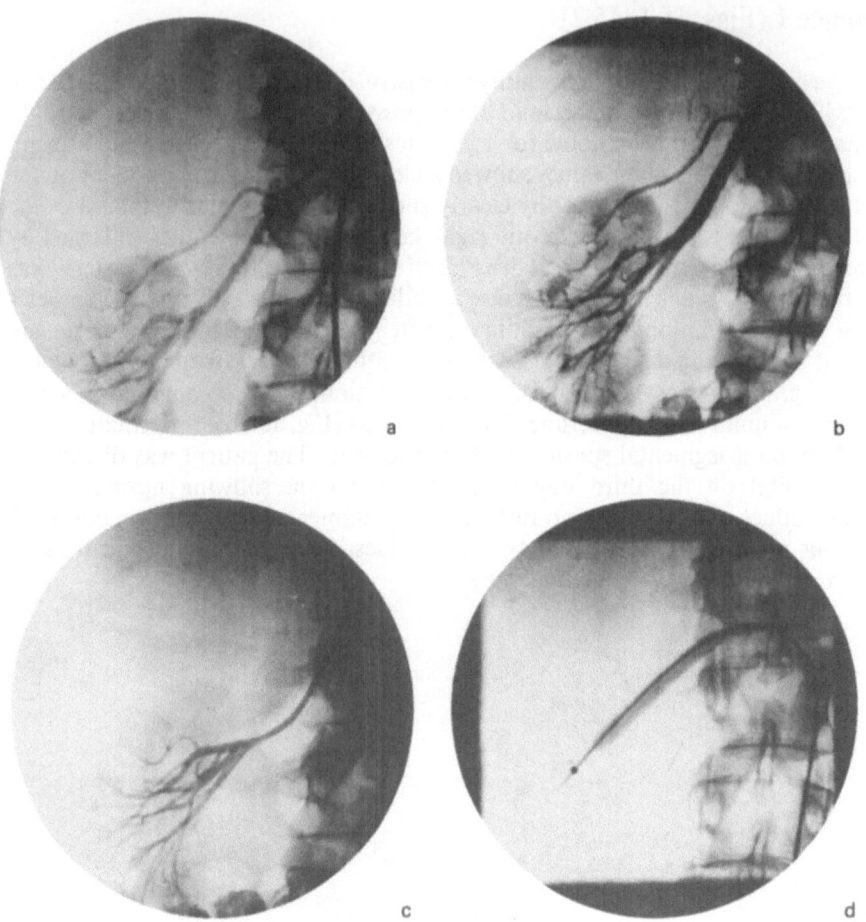

Fig. 15.2a–d. Control images during PTRD. **a** Right renal angiography prior to passage of the stenosis. **b** Control angiography after successful dilatation. **c** Angiography after safe passage of the renal artery stenosis using a sidewinder II catheter. **d** Image during the dilatation of the stenosis utilizing a balloon catheter.

Example 2 (Fig. 15.3)

A 46-year-old female in whom arterial hypertension showing values between 200/ 125 mmHg and 180/100 mmHg was detected 6 months previously. Antihypertensive drug treatment lowered blood pressure values. Renal scintigraphy and the determination of the renin values reliably indicated a renal artery stenosis on the right side. The patient was referred for PTRD.

The arterial pressure measurements showed a systemic aortic blood pressure of 240 mmHg and a poststenotic systolic pressure of 60 mmHg. Angiography visualized a severe central circular stenosis with poststenotic dilatation (Fig. 15.3). After investigating with a sidewinder catheter, the dilatation was performed with a polyethylene catheter 3 cm long and 8 mm in diameter. The pressure measurements after dilatation showed poststenotically the same pressure values as in the aorta. Control DSA was performed following dilatation, using the same dilating balloon

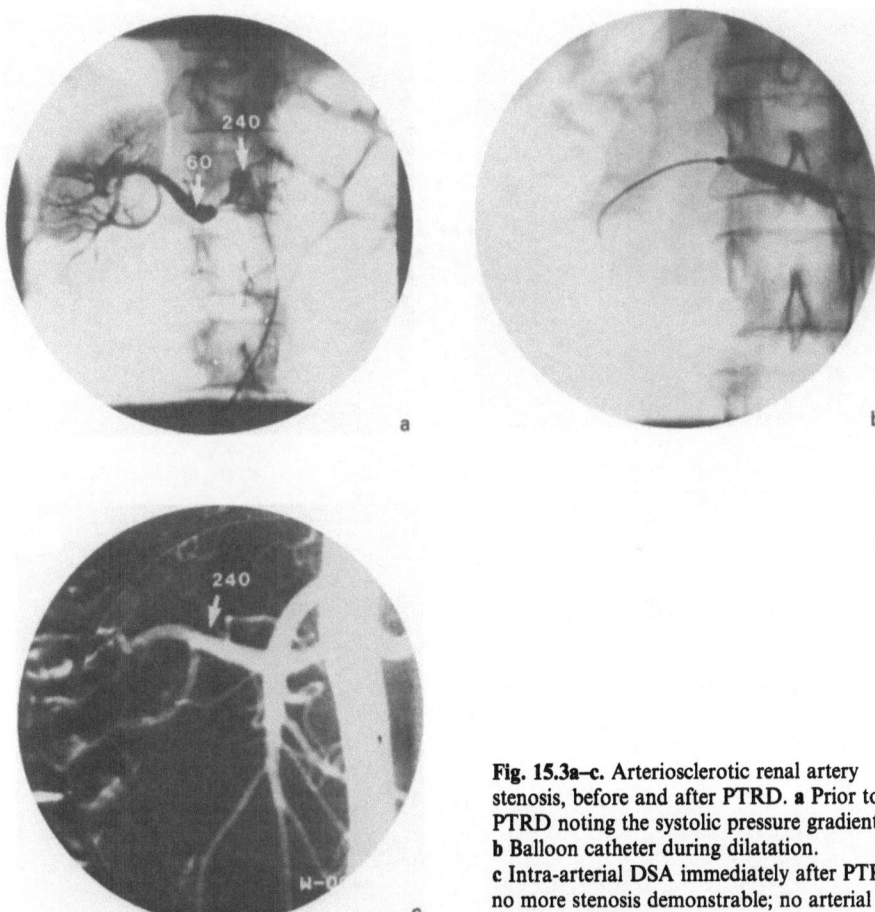

Fig. 15.3a–c. Arteriosclerotic renal artery stenosis, before and after PTRD. **a** Prior to PTRD noting the systolic pressure gradient. **b** Balloon catheter during dilatation. **c** Intra-arterial DSA immediately after PTRD; no more stenosis demonstrable; no arterial pressure gradient.

catheter. A decrease in systolic pressure values to 140/95 mmHg was noticed within 4 h after dilatation. The patient was normotensive without additional hypertensives. The follow-up investigation 6 weeks later showed borderline hypertension of 150/100 and 130/90 mmHg. Low-dose antihypertensive treatment resulted in well controlled normal blood pressure values.

Example 3 (Fig. 15.4)

An 18-year-old female who had suffered from arterial hypertension with systolic pressure values varying between 140 and 170 mmHg and diastolic values of 100–120 mmHg for several weeks. The angiogram demonstrated a bifurcation stenosis at the point of the branching-off of the right renal artery. Intra-arterial pressure measurements using an orthograde catheter showed an occlusion pressure at both stenoses. The lower stenosis was investigated by a sidewinder II catheter, the upper stenosis by a sidewinder I catheter. Dilatation of the stenoses was performed consecutively using a Grüntzig-type coaxial balloon catheter with a diameter of 5 mm. In the second branch a diagnostic catheter was placed.

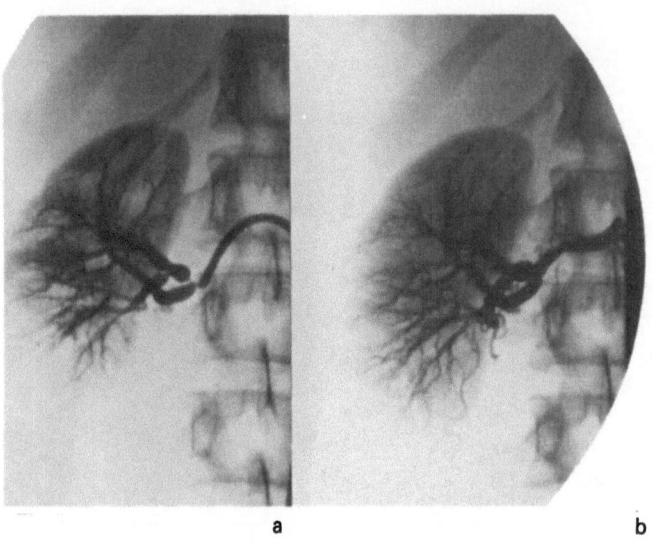

a   b

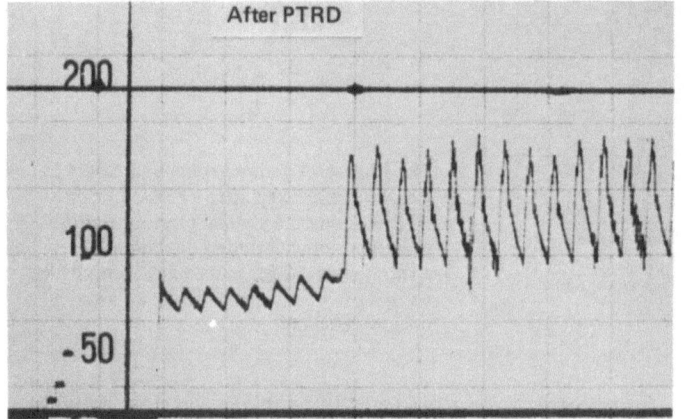

c

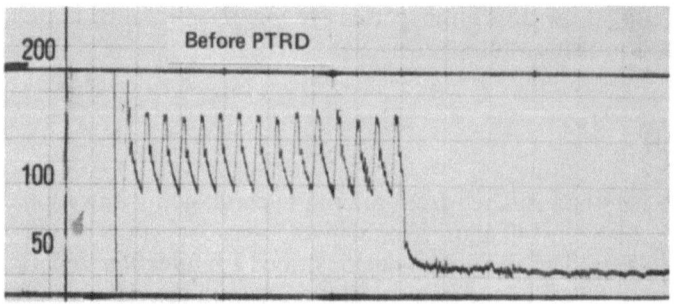

d

Fig. 15.4. a Renal angiography prior to dilatation with demonstration of a bifurcation stenosis of the right renal artery. **b** Control angiography after successful dilatation. The poststenotic dilatation at the upper and renal artery branch is still recognizable. **c** Pressure record of the aorta and poststenotically in the upper branch of the right renal artery prior to dilatation. **d** Pull-back of the upper branch of the right renal artery following dilatation; clear residual gradient.

The pull-back demonstrated no more pressure gradient in the region of the lower renal artery stenosis but a pressure gradient of 75 mmHg in the region of the upper renal artery stenosis (Fig. 15.4c, d). A control angiogram showed no remaining stenosis, and the dilatation generated normal blood pressure values. Antihypertensives were not necessary.

In such bifurcation stenoses the application of the so-called "kissing balloon technique" may be advisable. This procedure is performed by inserting two balloon catheters into the right renal artery, one positioned in the upper and one in the lower stenosis. Dilatation is executed simultaneously.

Example 4 (Fig. 15.5)

A 44-year-old male with renal insufficiency, increased creatinine values, and blood pressure values during antihypertensive treatment varying between 150/90 and 190/100 mmHg. Radionuclide scintigraphy indicated a left renal artery stenosis and a smaller left kidney. Intravenous DSA depicted a central arteriosclerotic renal artery stenosis on the left side.

A pretherapeutic angiogram (Fig. 15.5a) documented a left renal artery stenosis which could be sounded by a sidewinder II catheter (Fig. 15.5c). The dilatation was successfully performed utilizing a polyvinyl chloride balloon catheter (Grüntzig) 3 cm long and 8 mm in diameter (Fig. 15.5d). Arterial control angiography (Fig. 15.5b) carried out 6 weeks later showed no more stenosis but a renal artery of a smaller caliber than on the right side. The left renal artery was still smaller than the right. The pull-back showed no pressure gradient. The renal insufficiency was influenced favorably. Hypertension was still present.

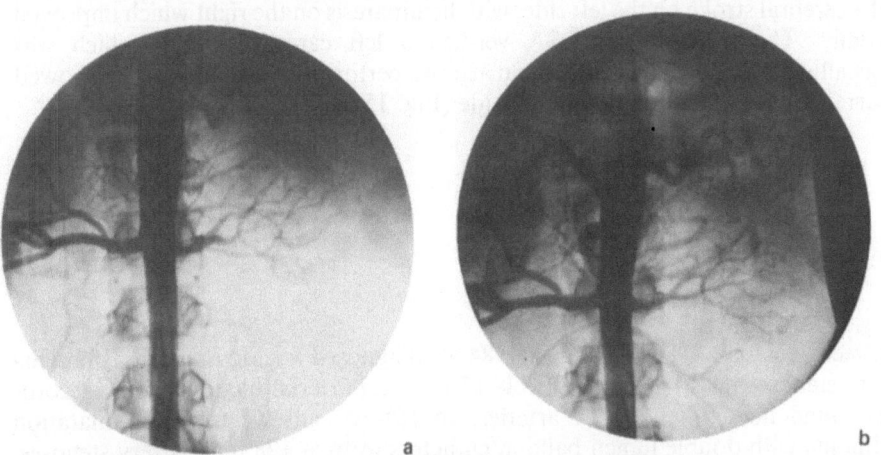

a   b

Fig. 15.5a–d. 44-year-old male with arteriorsclerotic renal artery stenosis on the left at renal insufficiency. **a** Angiogram prior to PTRD. **b** Control angiogram 6 weeks after successful PTRD. **c** Investigation of the stenosis using a sidewinder II catheter. **d** Baloon catheter during diltation.

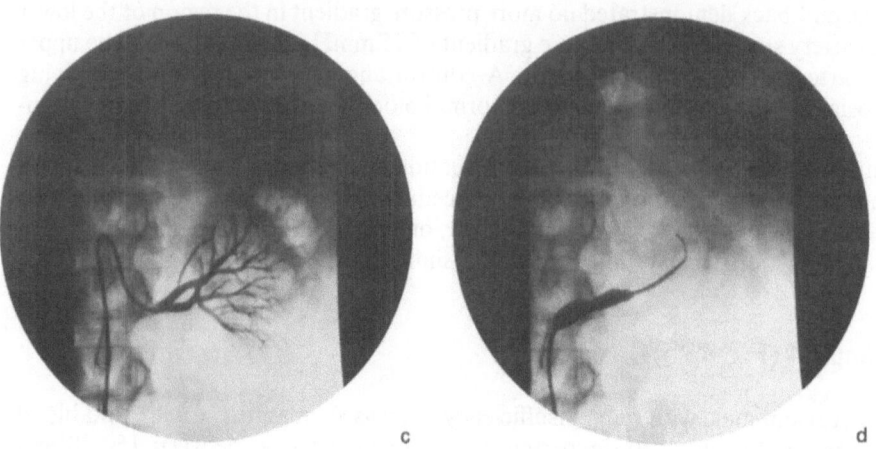

Fig. 15.5 (*continued*)

Example 5 (Fig. 15.6)

A 41-year-old manager with arterial hypertension and blood pressure values varying between 210/135 and 240/140 mmHg. He was an excessive smoker who weighed 95 kg and was 1.68 m tall. It was not possible to manage the hypertension by medicamentous treatment. Renal angiography showed proximal arteriosclerotic renal artery stenoses on both sides, the one on the left being more severe.

Dilatation of the left renal artery stenosis was performed in January 1978, and dilatation of the right artery stenosis in April 1978. We dilated with a Grüntzig-type coaxial balloon catheter system using a balloon catheter of polyvinyl chloride 2 cm long and 6 mm in diameter. Strict additional treatment involving three antihypertensives was necessary. The patient attained borderline hypertension, with blood pressure values that still varied. Five and a half years later the patient had a cerebral stroke on the left side, with hemiparesis on the right which improved partially. The intra-arterial DSA verified a left carotid stenosis which was surgically treated. A DSA of the renal arteries performed at the same time showed recurrence of the stenosis on the left side (Fig. 15.6c).

Personal Case Material

Between January 1978 and August 1984 we diagnosed angiographically 189 renal artery stenoses in 161 patients (Table 15.1). Intra-arterial blood pressure recordings found no gradient in 11 arteries. In 151 patients we used the dilatation technique with double lumen balloon catheters to treat 178 renal artery stenoses. We published our first results together with Lux and Richter in 1980 [22, 34]. There have been numerous reports on renal artery dilatation in patients with renal vascular hypertension in Europe and the United States.

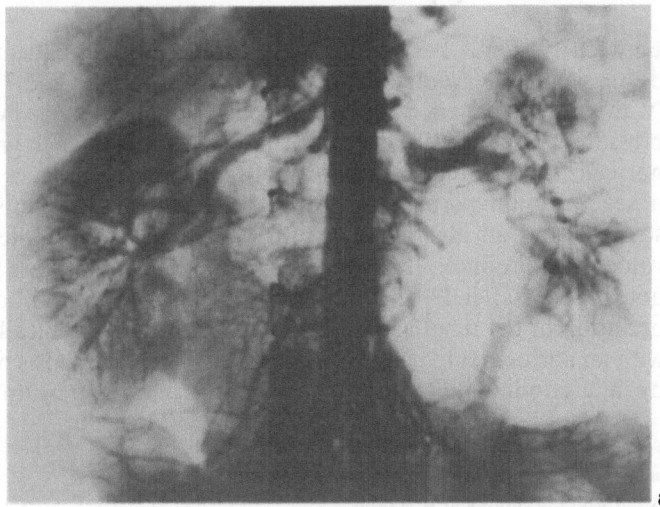

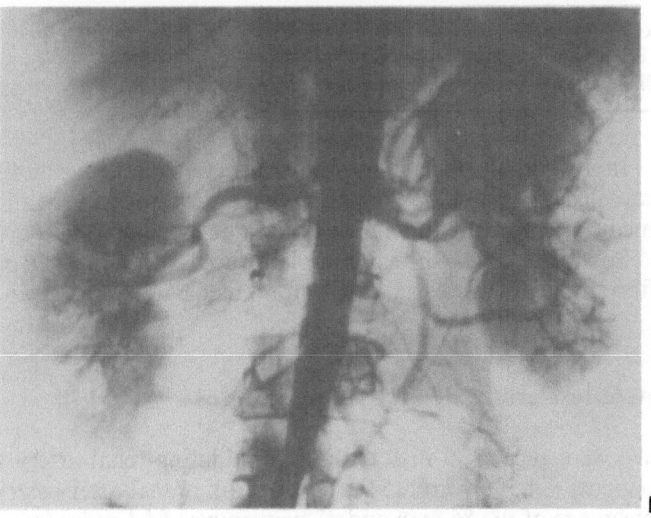

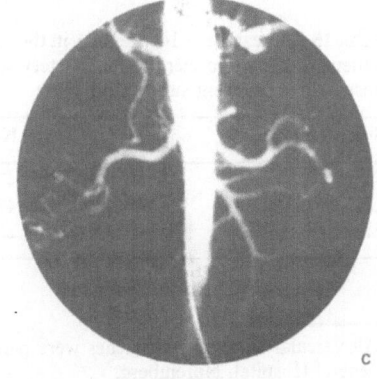

Fig. 15.6a–c. 41-year-old male with excessive arterial hypertension and the risk factors nicotine, overweight, and stress. **a** Angiography prior to PTRD with arteriosclerotic renal artery stenoses on both sides, but more severe on the left. **b** Control angiography of both sides following successful PTRD. **c** Control angiography 5 years and 6 months later, with intra-arterial DSA documenting a recurrence of the stenosis on the left.

Fibromuscular Dysplasia

Between 1978 and 1981 we treated 24 stenoses in 22 patients with fibromuscular dysplasia and an average age of 35.8 years (15 females and 7 males). In 20 patients (with 22 stenoses) good primary success was achieved, as evaluated by a reduced pressure gradient in the region of the stenosis, the angiographic result, and the normalization of blood pressure both with and without a reduced number and dosage of antihypertensives (Table 15.2). In one case the stenosis could not be sounded and an aortorenal bypass was applied. Normotensive blood pressure values were produced. In a second patient a sudden increase in blood pressure was noted 4 days after PTRD and before his discharge from hospital. A thrombotic occlusion of the renal artery was confirmed angiographically. Surgical treatment with an aortorenal bypass was successful.[1] The thrombosis may have been caused by failure to initiate treatment with coumarin or aggregation inhibitors.

Table 15.2. Location of 24 stenoses in 22 patients (age range 18–56 years, mean 35.8 years) with fibromuscular dysplasia

Site of stenosis	No.
Right	13
Left	7
Bilateral	2

In 16 out of 19 patients follow-up controls between 42 and 70 months later revealed normal blood pressure values without medication or with additional medicamentous treatment involving not more than two drugs.

Sos [42–44] has shown complete success in 27 of 31 patients with unilateral fibromuscular dysplasia in whom no medication was given.

Arteriosclerotic Renal Artery Stenoses

We were successful in sounding and dilating renal artery stenoses in 121 of 129 patients (94.5%) with 154 arteriosclerotic renal artery stenoses (Table 15.3). The mean age of the 86 men and 43 women was 54.1 years (age range 39–72 years). In 25 patients we found renal artery stenoses on both sides.

Table 15.3. Location of 146 stenoses in the 121 patients with arteriosclerotic renal artery stenoses who underwent successful PTRD

Site of stenosis	No
Right	47
Left	49
Bilateral	25

---

[1] All vascular surgical approaches were performed by Prof. Dr. Raithel, Dept. of Vascular Surgery, General Hospital, Nuremberg.

In most cases, the systolic pressure gradient in the region of the stenosis could be reduced to 30 mmHg by the first dilatation or, if necessary, by a second dilatation (Table 15.4).

Table 15.4. Pressure gradient (mmHg) before and after PTRD

	Before	After
1st PTRD[a]	125	28
2nd PTRD[b]	98	26

[a] $n = 37$ renal artery stenoses
[b] $n = 7$ renal artery stenoses

In eight patients neither passage of the renal artery stenosis nor mechanical dilatation of the stenosis was feasible. Aortorenal bypasses were only applied in three of these patients who were undergoing dialysis treatment due to age or the stage of renal insufficiency. Two patients suffered from a recurrent stenosis within the first year after a second dilatation. Thus, vascular surgical treatment was required in just 5 of the 129 patients (4%) with arteriosclerotic artery stenoses. In 118 patients undergoing follow-up controls 40–70 months after PTRD the results quoted in Table 15.5 were attained in respect of hypertension. They indicate that 49% of the patients with arteriosclerotic renal artery stenoses remained normotensive and that only in 19% did the blood pressure remain at pre-PTRD levels (regardless of additional antihypertensive treatment).

Table 15.5. Late results (42 months after PTRD) in 118 patients with arteriosclerotic renal artery stenoses

Normotensive	58 (49%)
Improved	37 (32%)
Unchanged	23 (19%)

Complications

Because renal angioplasty is more complex than peripheral angioplasty and the potential complications of renal angioplasty are serious, the procedure should be performed only in hospitals where a skilled vascular surgeon is immediately available. The complication rate following renal angioplasty varies between 5% and 10%. Most of the complications are minor but major complications may be encountered. The most frequent major complication reported in the literature is transient renal insufficiency [47]. The frequency of this complication can be decreased (as we ourselves have found) by performing the diagnostic arteriogram several days prior to the therapeutic procedure and with intravenous DSA at the time of renal blood sampling.

Subintimal dissection by a guide wire or catheter may result when attempting to cross the stenosis. A small intimal flap or an intimal dissection usually heals within 6 weeks. Thrombosis of the renal artery may occur immediately following balloon dilatation if no anticoagulation or aggregation inhibitors are used. The renal artery may be ruptured at the border of an arteriosclerotic focus or at the time of balloon dilatation. This is a rare complication observed only in cases of ostial stenoses. If rupture of the renal artery is noted immediately following deflation of the balloon, the balloon should be reinflated, thus occluding the proximal renal artery, and the patient taken to the operating room immediately.

Before PTRD is performed blood type is ascertained and matched for transfusion.

Distal embolization is an infrequent complication. Spasm or occlusion of arterial branches is usually caused by the tip of the guide wire moving back and forth within the renal artery branches during the procedure. If possible the guide wire should not be placed within the segmental branches of the renal artery. Focal spasm can be prevented by calcium-channel blockers or nitroglycerin. Nifedipine is the most potent vasodilator of the calcium antagonists, and can be given sublingually in a dose of 20 mg. Serapamil may be given parenterally through the arterial catheter at a dose of 2.5–5 mg. Nitroglycerin is either injected directly into the affected renal artery (50–200 mg) or given sublingually in a dose of 0.4–0.6 mg. In addition to the complications at the place of renal angioplasty, complications may occur at the puncture site.

In our own case material we encountered 12 complications in 161 patients (7.5%). Two patients required surgical intervention, and one died 2 days after PTRD and two operations (Table 15.6).

Table 15.6. Details regarding the 12 complications seen in 161 patients who underwent PTRD

1 perforation after dilatation of a renal artery ostial stenosis—vascular surgery → death after 2 operations
1 renal artery perforation 2 cm distal of the ostium—no surgery necessary
2 subintimal dissections—no surgery necessary
4 major arterial spasms
2 intrarenal emboli in segmental arteries
2 large hematomas at puncture site which needed surgery

Results of a Cooperative Study

In May 1982, during the 2nd symposium on PTA in Nuremberg, reports were made on the 2–4 year results following PTRD at 14 different centers [8]. In the total group of 792 patients, normal or ameliorated blood pressure values and reduction of necessary antihypertensives were much more often found in patients with fibromuscular renal artery stenosis than in patients with arteriosclerotic stenosis. Blood pressure was normalized or significantly improved in 78% of the patients with fibromuscular dysplasia and in 57% with arteriosclerotic renal stenosis.

So far these results correspond to the first stage of a treatment procedure in which further advances are to be expected. Better results may be achieved by improved technique [4, 8, 46], selection of optimum balloon catheters, long-term follow-up controls, and additional medicamentous treatment [53] in cooperation with the family doctor. The problem of an optimum additional antihypertensive drug treatment to avoid restenosis (time and dosage of aggregation inhibitors or anticoagulation) has not yet been solved.

A particular advantage of percutaneous dilatation of renal artery stenoses in comparison to vascular surgery is the feasibility of the procedure in patients aged above 45 years (owing to the low risk). It is reasonable to perform PTRD in patients with renal insufficiency and renal stenosis, but one cannot expect the results to be as good as in young patients with fibromuscular dysplasia.

The present outcome shows that the same results may be achieved as with vascular surgery without the risks of an operation and anesthesia [8, 39, 44, 48].

A therapeutic procedure with little risk may cause more frequent use of angiography and especially DSA in patients suffering from increased diastolic blood pressure. This will induce a treatment aiming at complete recovery over and above the excellent possibilities offered by drug therapy in combatting hypertension.

References

1. Arlart IP, Ingrisch H (1984) Renovaskuläre Hypertonie. Thieme, Stuttgart
2. Baert AL, De Somer F, Wilms G, De Maeyer P (1983) Digitale intravenöse Subtraktionsangiographie als Screeningsmethode bei Patienten mit Verdacht auf renovaskuläre Hypertonie. Röntgenblatter
3. Bussmann WD, Dowinsky S, Rummel D, Faßbinder W, Grützmacher P, Starke E, Kaltenbach M, Schoeppe W (1982) Percutaneous transluminal angioplasty in the treatment of renovascular hypertension. In: Kaltenbach M et al. (eds) Transluminal coronary angioplasty and intracoronary thrombolysis. Springer, Berlin Heidelberg New York, pp 431–439
4. Castaneda-Zuniga WR, Formanek A, Tadavarthy M et al. (1980) The mechanisms of balloon angioplasty. Radiology 135:565
5. Colapinto RF, Stronell RD, Harries-Jones EP et al. (1982) Percutaneous transluminal dilatation of the renal artery: Follow-up studies on renovascular hypertension. AJR 135:727–732
6. Crummy AB, Strother CM, Sacket JF, Ergun DL, Shaw CG et al. (1980) Computerized fluoroscopy: Digital subtraction for intravenous angiocardiography and arteriography. AJR 135:1131
7. Dotter CT, Judkins MP (1964) Transluminal treatment of arteriosclerotic obstruction: Description of a new technique and a preliminary report of its application. Circulation 30:654
8. Dotter CT, Grüntzig AR, Schoop W, Zeitler E (eds) (1984) Percutaneous transluminal angioplasty—technique, early and late results. Springer, Berlin Heidelberg New York Tokyo
9. Eigler FW (1970) Operative Behandlung der Hypertonie. MMW 47:2152
10. Geyskes GG, Puijlaert CBAJ, Oei HY, Mees EJD (1983) Follow up study of 70 patients with renal artery stenosis treated by percutaneous transluminal dilatation. Br Med J 287:333–336
11. Greminger P, Kuhlmann U, Vetter W, Grüntzig A, Schneider E, Pouliadis G, Wehling M, Neyses L et al. 1982) Langzeitverläufe nach perkutaner transluminaler Dilatation von Nierenarterienstenosen. VASA 11:362
12. Grüntzig A, Hopff H (1976) Perkutane Rekanalisation chronischer arterieller Verschlüsse mit einem neuen Dilatationskatheter (Dotter-Prinzip). Fortschr Röntgenstr 124:80
13. Grüntzig A, Kuhlmann U, Vetter W, Litolf U, Meier B, Siegenthaler W (1978) Treatment of renovascular hypertension with percutaneous transluminal dilatation of renal artery stenoses. Lancet I:801
14. Ingrisch H, Holzgreve H, Middeke N, Frey KW (1980) Moderne röntgenologische Diagnostik und Therapie des Hochdruckes bei Nierenarterienstenosen. Klin Wochenschr 58:1105

15. Ingrisch H, Frey KW (1980) Diagnostische Angiographie und therapeutische Dilatation von Nierenarterienstenosen in einer Sitzung. Neues radiologisches Vorgehen. Deutscher Röntgenkongreß Köln, May 1980
16. Ingrisch H, Fink U, Leisner B (1982) Röntgenologische und nuklearmedizinische Diagnostik von Nierenarterienstenosen im Hinblick auf deren perkutane transluminale Angioplastie (PTA). Vasa 11:347
17. Ingrisch H, Hegele T, Frey KW (1982) Angiographic control of renal artery stenoses 6 months following percutaneous transluminal angioplasty. Cardiovasc Intervent Radiol 5:249
18. Katzen BT, Chang J, Lukowsky GH, Abramson EG (1979) Percutaneous transluminal angioplasty for treatment of renovascular hypertension. Radiology 131:53
19. Katzen BT, Chang J, Knox WG (1979) Percutaneous transluminal angioplasty with the Grüntzig balloon catheter. A review of 70 cases. Arch Surg 114:1389–1399
20. Kuhlmann U, Grüntzig A, Vetter W, Lütolf U, Meier B, Siegenthaler W (1978) Percutaneous transluminal dilatation: A new treatment of renovascular hypertension? Klin Wochenschr 56:703
21. Löhr E (1983) PTA of renal arteries—PTRD—technique, indication, complication and results. In: Dotter C, Grüntzig A, Schoop W, Zeitler E (eds) Percutaneous transluminal angiopasty. Springer, Berlin Heidelberg New York
22. Lux E, Seybold D, Grosse-Vorholt R, Zeitler E, Gessler U (1980) Perkutane transluminale Katheterdilatation von Nierenarterienstenosen bei Patienten mit renovaskulärer Hypertonie. Fortschr Med 98:563
23. Mahler F, Krneta A, Haertel M (1979) Treatment of renovascular hypertension by transluminal renal artery dilatation. Ann Int Med 90:56
24. Mahler F, Glück Z, Probst P, Weidmann P, Nachbur B (1982) Perkutane transluminale Dilatation von Nierenarterienstenosen. Technik und Resultate. Vasa 11:353
25. Martin EC, Mattern RF, Baer L, Fankuchen EI, Casarella WJ (1981) Renal angioplasty for hypertension: Predictive factors for long term success. AJR 137:921–924
26. Mathias K, Rau W, Kauffmann G (1979) Katheterdilatation einer Arterienstenose nach Nierentransplantation. Dtsch Med Wochenschr 104:437
27. Meaney TF, Weinstein MA, Buonocore E (1980) Digital subtraction angiography of the human cardiovascular system. AJR 135:1153
28. Millan VG, Wetzner SM, Madias NE (1978) Transluminal renal artery dilatation by balloon catheter. RSNA Congress, Chicago, USA, Paper No. 189
29. Mistretta CA, Crummy AB, Strother CM (1981) Digital angiography: A perspective. Radiology 139:273
30. Olbert F, Nell M, Baumruck H (1984) Exposure of physicians and patients to radiation during transluminal dilatation and recanalization according to Dotter. In: Dotter CT, Grüntzig AR, Schoop W, Zeitler E (eds) Percutaneous transluminal angioplasty. Springer, Berlin Heidelberg New York Tokyo, pp 24–25
31. Pereiras RV, Rodrigues A, Videros DC, Materson BJ, Hutson DG, Zamora MT (1978) Percutaneous balloon transluminal angioplasty of stenosis of the renal arteries secondary to fibromuscular dysplasia. RSNA Congress, Chicago, USA, Paper No. 36
32. Puijlaert C (1979) Preliminary report in dilatation of renal artery stenosis in hypertension with the aid of a balloon catheter. J Belge Radiol 62:340
33. Puijlaert C, Boomsma J, Ruijs J, Geyskes G, Franken A, Hoekstra A, Oei H (1981) Transluminal renal artery dilatation in hypertension: Technique, results and complications in 60 cases. Urol Radiol 2:201–210
34. Richter E-I, Grüntzig A, Ingrisch H, Mahler F, Mathias K, Roth F-J, Sörensen A, Zeitler E (1980) Percutaneous dilatation of renal artery stenoses. Ann Radiol (Paris) 23:275
35. Richter E-I, Krönert E, Zeitler E (1983) Technique, indications, complications and results of percutaneous transluminal renal artery dilatation (PTRD). In: Dotter C, Grüntzig A, Schoop W, Zeitler E (eds) Percutaneous transluminal angioplasty. Springer, Berlin Heidelberg New York
36. Richter E-I, Zeitler E (1983) Additional drug treatment at PTA. In: Dotter C, Grüntzig A, Schoop W, Zeitler E (eds) Percutaneous transluminal angioplasty. Springer, Berlin Heidelberg New York
37. Schwarten DE (1980) Percutaneous transluminal angioplasty of renal artery. Cardiovasc Intervent Radiol 2:197
38. Schwarten DE, Yune HY, Klatte EC et al. (1980) Clinical experience with percutaneous transluminal angioplasty (PTA) of stenotic renal arteries. Radiology 135:601
39. Schwarten DE (1981) Percutaneous transluminal renal angioplasty. Urol Radiol 2:193–200
40. Seyferth W, Marhoff P, Zeitler E (1982) Transvenöse und arterielle digitale Videosubtraktionsangiographie (DVSA). Fortschr Röntgenstr 136:301
41. Sniderman KW, Sos TA, Sprayregen S et al. (1980) Percutaneous transluminal angioplasty in renal transplant arterial stenosis for relief of hypertension. Radiology 135:23

42. Sos TA et al. (1983) Percutaneous transluminal renal angioplasty. Int Angiol 2:59
43. Sos TA, Sniederman KW, Pickering T, Vaughan ED Jr, Case D, Laragh JH (1982) Percutaneous transluminal renal angioplasty: Experience in over 100 arteries. In: Kaltenbach M et al. (eds) Transluminal coronary angioplasty and intracoronary thrombolysis. Springer, Berlin Heidelberg New York, pp 412–425
44. Sos TA, Pickering TG, Sniderman K, Saddekni S, Case DB, Silane MF, Vaughan ED, Laragh JH (1983) Beneficial effects of percutaneous transluminal renal angioplasty on blood pressure in patients with renovascular hypertension due to atheroma and fibromuscular dysplasia. N Engl J Med 309:274–279
45. Tegtmeyer CJ, Dyer R, Teates CD et al. (1980) Percutaneous transluminal dilatation of the renal arteries. Techniques and results. Radiology 135:589–599
46. Tegtmeyer CJ, Elson J, Glass TA et al. (1982) Percutaneous transluminal angioplasty: The treatment of choice for renovascular hypertension due to fibromuscular dysplasia. Radiology 143:631–637
47. Tegtmeyer CJ, Kofler TJ, Ayers CA (1984) Renal angioplasty: Current status. AJR 142:17–21
48. Van Dongen RJ (1971) Ergebnisse der Wiederherstellungschirurgie bei renovaskulärem Hochdruck. In: Denck H, Flora G, Hilbe G, Piza F (eds) Renovaskuläre Hypertonie. Verlag Wiener Med Akademie 223
49. Vaughan ED, Bühler FR, Laragh JH et al. (1973) Renovascular hypertension renin measurements to indicate hypersecretion and contralateral suppression, estimate renal plasma flow and score for surgical curability. Am J Med 55:402
50. Vogler E (1974) Radiologische Diagnostik der Harnorgane. Thieme, Stuttgart, p 321
51. Vollmar J (1975) Rekonstruktive Chirurgie der Arterien. Thieme, Stuttgart
52. Zeitler E, Grosse-Vorholt R, Gessler U, Krönert E, Lux E (1982) Percutaneous transluminal dilatation (angioplasty) in renal arteries. In: Kaltenbach M et al. (eds) Transluminal coronary angioplasty and intracoronary thrombolysis. Springer, Berlin Heidelberg New York, pp 426–430
53. Zeitler E (1978) Drug treatment before and after percutaneous transluminal recanalization (PTR). In: Zeitler E, Grüntzig A, Schoop W (eds) Percutaneous vascular recanalization. Springer, Berlin Heidelberg New York, p 73
54. Zollikofer C, Castaneda-Zuniga WR, Amplatz K (1983) Results of animal experiments with balloon dilatation. In: Dotter CT, Grüntzig A, Schoop W, Zeitler E (eds) Percutaneous transluminal angioplasty. Springer, Berlin Heidelberg New York

Chapter 16

Endourology for Trauma

William G. Guerriero

Introduction

Endourology is visualization of the urinary tract for diagnosis and treatment using high-quality optics and miniaturized manipulative nephroscopic instruments. Endourology for the treatment of urologic trauma is performed rarely, except for the management of renal bleeding and arteriovenous fistula. Until 1977 few cases of percutaneous access to the kidney had even been recorded. Since then, thousands of nephrostomies have been inserted percutaneously and manipulation of stones, tumors, and strictures of the upper urinary tract has become common.

Angiography predates percutaneous access by at least 10 years, and vascular manipulative procedures for the treatment of sequelae of urologic trauma are much more common than percutaneous manipulative procedures. In the management of trauma, angiographic catheters are used to provide diagnostic radiographs of the kidney and to establish the extent of renal injury or to identify renal pseudoaneurysms, areas of devascularization, and arteriovenous fistulas. Computed tomography has recently been used to define the extent of injury in kidneys injured with blunt trauma, but has not, at present, superseded arteriography, rather being a complementary technique. The definitive study for renal trauma remains selective renal arteriogram.

Renal injuries may be classified as penetrating or secondary to blunt trauma. They also may be separated into major and minor categories as illustrated in Figs. 16.1 and 16.2. Minor injuries are those injuries which will heal without surgical intervention and do not carry a risk of morbidity to the patient. Over 80% of injuries to the kidney fall into this category. As can be seen in Fig. 16.1, minor renal injuries are renal contusion, shallow cortical laceration, and forniceal disruption. Regardless of treatment of these injuries, the patient will not develop sequelae such as hypertension, and to my knowledge no case of arteriovenous malformation or cortical damage significant enough to impair renal function has occurred as a result of renal contusion.

Major renal injuries may heal without treatment but carry a significant risk of morbidity. They consist of deep cortical laceration into the medulla of the kidney

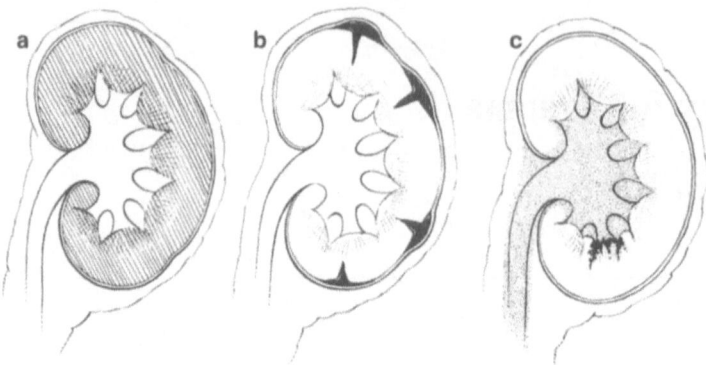

Fig. 16.1a–c. Classification of renal trauma: minor injury. **a** contusion of the kidney; **b** shallow cortical laceration; **c** forniceal disruption.

with or without extravasation and with or without displaced fragments. Displacement of fragments from a cortical laceration significantly increases the possibility that these injuries will necessitate surgery as the hematoma is poorly contained within Gerota's fascia. For this reason, these injuries should be separated from nondisplaced cortical lacerations to emphasize their risk to the patient. Multiple deep cortical lacerations or shattered kidney is a serious risk to the patient but is particularly worrisome if the fragments are not contained. Vascular injuries to the kidney, such as renal pedicle injury, are a threat to the patient's life if bilateral and

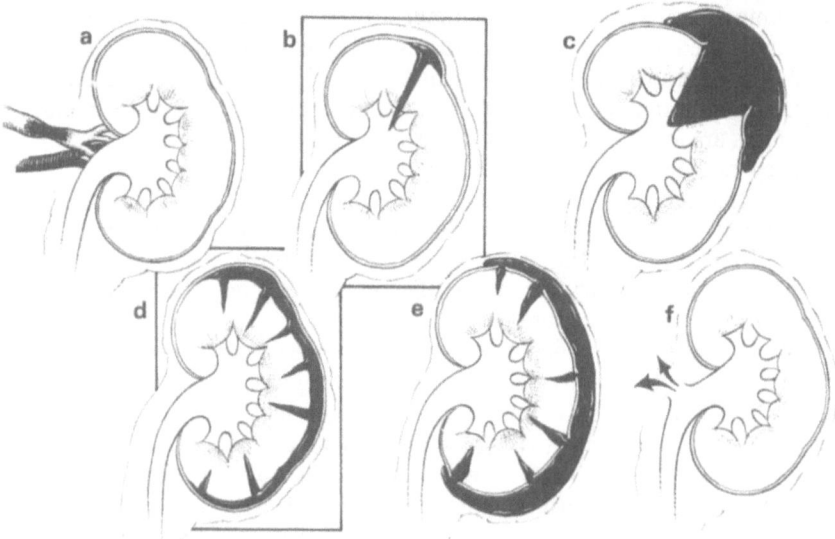

Fig. 16.2a–f. Classification of renal trauma: major injury. **a** renal pedicle injury; **b** deep laceration (into medulla) with contained fragment; **c** deep laceration with disrupted fragments; **d** multiple lacerations (shattered kidney) with contained fragments; **e** multiple lacerations (shattered kidney) with disrupted fragment; **f** collecting system injury.

a risk to renal function if unilateral. These injuries may be discovered only with angiography, and any evidence of poor functioning of the kidney or nonfunction of the kidney by intravenous pyelogram or scan should be an indication for immediate arteriography. Arteriovenous malformation and renal pseudoaneurysm occur in any kidney which is injured severely, particularly in those instances in which there is a deep laceration through the cortex of the kidney. Though arteriovenous fistula might occur with a shallow cortical laceration, I personally have never seen such a case.

Injury to the collecting system, such as rupture of the renal pelvis or avulsion at the ureteropelvic junction, is not uncommon with blunt trauma or penetrating injury to the kidney. When injuries to the collecting system occur as a result of external violence, surgical treatment is mandatory, though in the near future I would not be surprised to see a series of cases in the literature managed with percutaneous nephrostomy and stent.

Associated organ injury is common with major renal injury and this must be kept in mind in the management of these conditions.

Definition of the extent of injury is mandatory before a patient may be selected for expectant treatment and before surgical or endourologic treatment can be planned. This is particularly true in the case of blunt renal trauma, where there may be little external sign of injury. Radiographic studies such as intravenous pyelogram with tomography should be performed in all patients with suspected renal trauma. If this study does not adequately define the nature of the patient's injury, an arteriogram and/or computed tomography would be indicated. Ultrasound does not offer much in the evaluation of renal trauma except for following the status of hematomas. Most patients who have significant renal trauma will also have ileus after ingesting large amounts of food and sometimes alcoholic beverages prior to injury. Ileus and poor preparation markedly decrease the quality of renal ultrasound.

All gunshot wounds and anterior stab wounds are explored in our institution, and except for arteriovenous fistulas which might develop in the healing period, the extent of renal damage may be defined at the time of surgery. Flank and posterior stab wounds are followed closely with ultrasound and physical examination if the initial intravenous pyelogram is normal, i.e., without extravasation and with intact renal outlines and good visualization of the collecting system. If a major renal injury is suspected after a posterior or flank stab wound, the patient undergoes a CT scan or an arteriogram to define the extent of injury, or surgical exploration if he is unstable.

Arteriovenous Fistula

Arteriovenous fistula or renal pseudoaneurysm is rarely discovered at the time of the initial evaluation of the patient for trauma unless the patient has a renal arteriogram. Suspicion of renal injuries of this type should occur if the patient has persistent gross hematuria or develops an abdominal bruit, which occurs in 75% of cases [4], or develops hypertension, high output heart failure, or an enlarging heart with no obvious cause. A mass in the flank as the result of an arteriovenous fistula or renal pseudoaneurysm is very uncommon. Areas of poor function may, however, be seen on renal scan, which would give some clue as to the presence of fistula. Arteriovenous fisula may become clinically significant at any time post-injury, but is usually discovered within the first year.

To recognize an arteriovenous fistula, one must be suspicious and observe the patient closely. One should remember that one-third of patients will have hypertension or significant hematuria. A blood pressure recording should be made every 3 months for 2 years after significant renal injury. Since one-half of these patients will eventually develop cardiomegaly, a chest X-ray is indicated at least yearly. Of most importance is continued auscultation of the costovertebral angle, as with significant fistula most of these patients will have a bruit. If arteriovenous fistula is suspected, a renal arteriogram must be performed to make the diagnosis.

Arteriovenous fistulas may be congenital or seen with renal carcinoma. They may be idiopathic or acquired. Congenital fistulas are cirsoid in appearance and usually are multiple and interconnecting. Idiopathic fistulas are single, as are acquired fistulas. Acquired fistulas may occur after a surgical procedure on the kidney, such as partial nephrectomy or open renal biopsy, or after blunt or penetrating trauma. The vast majority of acquired fistulas described in the literature are secondary to needle biopsy of the kidney.

Eighteen percent of patients who underwent needle biopsy of the kidney had arteriovenous fistula in Tynes' series [8], but 95% of needle biopsy fistulas healed spontaneously in 3–30 months in Maldonado's series [6], and 20 of 24 fistulas closed spontaneously in McAlhany's series [7].

Criteria for intervention in cases of arteriovenous fistula have not been developed [3] but most authors agree that asymptomatic fistulas should be followed expectantly. Since 75% of these fistulas have bruits, auscultation of the costovertebral angle area, frequent blood pressure determination, and renal function tests are indicated. Arteriograms are expensive and may cause morbidity, and should therefore be performed only if the patient develops signs or symptoms that would suggest that treatment is necessary or to confirm that the fistula has gone 2–3 years post-biopsy.

Suggested criteria for surgical or endourologic intervention include persistent gross hematuria with pain or repeated transfusion, severe hypertension not easily controllable with medication, enlargement of the heart and heart failure, decreasing renal function, and expanding perirenal hematoma [4].

Numerous agents have been used to embolize the kidney, including oxidized cellulose, muscle, silicone beads, absorbable gelatin sponge, wool-wrapped steel coil, Ivalon, silicone balloons, and autologous clot [10].

Autologous clot is particularly attractive as an embolic particulate as most of these fistulas are peripheral, and it is difficult to minimize the amount of renal cortex made ischemic by the embolus. Lysis of the clot occurs rapidly in normal blood vessels but not as promptly in the fistula. Thus, even though repeated embolizations may be necessary, renal function is less likely to be impaired permanently with autologous clot embolization (Figs. 16.3, 16.4). Also, passage of the clot through the fistula is less serious than if a poorly absorbable material such as gelatin is used [5].

Clot does not work well in large fistulas. For lesions of this type, the Gianturco stainless steel coil, which comes in various sizes, is appropriate. This coil can be placed from the arterial or venous side and has been particularly helpful for fistulas secondary to tumor and for congenital fistulas [9]. The coil should be matched with the vessel to form a compact plug. The coil is placed as far into the fistula as

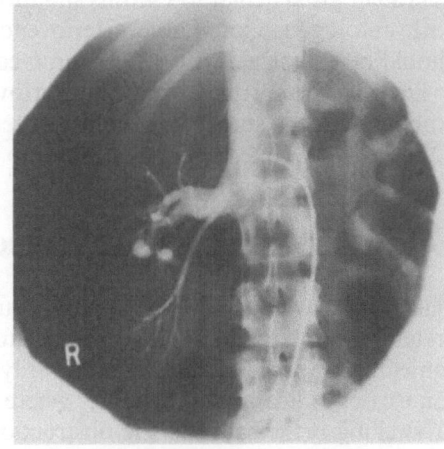

Fig. 16.3. Arteriogram showing post-traumatic arteriovenous fistula.

possible to minimize cortical ischemia. Controlled release of the coil allows for its retrieval if placement is not optimal.

Rarely nephrectomy or partial nephrectomy may be needed with large needle biopsy fistulas. This is a disaster as almost all of these patients have glomerulo-nephritis, amyloidosis, or collagen diseases that make any loss of functional renal parenchyma intolerable.

Arteriovenous fistula which is a result of trauma may also close spontaneously [3], but usually these fistulas are associated with other major renal injury, such as deep cortical laceration or shattered kidney; such patients have a high incidence of nephrectomy and partial nephrectomy. Cosgrove [2] has reported that stab wounds with fistula usually require an operative procedure for cure. Angorn [1], however, had three of eight stab wound fistulas close spontaneously.

It would be best to consider each case of traumatic arteriovenous fistula separately. If the fistula is small and not associated with other indications for surgery, such as deep cortical laceration with a displaced fragment or falling hematocrit and expanding hematoma, one should treat the patient expectantly.

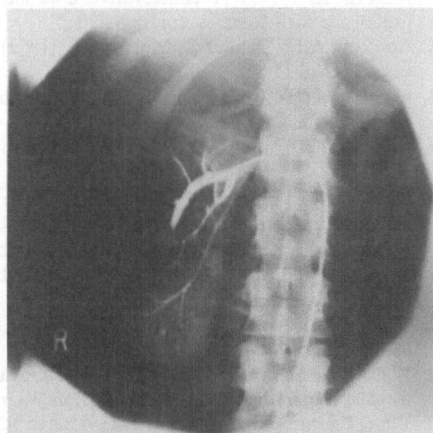

Fig. 16.4. Arteriogram showing arteriovenous fistula postembolization with autologous blood clot.

Persistent gross hematuria in this situation may be an indication for embolization with autologous clot. Large arteriovenous fistulas probably will not close and should be embolized with a Gianturco coil.

External hemorrhage and/or arteriovenous fistula may be controlled with embolization but surgery is usually a necessary and safer alternative when bleeding is not into the collecting system but into the flank.

Other Endourologic Techniques for Trauma

Placement of a nephrostomy percutaneously when there is late discovery of lower ureteral injury and attempts to pass a ureteral stent in an antegrade fashion may sometimes be successful, thus temporarily avoiding an open surgical procedure. In some cases of ligation of the ureter where absorbable suture or a pelvic hematoma or swelling is the cause of the obstruction to the ureter, the condition may cure itself spontaneously, though one should remember that this does not happen in most cases.

Nephrostomy is also indicated in cases of vesicovaginal fistula, and again, an attempt should be made to pass a stent across the fistula site in an antegrade fashion to promote healing.

One of the by-products of endourologic surgery for stones has been the realization that inadvertent traumatic perforation of the collecting system or kidney is not usually a serious complication as long as the kidney is drained with a nephrostomy tube. Whether or not arteriovenous fistulas or ureteral strictures will occur with these techniques is not known as enough cases have not been followed long enough to determine whether perforation of the kidney for placement of a nephrostomy tube or dilatation of the ureter, ureteroscopy, and extraction of stones will lead to complications. Endoscopic procedures for trauma are in their infancy. Perhaps other techniques will soon be developed to benefit the trauma patient.

References

 1. Angorn IB (1977) A conservative approach to traumatic intrarenal arteriovenous fistulae: experience with 13 cases. Injury 8:290
 2. Cosgrove MD, Mendez R, Morrow JW (1973) Traumatic renal arteriovenous fistula: report of 12 cases. J Urol 110:627
 3. Halpern M (1969) Spontaneous closure of traumatic renal arteriovenous fistulas. Am J Roentgenol 107:730
 4. Iloreta AT, Blaufox MD (1979) Natural history of post-biopsy renal arteriovenous fistula: a 10-year follow-up. Nephron 24:250–253
 5. Kaufman SL, Freeman C, Busky SM, White RI Jr (1976) Management of postoperative renal hemorrhage by transcatheter embolization. J Urol 115:203
 6. Maldonado JE, Sheps SG (1966) Renal arteriovenous fistula. Postgrad Med 46:263
 7. McAlhany JC, Black HC, Hanback LD, Yarbrough DR (1971) Renal arteriovenous fistula as a cause of hypertension. Am J Surg 122:117
 8. Tynes WV, Devine CJ Jr, Devine PC, Poutasse EF (1970) Surgical treatment of renal arteriovenous fistulas: report of 5 cases. J Urol 103:692–698
 9. Wallace S, Schwarten DE, Smith DC, Gerson LP, Davis LJ (1978) Intrarenal arteriovenous fistulas: transcatheter steel coil occlusion. J Urol 120:282
10. White RI, Strandberg JV, Gross GS, Barth KH (1977) Therapeutic embolization with long-term occluding agents and their effects on embolized tissues. Radiology 125:677

Chapter 17

Renal Neoplasms

Milton Elkin, Helen T. Morehouse, and
Janet C. Hoffman-Tretin

Introduction

This chapter will deal with the radiology of malignant renal neoplasms in adult patients, with prime attention being paid to the more common types and their chief differential diagnostic considerations. The burgeoning technologies of diagnostic radiology have made possible the accumulation of many findings regarding renal neoplasm, which, when considered together, permit greater specificity in diagnosis. However, the approach to diagnosis is not to gather the most data possible, but rather to proceed with data accumulation in a planned, orderly way so as to reach a level of diagnostic confidence that will result in proper patient management. It is upon the basis of such a structure that this chapter has been devised. Going under the name of decision trees or algorithms, the method is simply the use of the available technologies in a sequence that depends not only on the initial clinical presentation that suggested the possibility of renal neoplasm but also the results of radiologic examinations already done, factoring in considerations concerning the costs of the technologies. Costs are not only financial but also the patient risks.

Classification

In the adult, adenocarcinoma of the parenchyma and transitional cell carcinoma of the urothelium make up over 95% of primary renal malignant neoplasms, with the parenchymal tumor being about 5 to 6 times more common than that of the pelvicalyceal mucosa. Renal lymphoma as well as metastases to the kidney from remote sites will also receive attention in our discussion. Only passing reference will be made to the rare tumors, such as Wilms' tumor in the adult patient, sarcoma of the renal capsule, and sarcoma of the renal parenchyma. Agreement is not yet universal that oncocytoma qualifies as a distinct renal neoplasm and, if so, whether it is always benign or only usually benign; this is of enough interest to warrant our consideration.

Renal Cell Carcinoma

Renal cell carcinoma is an adenocarcinoma originating from the epithelium of the renal tubules. It accounts for about 80%–85% of all primary renal malignancies in the adult. Median patient age at the time of diagnosis is 55–60 years, with a wide range, the neoplasm occurring infrequently in young adults and even children. Lieber et al., in a review of 3768 cases of renal adenocarcinoma treated at the Mayo Clinic, reported that 3.5% occurred in patients from 20 to 40 years old [48]. For patients of all ages the 5-year survival rate has been reported as 40%–45% and the 10-year rate as 25%–30%. Patients in the 20- to 40-year-old age group have similar survival rates. Renal cell carcinoma is twice as common in men as in women. The prognosis is reportedly more favorable in women than men, with a 55% 5-year survival for women as compared with 44% for men [48]. The neoplasm usually appears as a distinct solid renal mass with abundant vascularity and sometimes with a pseudocapsule. Areas of necrosis and hemorrhage contribute to its multicolored cut surface. Its histologic composition is that of solid collections of neoplastic cells with granular cytoplasm or clear cytoplasm, the proportions of granular cells or clear cells having no prognostic significance. About 10%–15% of renal adenocarcinomas are of the papillary–tubular type, showing tubular and papillary histologic configurations. These tumors are usually hypovascular.

Rarely, renal adenocarcinoma contains neoplastic spindle cells; such lesions are referred to as sarcomatoid renal cell carcinoma or spindle cell renal cell carcinoma. These tumors are less vascular and more infiltrative than the usual renal adenocarcinomas.

Infrequently (in less than 5% of cases) renal cell carcinoma presents grossly as an atypical cyst, i.e., thick-walled with fluid content which is usually hemorrhagic but sometimes clear. Varied mechanisms of development have been ascribed to these cystic carcinomas. Very likely most represent a late result of necrosis of the renal neoplasm. Some have probably begun histologically as malignant neoplasms with cystic spaces and have continued to develop as a cystic mass. The third type, the secondary development of adenocarcinoma in the epithelial lining of a simple renal cyst, is very rare.

Calcification, mottled or in plaques, can occur in any of the types of renal adenocarcinoma and does so overall in probably 10%–15%. The presence of calcification has in some reported series indicated improved patient survival and in others a worse prognosis. The evidence is not clear-cut either way.

Renal adenocarcinoma is prone to extend directly into intrarenal veins and grow as a tumor thrombus in the main renal vein and then into the inferior vena cava. Inasmuch as the right renal vein is much shorter than the left renal vein, involvement of the inferior vena cava by tumor is more common in lesions of the right kidney than in those of the left. Metastases occur most commonly to lungs, lymph nodes, bone, adrenals, and liver [28].

Transitional Cell Carcinoma

Transitional cell carcinoma, arising in the epithelium of the pelvicalyceal system, makes up about 12%–15% of primary malignant renal tumors in the adult. Most often they are discovered in patients older than 60 years, with a male–female ratio of 2:1 [71]. The neoplasm usually first appears as a polypoid growth protruding into the pelvicalyceal cavity; infrequently it grows as an irregular, spreading sheet of solid neoplasm in the mucosa, simulating inflammatory changes of the mucosa.

With involvement of the renal parenchyma, the neoplasm infiltrates the kidney substance, often widely, and with little change in the renal contour, an appearance quite different from the mass of an adenocarcinoma. Calcification occurs only rarely. Transitional cell carcinoma can invade the renal vein and the inferior vena cava, although it does so less frequently than renal adenocarcinoma.

It is important to remember that urinary tract transitional cell carcinoma is a multicentric lesion, presenting synchronously or metachronously in about one-third of the patients. During the diagnostic workup of the renal tumor, attention must be given to the possibility of involvement of other parts of the urinary tract. Similarly, in a patient who has been treated for transitional cell carcinoma of the bladder, even by total cystectomy, follow-up care should include consideration of the possibility of renal involvement, even though this is infrequent. Also, of those patients in whom the neoplasm of the renal pelvis has been treated by nephrectomy and subtotal ureterectomy, about 15% will later show evidence of transitional cell carcinoma of the ureteral stump.

Lymphoma

Most likely lymphoma does not originate in the kidney but is brought there by hematogenous or possibly lymphatic dissemination from a primary site elsewhere or by direct invasion of the kidney from adjacent, involved lymph nodes. Bilaterality is common. Lymphoma can occur as a single localized mass within the kidney, as a mass involving practically the entire kidney, as a mass extending directly into the kidney from nearby lymph nodes, or, commonly, as multiple lymphomatous nodules of varying size in the kidney. In some patients with disseminated lymphoma, renal involvement is only microscopic.

Calcification is rare in untreated lymphoma, but does appear occasionally after treatment by drugs and/or irradiation. Renal lymphoma is hypovascular, usually shows no necrosis, and does not tend to extend into the lumen of the renal vein or inferior vena cava.

Metastasis to the Kidney

Statistics from autopsy studies show that metastases to the kidney occur more commonly than do primary renal malignancies. However, this is not the clinical experience, because patients with widespread metastatic disease are understandably not studied specifically for deposits in the kidneys.

Primary sites are very variable, lung and breast being most common. Autopsy studies show that with renal metastases both kidneys are involved in about 50% of cases. A metastasis may appear as a distinct renal mass or it may be infiltrative, bearing a radiologic resemblance to lymphoma, transitional cell carcinoma invading the parenchyma, or sarcomatoid renal cell carcinoma. It was once believed that metastases to the kidney do not extend into the lumen of the renal vein; however, several instances of such extension have occurred in our experience.

Uncommon Renal Malignancies

Wilms' tumor occurs primarily in children under 10 years of age. The term adult-type Wilms' tumor is used for patients older than 15 years. A review of 35 documented instances of adult Wilms' tumor showed an average age of 40 years and a median age of 33 years [35]. Clinical presentation usually suggests renal cell carcinoma, as do the radiologic findings, although the vascularity of the Wilms' tumor is different from that of the usual adenocarcinoma. In Wilms' tumor the arteries are thin, stretched, and well-defined, without the marked variability in size, hypervascularity, and arteriovenous shunting of the usual adenocarcinoma.

Sarcomas of the renal capsule occur chiefly in the elderly, are often large at the time of discovery, and can go on to grow to an enormous size, usually containing zones of necrosis and myxomatous degeneration. They often appear encapsulated and are thus surgically removable despite their large size. Unfortunately, the presence of a capsule does not indicate a good prognosis; most patients succumb to the disease within a few years of diagnosis. The distinctive pathologic features which allow a radiologic diagnosis are (a) the neoplasm surrounds and deforms, but does not invade the kidney and (b) the blood supply to the tumor is by way of capsular vessels rather than intrarenal arteries.

Sarcomas of the renal parenchyma are very rare; they include such histologic types as leiomyosarcoma, fibrosarcoma, liposarcoma, and even primary osteogenic sarcoma. They are usually infiltrative and their vascularity is usually less profuse than that of the typical adenocarcinoma. Liposarcoma contains fatty elements. Osteogenic sarcoma contains bone.

Squamous cell carcinoma of the pelvicalyceal system is an infrequent, highly aggressive malignancy arising from metaplasia of the pelvic mucosa secondary most often to the irritation of calculi or infection. By the time of diagnosis, the neoplasm has usually involved the renal parenchyma and extrarenal tissues.

Oncocytoma

There is no agreement among pathologists as to the entity of renal oncocytoma. Some consider reported cases of renal oncocytoma to represent adenocarcinomas of low malignancy.

Renal oncocytoma is described as a specific type of well-defined, benign adenoma consisting of a homogeneous cell type, oncocytes [37]. Oncocytes, believed to originate from proximal tubular cells, are eosinophilic epithelial cells, arranged in tubular and alveolar patterns. Grossly, oncocytomas are uniformly tan in color without hemorrhage or necrosis.

Symptoms and Signs

The triad of hematuria (gross or microscopic), flank pain, and abdominal or flank mass are commonly offered as pointers toward renal malignancy. However, less than 15% of patients with such malignancy have all the elements of the triad at the time of presentation. Any one of the three in itself should stimulate the consideration of renal neoplasm.

The discovery of a metastasis elsewhere, e.g., lung, liver, or brain, with appropriate histologic appearance can trigger the search for a primary renal tumor.

Abdominal radiography or intravenous urography done for an unrelated reason, e.g., workup of benign prostatic hypertrophy, trauma, hypertension, or urinary tract infection, may disclose an abnormality that suggests the possibility of renal malignancy. Such abnormalities include renal mass, parenchymal calcification, pelvicalyceal filling defect, obstruction of all or part of the pelvicalyceal system, and nonexcretion of contrast medium in the absence of a known cause. Similarly, an ultrasonographic examination or a CT scan of the abdomen done for an unrelated reason may disclose renal mass, calcification, or obstruction.

Radiologic Diagnostic Evaluation

Intravenous Urography

Most often the initial radiologic study in the workup of a possible renal neoplasm is intravenous urography including tomography.

Renal Mass

The finding of a renal mass suggests a number of possibilities, the most common including neoplasm, cyst, inflammatory process (such as lobar nephronia, abscess, and tuberculoma), hypertrophy of a renal column (septum of Bertin), obstructed duplicated collecting system (usually the upper segment of a duplex system), and angiomyolipoma.

The presence of calcification, clumped or mottled, within the mass strengthens the possibility of malignant neoplasm, although this finding also occurs often in tuberculoma and infrequently in adenoma, angiomyolipoma, and chronic infection, e.g., xanthogranulomatous pyelonephritis. Curvilinear calcification within the mass also favors the diagnosis of neoplasm. A smooth, thin, complete or incomplete rim of calcification at the periphery of the mass suggests the diagnosis of cyst, but in about 20% of patients with this finding, the lesion turns out to be renal parenchymal carcinoma. If the calcific rim is thick or clumped, renal cancer is the most likely diagnosis, although renal cysts, especially if infected or hemorrhagic, can have this appearance.

Calyceal amputation, irregular destruction of calyces, and irregular extravasation of contrast medium into the mass are other urographic signs for the diagnosis of renal carcinoma.

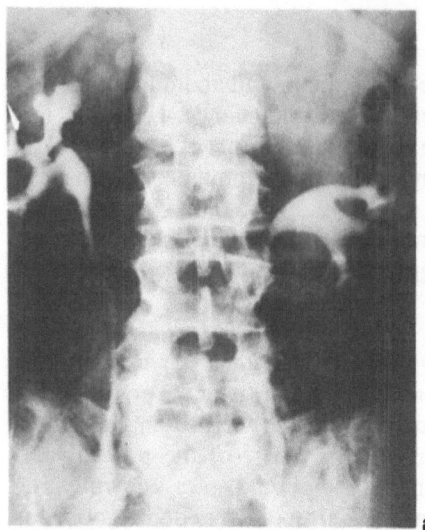

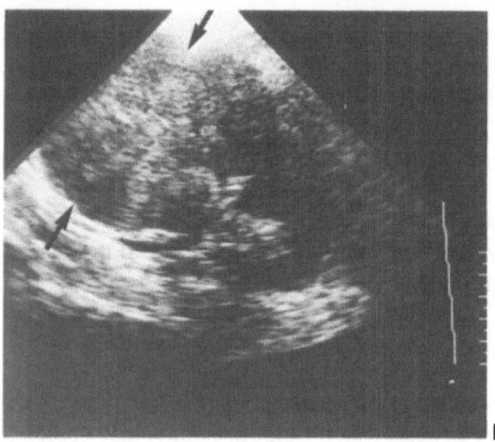

Fig. 17.1a,b. Renal cell carcinoma of upper pole. A 60-year-old woman presented with one episode of painless, gross hematuria. a Intravenous urogram shows inferior and lateral displacement of the left renal collecting system, simulating the drooping lily appearance associated with hydronephrosis of the upper segment of a duplex pelvis. Note, however, that the left ureter is not deviated. b Coronal sonogram of the left kidney demonstrates a moderately echogenic solid mass (*arrows*) of the upper pole.

Clinical evidence of infection, such as fever, pyuria, and bacteriuria, favors the possibility of abscess, either in the stage of induration (lobar nephronia) or frank liquefaction. Tuberculoma large enough to present as a gross renal mass is unusual; in such a case, the presence of associated evidence of urinary tract tuberculosis, such as pelvicalyceal strictures, ureteral strictures, and a small, thick-walled urinary bladder, would suggest the correct diagnosis.

The mass effect of hypertrophy of a renal column causes spreading of the calyceal system, most commonly between the upper and middle groups of calyces, without evidence of calyceal amputation or destruction and without protrusion of the renal contour.

Hydronephrosis of the upper segment of a duplex pelvis appears as a mass of the upper pole of the kidney, typically with a drooping lily appearance of the pelvicalyceal system of the lower segment. An important additional radiologic sign is the deviation, usually laterally, of the opacified orthotopic ureter being displaced by the nonopacified, dilated ectopic ureter. A solid upper pole renal mass can on occasion produce a urographic appearance simulating that of an upper segment hydronephrosis (Fig. 17.1).

If an angiomyolipoma contains large amounts of fat, the areas of lucency may be discernible on the scout film or on the tomograms, suggesting the diagnosis of hamartoma. Otherwise, there are no urographic findings to distinguish the mass from that of a renal neoplasm.

Typically, the mass of a renal cyst is smoothly rounded with a well defined smooth interface between the relatively lucent cyst and the relatively radiodense nephrogram of renal parenchyma, as seen best on the tomograms during urography. Lobulation of the mass suggests a solid lesion rather than a cyst. However, differentiation of cyst from neoplasm is usually impossible on the urographic study.

Pelvicalyceal Filling Defect

The urographic finding of a fixed, irregular, soft-tissue filling defect in the pelvicalyceal system suggests transitional cell carcinoma. The chief differential possibilities include nonopaque calculus or calculi, extruded ischemic pyramid tissue in papillary necrosis, blood clot, extension of a parenchymal neoplasm (renal cell carcinoma) into the calyceal system, and fungus ball. Nonopaque calculus or extruded ischemic pyramid tissue often moves with change in position of the patient, and the borders of the filling defect are sharp, sometimes angular. However, the various pelvicalyceal defects may be quite similar, without clear urographic differentiation. Sometimes transitional cell carcinoma carpets the mucosal surface irregularly, simulating inflammatory disease, or produces relatively smooth luminal narrowings simulating fibrotic strictures.

Generalized Renal Enlargement

Infiltrative renal neoplasm may involve practically the entire renal parenchyma without formation of a discrete renal mass. This occurs most commonly with sarcomatoid renal cell carcinoma, lymphoma, and transitional cell carcinoma invading the renal parenchyma. In such cases, urography may show no excretion of contrast medium. The differential possibilities include renal vein thrombosis and acute bacterial nephritis.

Hydronephrosis

Generalized or segmental hydronephrosis can result from a neoplasm, secondary to obstruction from intraluminal transitional cell carcinoma or from luminal narrowing or distortion due to neoplasm of the parenchyma. In such cases, the differential possibilities include calculus disease, ureteropelvic junction abnormality, and inflammatory stricture.

"Nonfunction"

Lack of any contrast medium excretion at the time of urography can infrequently be secondary to renal neoplasm, as with widespread replacement of renal parenchyma by tumor, with urography offering minimal specific help as to the cause.

The differential possibilities are many, including renal artery abnormality (e.g., embolus), congenital anomaly (e.g., dysplasia), and infection (e.g., pyonephrosis).

Normal Urography

The neoplasm may be so small or its effects on the pelvicalyceal system or renal contour so subtle that the urographic abnormalities are overlooked. Thus, despite negative urography, radiologic investigation should continue if there is a strong clinical suspicion of neoplasm.

Retrograde Pyelography

Retrograde pyelography is done to better delineate pelvicalyceal lesions suspected on urography or to clarify incomplete visualization of the renal collecting system at urography.

Complications of retrograde pyelography have included sepsis, pyelonephritis, ureteral obstruction secondary to edema or spasm, and injury, usually minor, to the ureter and renal tissues. The risk of the procedure is increased in the presence of urinary tract infection. Absorption of contrast medium by the urothelium may also theoretically precipitate a hypersensitivity reaction [66].

Ultrasonography

General Principles

Medical sonography is an imaging modality in which the variable interactions of high frequency sound waves with tissues and biological fluids can be used to create a tomographic representation of internal anatomy. Sound is a mechanical wave form which transmits energy by changes in the acoustic variables of pressure, density, temperature, and particle motion along a given linear path. In medical usage, short pulses of sound energy with a frequency of approximately 1–10 MHz are transmitted into the patient by a transducer which also serves as a receptor of reflected acoustic signals. Within the body the sound may be transmitted, attenuated (absorbed or scattered), or reflected, depending upon the density and elastic properties of the tissues through which it passes as well as the acoustic interfaces it encounters. An acoustic interface is a boundary between two substances of different acoustic properties. The acoustic signals returning to the sonographic transducer can be processed and presented in various modes. A B-mode or two-dimensional image is created as the transducer is swept over the skin surface; there is a built-in assumption of a constant speed of sound in soft tissue. The time for transmission and reflection (round trip of the sound pulse) is correlated with depth from the transducer face.

The sonographic image is influenced not only by the acoustic properties of tissues but also by the frequency of wavelength of the sound and the width of the sonographic beam. The axial resolution, the resolution along the linear path of the sound beam, improves as the wavelength decreases and the number of cycles in the ultrasound pulse (or the frequency) increases. However, as frequency increases, attenuation of the sound beam also increases, diminishing the range of penetration. The lateral resolution, the resolution along an axis perpendicular to the direction of the sound beam, improves as the width of the sound beam decreases. In most ultrasound transducers the sound beam is focused so that its natural divergence is delayed for some distance beyond the transducer face. Lateral resolution is best in the narrowest portion (focal zone) of the sound beam.

The acoustic signals returning to the transducer face are differentially amplified by a manually adjusted "time gain compensation curve" to compensate for progressive normal attenuation as the sound penetrates a greater depth of soft tissue. Another "gain" or amplification control also allows uniform enhancement of the entire image [16, 39].

In addition to the static two-dimensional B-mode image produced by an articulated arm scanner, "real-time" sonographic units can produce a pie-shaped or rectangular moving display of two-dimensional anatomy. This is accomplished by continuously updating the two-dimensional sonographic image at a frame rate consistent with visual perception of motion. Real-time scanning has the basic advantages of portability, ease of transducer positioning, display of motion in anatomic structures, and reduced technical expertise required in operation. The resolution of current real-time units is comparable to that of the static imager [16, 39, 67].

The major features of intrarenal anatomy demonstrated by sonography are the cortex, medulla, and renal sinus. The renal cortex is normally characterized by homogeneous, low-level echoes. The renal medullary pyramids are echo-poor, triangular structures arranged in a spoke-wheel distribution just peripheral to the intensely echogenic renal sinus. Normal variations in the contour and thickness of the renal parenchyma (e.g., prominent septum of Bertin) may simulate an abnormality.

Renal Mass

Sonography of a renal mass is commonly done after its initial demonstration by intravenous urography. The role of sonography is not only to distinguish cystic and solid lesions, but also (a) to identify atypical cysts or cystic tumors requiring further evaluation, (b) to suggest, where possible, histologic diagnosis (angiomyolipoma, multilocular cysts), (c) to provide staging information for malignant tumors, and (d) to suggest the presence of a pseudotumor. Additional indications prompting sonography of a renal tumor include a palpable flank mass, abnormal renal axis on intravenous urography, nonvisualization of a kidney on intravenous urography, screening for a renal mass in a patient in whom radiographic contrast medium is contraindicated, or screening for an occult malignancy.

In selected instances some authors [34] have advocated the use of sonography or computed tomography in patients with hematuria in whom intravenous urography is normal. A renal mass is also occasionally detected as an incidental finding on sonographic examination for an unrelated cause (Fig. 17.2). Renal sonography performed because of suspected inflammatory disease may occasionally reveal tumor, and, conversely, renal inflammatory masses detected on sonography may mimic renal neoplasms.

Cyst

Sonography has largely replaced nephrotomography as the initial study following urographic demonstration of a renal mass.

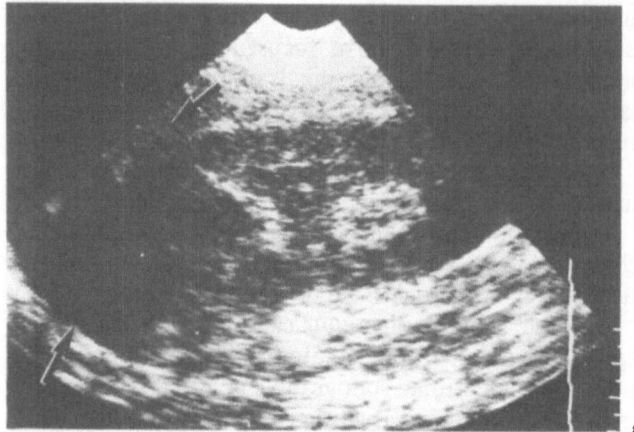

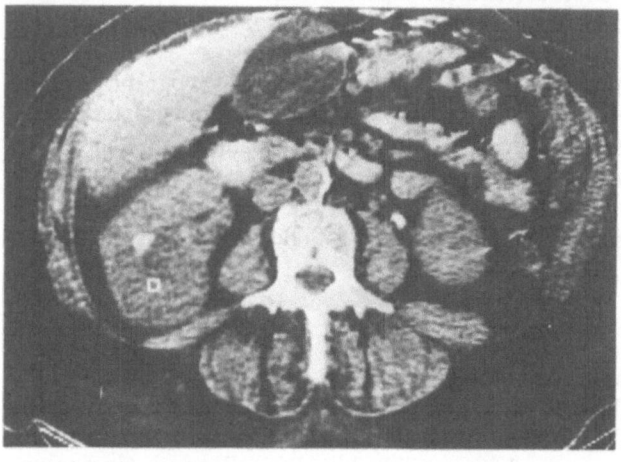

Fig. 17.2a,b. Unsuspected renal cell carcinoma detected by sonography. A 60-year-old woman with chronic renal insufficiency underwent sonography for evaluation of renal size. **a** Longitudinal sonogram shows an echo-poor but solid right upper pole renal mass (*arrows*). **b** Computed tomography confirms the finding of a neoplasm (cursor) projecting posteriorly and confined by the renal capsule (stage 1).

In reported autopsy series, renal cysts are found in 3%–5% in patients of all ages [11] and in 50% of patients 50 years of age or older [36]. Cysts can be cortical, intrarenal, or parapelvic in location. A parapelvic cyst can mimic renal pelvic dilatation or renal sinus lipomatosis [29]. In 1976 Green et al. [25] defined the basic criteria for a simple renal cyst: (1) anechoic interior, (2) well-defined, smooth, millimeter thin walls, and (3) enhanced through-transmission of acoustic energy (as evidenced by a bright slowly diverging beam of echoes visualized distal to the cyst). Renal cysts may normally be indented by adjacent structures. No further evaluation is required for an asymptomatic patient in whom the features of a simple renal cyst have been confirmed by sonography.

An "atypical cyst" denotes a cystic mass which deviates in some way from the above strict criteria. Further evaluation by either computed tomography or percutaneous cyst puncture is generally indicated for an atypical cyst. Low-level echoes or an actual fluid–sediment level may be present, generally indicating hemorrhage or infection. Septations can appear as bright, thin linear echoes within the cyst lumen. Although the presence of one or two septa has been observed in occasional renal cysts and such a finding is not considered by some authorities to be an indication for further evaluation, it is advisable to view this appearance as evidence of atypicality and proceed with further workup. A thickened cyst wall, either nodular or smooth, suggests an inflammatory process or tumor. Adenocarcinoma presenting as a papillary mass arising from a cyst wall has been described [77]. Calcification within the cyst wall or septa appears as an intensely echogenic focus with distal acoustic shadowing. The exact configuration of the calcification can be better demonstrated by computed tomography. Limited distal through-transmission may indicate the presence of solid material within the cyst or an echo-poor solid mass simulating a cyst [2, 64].

Various studies [6, 25, 77] indicate that approximately 2% of masses diagnosed as simple renal cysts on sonography proved to be hematoma, localized hydronephrosis, renal artery aneurysm, infected cyst, or abscess. The chance of missing an infected cyst or abscess should be less likely now than in the past because of the improved ability of current equipment to demonstrate low level echoes within a cystic mass. A cyst smaller than 2 cm may still occasionally be technically difficult to evaluate. Patient obesity, adjacent bowel gas, and limited sonographic "windows" between bony structures may also limit the sonographic examination.

Solid Mass

A variety of sonographic appearances have been described for renal cell carcinoma. A solid renal mass is generally presumed to represent carcinoma although certain features, e.g., intense echogenicity for angiomyolipoma, or clinical settings, e.g., known diagnosis such as lymphoma, may suggest other possibilities. A solid mass is characterized by the presence of internal echoes and minimal or no enhanced through-transmission. Tumor walls may or may not be poorly defined. Carcinoma may be more or less echogenic than normal renal parenchyma (occasionally even stimulating an intensely echogenic angiomyolipoma) and homogeneous or heterogeneous in consistency. The tumor may be solid with irregular cystic components or largely fluid with solid components. At gross pathology, approximately 4% of renal cell carcinomas are cystic. Recent studies indicate that no correlation exists between the degree of necrosis or vascularity of a renal tumor and the sonographic pattern [17, 57].

Coleman et al. [17] indicate that renal cell carcinoma may have echogenicity comparable to normal renal parenchyma, although frequently subtle differences may still allow the correct diagnosis. Interruption of normal renal architecture, i.e., medullary and cortical pattern, or distortion of the renal sinus may be a helpful indication of a subtle renal mass on sonography. While "isoechoic renal masses" appear to be an uncommon problem, especially with optimal technique, masses detected on intravenous urography which are not demonstrated sonographically should be further evaluated with radionuclide imaging or CT scanning.

The sonographic examination of a renal mass suspected of being malignant should include evaluation of the renal vein and inferior vena cava for tumor thrombus (Fig. 17.3), the liver for metastases, the opposite kidney for additional lesions, and the para-aortic and paracaval regions for adenopathy. Perirenal and pararenal space extension of tumor is not demonstrable by sonography; this is best done by computed tomography.

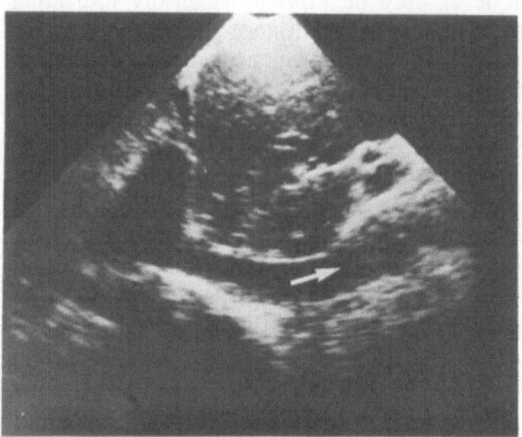

Fig. 17.3. Extension of renal cell carcinoma to the inferior vena cava. A 55-year-old man with weight loss and right flank pain. Longitudinal supine sonogram demonstrating a soft-tissue mass within the inferior vena cava (*arrow*), consistent with tumor thrombus.

Lymphomatous involvement of the kidney may appear as multiple small echo-poor masses, discrete large echo-poor solid masses resembling cysts, or enlarged kidneys with altered parenchyma. Direct extension into the renal parenchyma from pararenal lymphomatous masses may also be demonstrated. The relatively homogeneous histologic pattern of lymphoma probably accounts for the occasional anechoic appearance which must be distinguished from fluid [27, 73].

The differential diagnosis of a solid or complex renal mass on sonography includes not only neoplasm but also pseudotumor (simulated mass representing normal renal tissue), hemorrhagic infarction, lobar nephronia, and inflammatory lesions such as abscess. Prominent septa of Bertin (hypertrophied renal columns), a type of renal pseudotumor, appear sonographically as an extension of normal renal parenchyma interrupting the renal sinus echoes laterally, often in the superior half of the kidney. These columns are usually less than 3 cm in thickness. A similar appearance of the opposite kidney supports the diagnosis of a prominent column but need not be present. A partial renal duplication on intravenous urography is frequently associated [46, 53]. Further evaluation with nuclear scan or computed tomography may occasionally be necessary to confirm a suspected pseudotumor. Fetal lobations and localized hypertrophy secondary to infection or trauma are other examples of pseudotumors. Focal zones of decreased echogenicity may occur with lobar nephronia (focal pyelonephritis) or acute infarction. Renal abscess may simulate a necrotic renal tumor with thick, shaggy walls and a fluid-filled center.

Sonography may also be helpful in distinguishing primary renal and adrenal masses or in suggesting an extrarenal origin of a large retroperitoneal mass secondarily involving the kidney.

Accuracy of Sonography

The accuracy of sonography in distinguishing simple renal cysts from other renal masses has been reported as 90%–98% [6, 49, 64]. However, in no case in these series was a renal tumor misdiagnosed as a simple cyst. Renal masses were not visualized in 4%–7% (older series) [6, 49], indicating the need for further evaluation by other imaging modalities. By applying the previously stated strict criteria for simple renal cysts, 8%–47% of simple renal cysts were interpreted as atypical on sonography, again suggesting the need for further evaluation. The reported accuracy of sonography in identifying solid renal masses has ranged from 90%–100% [6, 49, 62]. Behan et al. [6] and Lingard and Lawson [49] found sonography to be a reliable means of distinguishing pseudotumors from true masses (94% accuracy in the series of Lingard).

While high resolution CT scanning is an extremely accurate means of distinguishing cystic and noncystic renal masses, sonography may occasionally be helpful in resolving an equivocal appearance [49].

Pelvicalyceal Filling Defects

Urographic findings prompting sonography in patients in whom transitional cell carcinoma is eventually diagnosed include a pelvicalyceal filling defect, incomplete filling of the pelvicalyceal system, or nonexcretion from the kidney. A nonopaque renal calculus demonstrates the sonographic features of intense echogenicity and distal acoustic shadowing. Blood clot may occasionally be highly echogenic, unlike tumors, although both are usually of moderate echogenicity. Mobility and change in appearance over a short period indicate blood clot rather than neoplasm.

Transitional cell carcinoma appears as a soft-tissue density splaying the echogenic renal sinus echoes (Fig. 17.4) and with similar echogenicity to normal renal cortex [3, 76]. While Subramanyam et al. [76] indicate that echogenic renal sinus

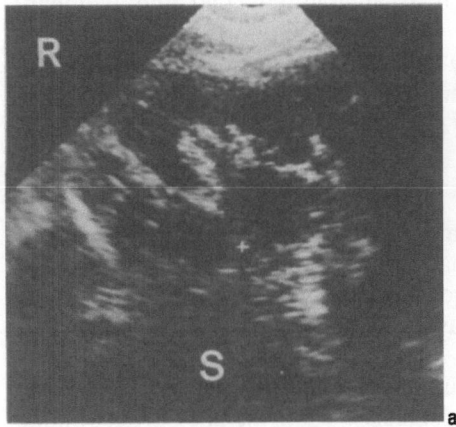
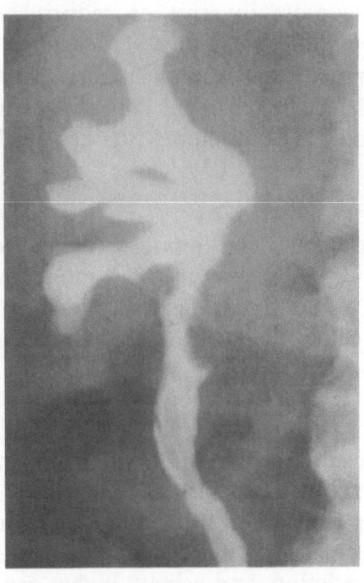

Fig. 17.4a,b. Transitional cell carcinoma. A 70-year-old diabetic and hypertensive man with microscopic hematuria. A filling defect at the medial aspect of the renal pelvis was seen on the intravenous urogram. **a** Transverse sonogram, with the patient in oblique projection, demonstrates a solid mass (between cursors) within the right renal pelvis and proximal ureter. *R*, right; *S*, spine. **b** Right retrograde pyelogram demonstrates the extent of the mucosal neoplasm.

components intervene between the tumor and renal parenchyma, this obviously would not be the case with invasion of renal parenchyma. Masses such as parapelvic cysts or renal cell carcinomas as well as renal sinus lipomatosis may also be identified sonographically as the cause of an impression on the renal collecting system. A nonexcreting kidney with transitional cell carcinoma may demonstrate hydronephrosis and an intraluminal soft tissue mass on ultrasonographic examination.

Computed Tomography

Introduction

Computed tomography is an excellent noninvasive technique for assessment of tumors of the upper urinary tract and is the current modality of choice with which to determine the presence or absence of disease in the retroperitoneum. A complete study of the kidney for malignancy by computed tomography includes scans of the renal fossa before and after intravenous injection of contrast material. This can be performed via a peripheral vein by infusion of a dilute concentration (30%) to opacify vascular structures, or by "bolus" injection of a smaller amount of high density contrast (76%) and rapid (dynamic) scanning of the area(s) of interest [42].

Computed tomography can usually differentiate between benign renal cyst and parenchymal malignancy for diagnosis of the indeterminate mass [4]. Parenchymal malignancies can be accurately staged by computed tomography [26, 68, 83], obviating more invasive procedures such as angiography [54] and lymphangiography.

Computed tomography can also clearly delineate the location and density of a filling defect in the renal collecting system [63], helping to diagnose and stage transitional cell carcinoma preoperatively [5].

Cyst

A cyst on computed tomography is a homogeneous water-density mass (-10 to $+10$ HU), without contrast medium enhancement or detectable wall thickness, making a smooth interface with adjacent renal parenchyma. A mass meeting these criteria can be diagnosed with confidence as a cyst, and there is no need for further workup [50].

The CT diagnosis of renal cyst is usually straightforward and accurate. However, technical artifacts can blur the diagnosis. These include partial volume averaging of the density measurements in a mass smaller than the beam width [72], poor resolution due to patient motion, and inaccurate density measurements resulting from beam hardening due to interposed bone or obesity of the patient. These technical problems can be corrected by repeating the scan with thinner cuts, patient sedation, and using a higher generation scanner [4].

Atypical (Indeterminate) Cystic Mass

A cystic mass, its fluid content demonstrated by sonography, is indeterminate on computed tomography if it exhibits one or more of the following features: does not measure water density, is inhomogeneous, has septations, enhances with contrast medium, has a detectable or thick wall, forms an irregular margin with normal renal parenchyma, or has calcifications [82]. The differential diagnostic possibilities of an indeterminate cystic mass include simple cyst, infected cyst, hemorrhagic cyst, cystic malignancy, multilocular cystic nephroma, abscess, intrarenal aneurysm, and echinococcal cyst.

A fresh hemorrhagic cyst has an attenuation value greater than normal renal parenchyma before enhancement (e.g., 50–90 HU) and does not change density after enhancement [78]. A high attenuation value may be due to fresh hemorrhage into the cyst or increased protein content of the cyst as a result of previous hemorrhage [22]. The material in the cyst is usually homogeneous but may have a fluid-fluid level. With aging and breakdown of the hemorrhagic contents, the attenuation value diminishes so that within a month or so the CT number can be that of water (Fig. 17.5). A dense mass should be further evaluated with aspiration

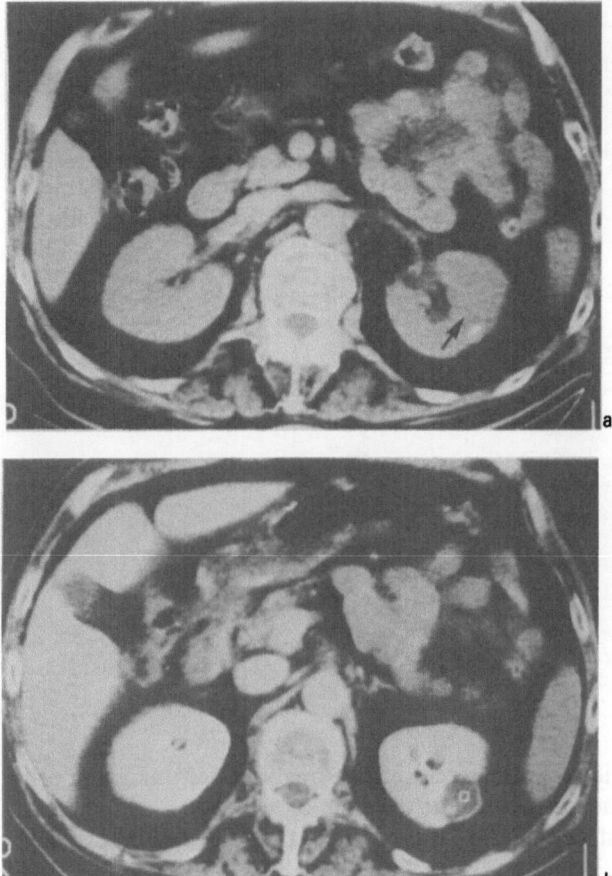

Fig. 17.5a,b. Hemorrhagic cyst. A 56-year-old man experienced left flank pain and gross hematuria after lifting a heavy object. Computed tomography was done 6 weeks later. **a** CT without contrast enhancement shows an ill-defined, slightly hypodense mass (10 HU) (*arrow*) in the posterolateral aspect of the left kidney. There is a small fleck of calcification associated with the mass. **b** CT with contrast enhancement shows the cystic mass with a thick, enhancing wall but no enhancement of its contents (8 HU). Surgical exploration revealed a renal cyst with an epithelial-lined, thick wall and containing old blood.

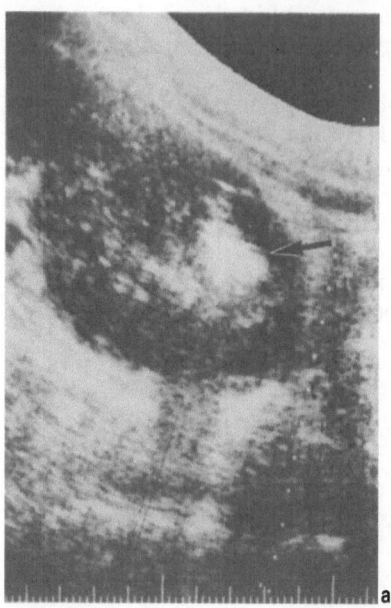

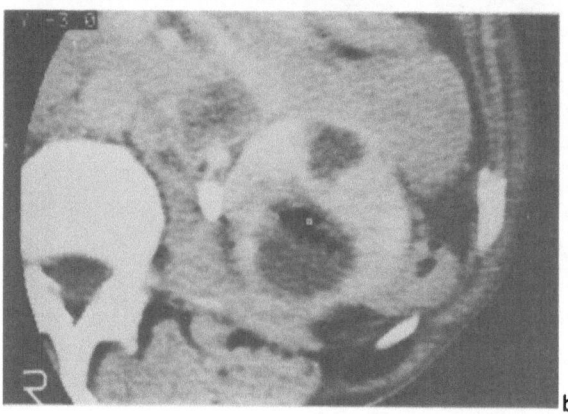

Fig. 17.6a,b. Gas in renal abscess. A 62-year-old diabetic man with fever and urinary tract infection. **a** Oblique sonogram of the left kidney shows an intensely echogenic focus in the kidney (*arrow*) with distal acoustic shadowing. This was initially interpreted as calcification in a renal mass. **b** CT with contrast enhancement shows several renal abscesses, one with many small gas bubbles (cursor).

needle biopsy. If bloody fluid is aspirated, it must be analyzed for malignant cells and fat. Air-cystography should be done at the time of aspiration; a rough cyst wall increases the suspicion of malignancy and such a mass must be explored surgically [12].

A cystic inflammatory mass, such as an abscess, measures more than water but less than normal renal parenchyma, does not enhance, and has a thick enhancing wall [30]. Diagnosis can be made readily by percutaneous aspiration and immediate gram stain as well as culture of the contents. The demonstration by CT of gas within the mass supports the diagnosis of abscess (Fig. 17.6).

Cystic necrotic tumor has a low density center that may enhance, an irregular margin with the normal parenchyma, and a thick wall. Calcifications may be present within the mass or at its periphery (Fig. 17.7) [18]. Angiography may not be helpful in such cases, for these masses are usually hypovascular.

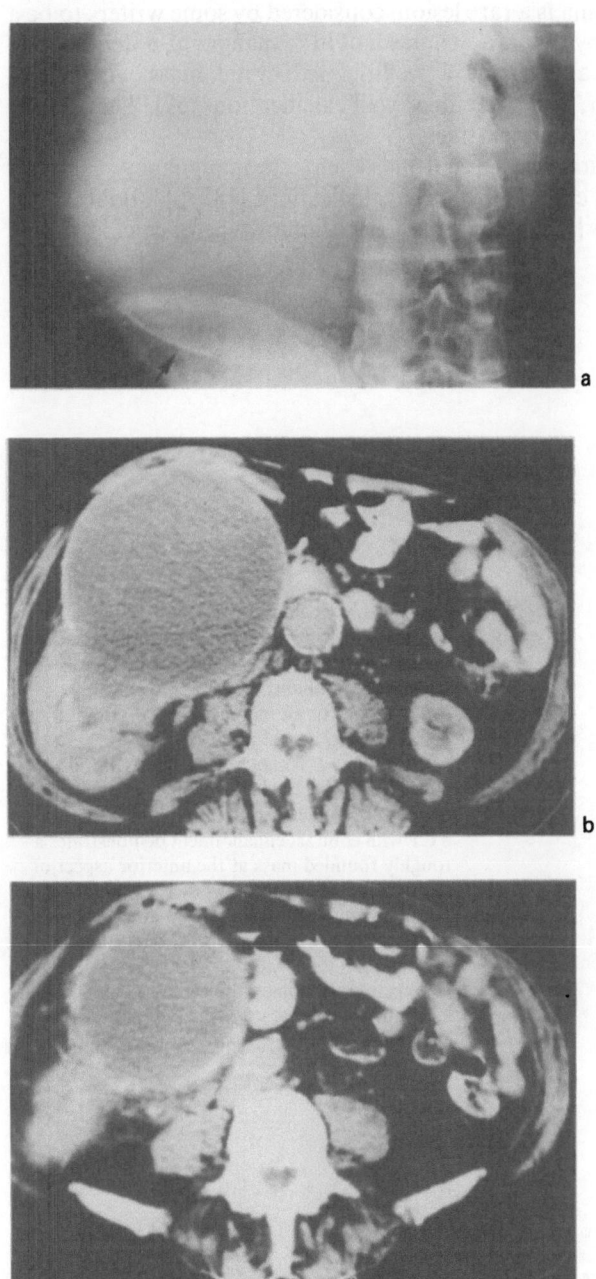

Fig. 17.7a–c. Cystic renal cell carcinoma. A large right upper quadrant mass was palpated during a routine physical examination in a 78-year-old man without gross hematuria or other urinary tract complaints. **a** Abdominal radiograph shows a large right abdominal mass with an incomplete peripheral calcified rim (*arrow*). **b** CT with contrast enhancement shows a fluid-filled mass (16–26 HU) with a thick wall containing calcification. The interface between the mass and renal parenchyma is irregular. There is also calcification of the aortic wall. **c** CT scan, at level more caudad than **b**, shows clumps of calcification in the wall of the cystic mass. Nephrectomy showed renal cell carcinoma with extensive necrosis. (By courtesy of Noel Nathanson, M.D., Brooklyn, New York)

Multilocular cystic nephroma is a rare lesion, considered by some writers to be a type of hamartoma [13] and by others a neoplasm of little malignant potential [52]. Computed tomography usually shows a well-defined cystic mass with many septations, lobulated contour, and sometimes wall calcifications [59]. The specific diagnosis is usually not made preoperatively.

The presence of calcifications in a renal mass suggests malignancy. Eight to eighteen percent of renal cell carcinomas have calcifications [18, 75]; about 2% of renal cysts have calcifications [75]. Although the location or type of calcification is

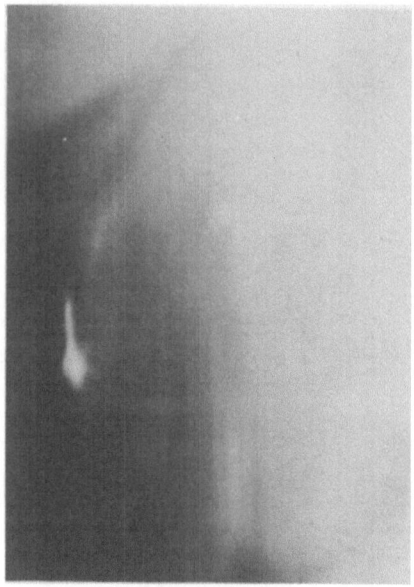

Fig. 17.8a,b. Renal cell carcinoma with peripheral calcification. A 59-year-old man underwent urography because of the finding of microscopic hematuria during physical examination for an inguinal hernia. Urography detected a right renal mass, containing calcifications. **a** Tomogram of the right kidney in oblique projection shows thick, irregular clumps of calcification in the wall of a mass. **b** CT with contrast enhancement demonstrates a roughly rounded mass at the anterior aspect of the right kidney, with a low density center (25 HU) and clumps of calcification in a thick wall. Without contrast enhancement, the center measured 20 HU. Pathologic examination of the nephrectomy specimen showed a well encapsulated adenocarcinoma with a cystic center containing clear, straw-colored fluid.

a

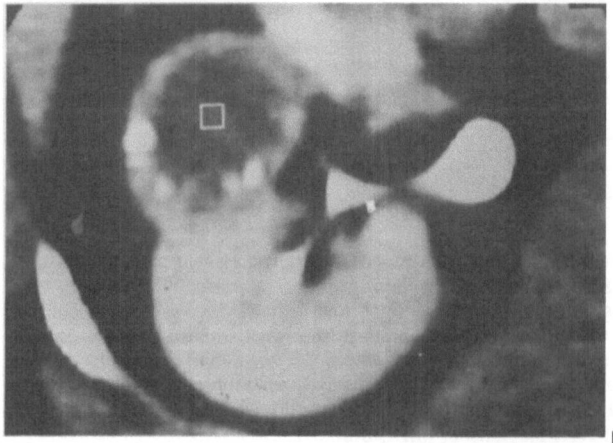

b

of uncertain diagnostic help, CT demonstration of calcification within the soft-tissue mass indicates malignancy (Fig. 17.9b). If the mass has a center of water density with a thin curvilinear rim of sharply defined calcification, the probable diagnosis is cyst; however, such a patient needs further workup, such as cyst puncture, since cystic carcinomas can have a rim of thin calcification (Fig. 17.7). If the calcific rim is thick or clumped, the most likely diagnosis is carcinoma (Fig. 17.8).

Solid Mass

Solid masses which measure slightly less than normal parenchyma before enhancement, display irregular enhancement, and have a lobulated contour are usually renal cell carcinoma [83]. Secondary signs of renal malignancy on computed tomography include enlargement of the renal vein, tumor thrombus in the renal vein or inferior vena cava, enlarged lymph nodes, perirenal extension, and metastatic disease in the retroperitoneum or other organs such as the lung, bone, and liver [68]. Dynamic computed tomography after bolus enhancement can demonstrate enhancement of malignant tissue on early scans, and clearly define the extent of the neoplasm in respect to the kidney, its surrounding spaces, and adjacent structures, thus increasing the accuracy of preoperative staging of renal cell carcinoma [42].

The presence of fat in angiomyolipoma allows specific diagnosis of this type of hamartoma by computed tomography; the muscular and vascular elements show contrast medium enhancement [21]. If the angiomyolipoma is large or contains much vascular tissue, resection or therapeutic embolization has been recommended to prevent hemorrhage. Rarely a Wilms' tumor contains fat tissue [61]. Liposarcoma and lipoma are other, relatively rare masses containing fat [38]. Thus, it has been recommended that serial follow-up CT studies be done on patients with asymptomatic fat-containing solid renal masses [9].

Adenomas are homogeneously enhancing masses, and cannot be differentiated from malignant neoplasms by CT. Oncocytoma appears on computed tomography as a well-defined solid mass with attenuation slightly greater than normal parenchyma, and enhances with contrast medium [47]. Calcification occurs infrequently in adenomas. Benign renal neoplasms are dealt with elsewhere in this book.

Metastatic disease to the kidney from a distant primary is commonly found at autopsy but is often too small to be detected on computed tomography. A homogeneous mass with minimal enhancement may be a metastasis [7]. However, second primary tumors in the kidney were found to be 4 to 5 times more common than CT-detectable metastases in patients with known malignancies [56].

Lymphoma involves the kidney as multiple nodules, invasion from nearby positive lymph nodes, solitary nodules, and diffuse infiltration, in order of decreasing frequency in autopsy series [69]. Computed tomography reveals similar frequencies of renal involvement by homogeneously enhancing masses [14]. The CT finding of accompanying enlarged retroperitoneal lymph nodes supports the diagnosis of lymphoma of the kidney [32]. Commonly both kidneys are involved.

An area of focal pyelonephritis (lobar nephronia) appears as a low density mass before enhancement and may show a "striated" appearance after enhancement [55]. Diagnosis is made by aspiration biopsy and culture or by response to appropriate antibiotic therapy.

CT Staging of Renal Cell Carcinoma

Preoperative staging of renal cell carcinoma by computed tomography can help the surgeon plan the operation as well as indicate the prognosis. CT has for the most part replaced angiography for staging (Figs. 17.9–17.11).

Staging of renal cell carcinoma has most commonly been in accordance with the criteria described by Robson et al. [70]:

Stage   I: Tumor confined within the renal capsule
           (5-year survival rate, 66%)

Stage   II: Involvement of the perirenal fat, but tumor remains within Gerota's
           fascia
           (5-year survival rate, 65%)

Stage III: Vascular involvement of either the renal vein or inferior vena cava, or
           lymph node involvement
           (5-year survival rate, 42%)

Stage   IV: Direct extension to adjacent organs other than the adrenal, or distant
           metastasis
           (5-year survival rate, 11%)

Recently, a more detailed TNM system for staging renal cell carcinoma has been proposed because the authors found a similar prognosis in patients with involvement of perinephric fat or involvement of the renal vein, but a worse prognosis in patients with regional nodal or inferior vena caval involvement [74]. Five groups were described:

Stage   I: Tumor confined within the renal capsule

Stage   II: Perinephric fat or renal vein involvement

Stage III: Inferior vena caval involvement

Stage   IV: Regional lymph node involvement

Stage   V: Distant metastasis or direct extension to adjacent organs other than
           the adrenal

Radical nephrectomy with regional lymph node resection is recommended in all operable cases and appears to improve survival. The benefit of preoperative radiation and chemotherapy is controversial. It has been suggested that preoperative renal artery embolization may increase general immunocompetence and possibly improve prognosis [80].

Gerota's fascia is clearly delineated by computed tomography in most patients, with use of a wide window setting (level 30, width 500). It may be difficult to detect fascial planes in children and very thin adults. Thickening of Gerota's fascia is a nonspecific finding [60], seen in inflammatory disease as well as in association with renal malignancy. Computed tomography can usually clearly delineate between stage I and II tumors, i.e., whether the tumor has broken through the renal capsule. However, this does not change the surgical approach [26].

A very large tumor is apt to efface perirenal fat and displace adjacent organs, suggesting that the lesion has extended beyond Gerota's fascia. However, at pathological examination Gerota's fascia is often not violated in such cases [26]. Tissue planes may be easier to determine with sagittal and coronal imaging.

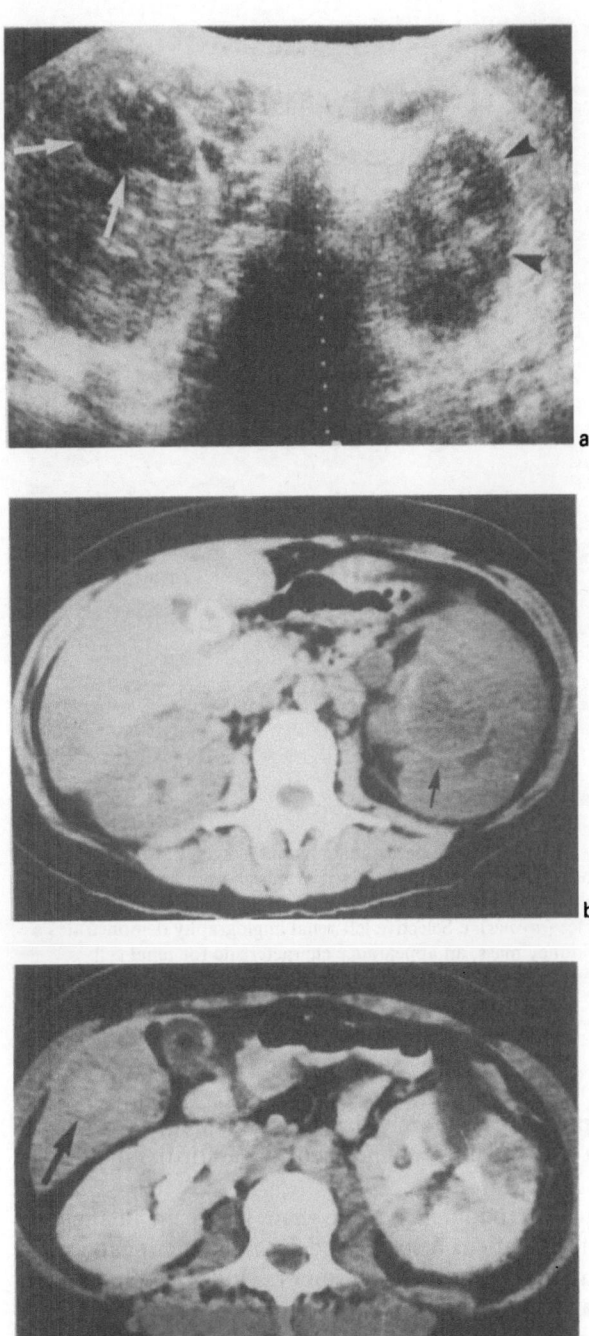

Fig. 17.9a–c. Renal cell carcinoma, stage IV. A 33-year-old woman with a left upper quadrant mass. **a** Transverse supine sonogram demonstrates metastases in the right lobe of the liver (*arrows*) and a left renal mass (*arrowheads*) containing calcifications. **b** Unenhanced CT shows a large left renal mass, with an incomplete ring of curvilinear calcification (*arrow*) within the mass. **c** Computed tomogram with contrast enhancement confirms the presence of liver metastases (*arrow*).

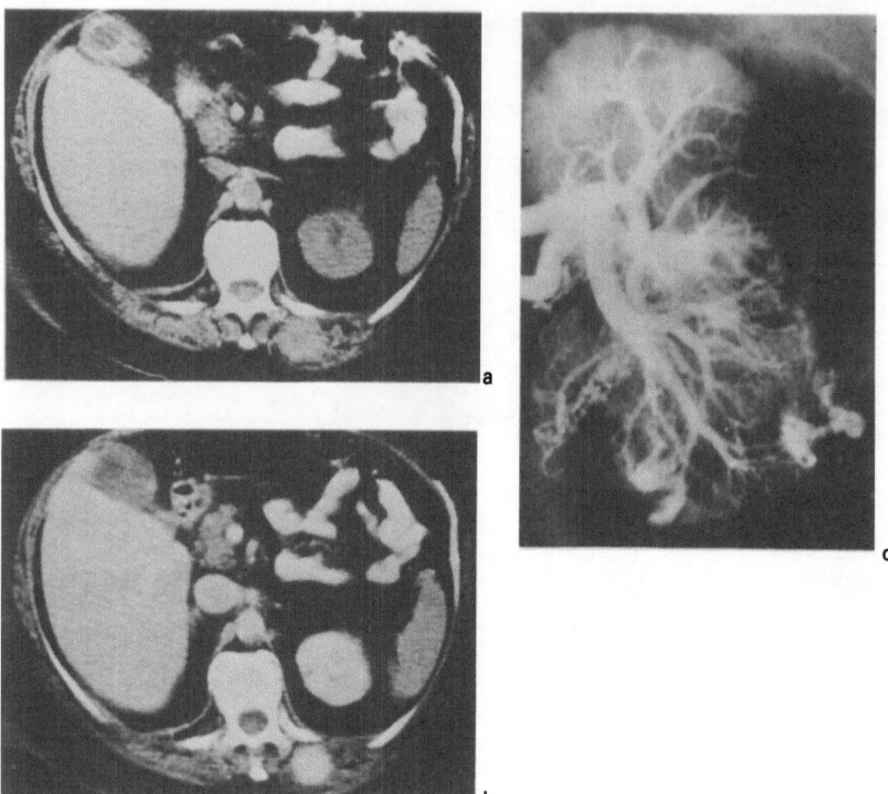

Fig. 17.10a–c. Renal cell carcinoma with metastasis to paraspinal muscles, stage IV. Intravenous urography on a 77-year-old woman being investigated for uterine fibroids showed a mass at the lower pole of the left kidney. CT **a** without and **b** with contrast enhancement shows an enhancing metastasis to the left paraspinal muscles (*arrows*). **c** Selective left renal angiography demonstrates a disorganized hypervascularity of the kidney mass, an appearance characteristic for renal cell carcinoma. Needle biopsy of the paraspinal mass showed a histology consistent with renal cell carcinoma.

Dynamic computed tomography can accurately demonstrate direct extension of tumor beyond Gerota's fascia by revealing enhancement of tumor tissue on early scans [42].

An isolated lymph node in the abdomen greater than 1.5 cm in diameter is considered to be abnormal. In the patient being staged for renal malignancy, it is assumed that this represents nodal involvement by tumor. However, the enlargement may be due to inflammation [83].

Tumor thrombus in the renal vein or inferior vena cava appears on contrast-enhanced computed tomography as an intraluminal filling defect, sometimes with localized enlargement of the vessel diameter and relative enhancement of the vessel wall.

Demonstration of tumor thrombus in the inferior vena cava can be facilitated by infusing contrast medium into a vein in the foot. The appearance of filling defects in the opacified cava due to the entrance of unopacified blood from its tributaries

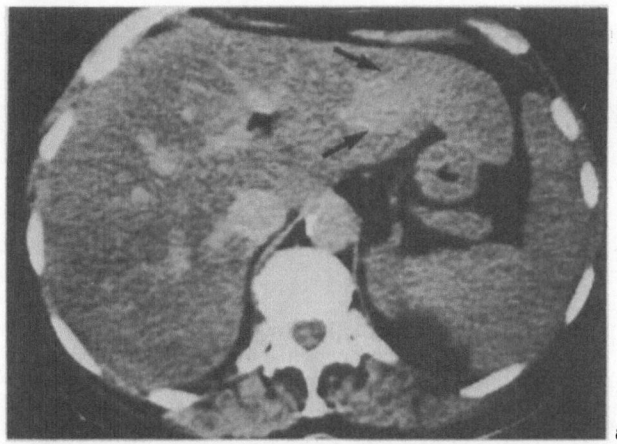

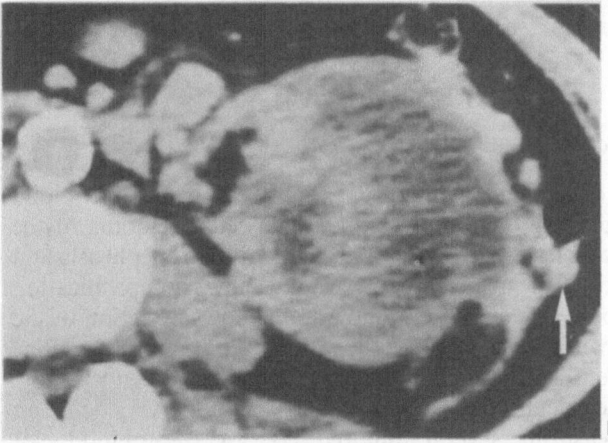

Fig. 17.11a,b. Renal cell carcinoma with metastasis to the liver as well as direct extension to colon, stage IV. Because of erythrocytosis discovered at the time of a general medical examination, this 74-year-old woman underwent intravenous urography, which disclosed a mass of the lower pole of the left kidney. **a** CT without contrast enhancement shows a fatty liver with consequent prominence of the blood vessels in the liver. The area of increased attenuation (*arrows*) of the lateral portion of the left lobe represents metastasis. **b** CT at the level of the left kidney shows the neoplasm with extension of the tumor through the lateroconal fascia to involve the wall of the descending colon (*arrow*). Subsequent surgery showed the serosa of the colon to be involved by tumor and also confirmed the liver metastases.

can be confusing and must be recognized as such lest false-positive diagnosis be made [83]. When this route is used, the contrast material must be flushed from the foot vein with normal saline immediately after the study to prevent thrombosis. It has been reported [42] that dynamic scanning increases the accuracy of computed tomography for the diagnosis of renal vein or.caval involvement by extension of the renal carcinoma (Fig. 17.12). Such extension is also diagnosable by ultrasonography. If a discrepancy is found between imaging modalities, or they are indeterminate, venography is suggested.

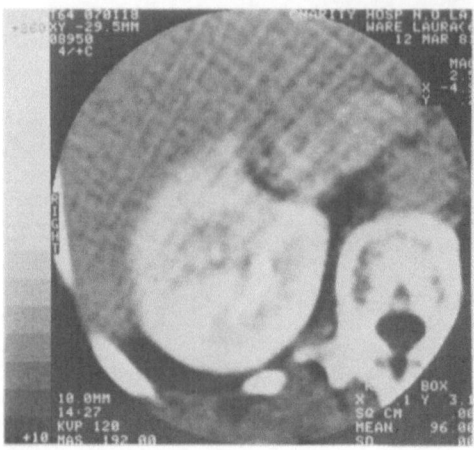

Fig. 17.12. Dynamic CT shows dense enhancement, during the capillary phase, of a tumor thrombus extending into the right renal vein (cursor) and inferior vena cava. (By courtesy of Erich K. Lang, M.D., and Radiology 1984; 151:149–155)

Pelvicalyceal Filling Defect

A filling defect in the renal collecting system on urography can be a stone, blood clot, sloughed papilla, fungus ball, or tumor. Transitional cell carcinoma of the renal pelvis may produce complete obstruction with marked hydronephrosis and loss of renal excretory function. In such a case, urography shows no opacification of the collecting system. However, computed tomography allows detection of the solid tumor within the hydronephrosis (Fig. 17.13). Computed tomography done before and after enhancement can be helpful for the differential diagnosis (Fig. 17.14) [58, 63]. A nonopaque calculus (a uric acid or matrix stone) is very dense on computed tomography, measuring several hundred HU. A fresh blood clot measures 50–90 HU and does not enhance. The attenuation of a sloughed papilla or fungus ball is similar to or less than that of renal parenchyma and will not enhance. Transitional cell carcinoma shows attenuation similar to that of renal parenchyma and will enhance [5].

Difficulties in interpretation of computed tomography of renal collecting system filling defects are usually due to partial volume averaging of density measurements of calculi smaller than the beam width and also to dense contrast medium in the collecting system surrounding the filling defect. These problems can be avoided by using a small beam width and small amounts of intravenous contrast material for enhancement.

The extent of transitional cell carcinoma in the kidney can be accurately determined by computed tomography, and the tumor can be staged preoperatively without retrograde pyelography or angiography [5]. The peripelvic fat helps to delineate the boundaries of the collecting system and perirenal anatomy is clearly demonstrated. Difficulties can arise in patients with superimposed chronic inflammation, because inflammatory changes can mimic tumor on CT.

If transitional cell carcinoma is treated while still limited to the mucosa, its prognosis is quite good, changing for the worse with involvement of the renal parenchyma. Rubenstein et al. reported the following method of staging transitional cell carcinoma of the kidney [71]:

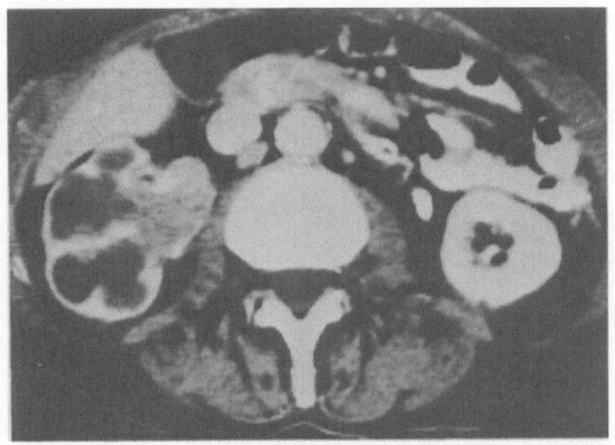

a

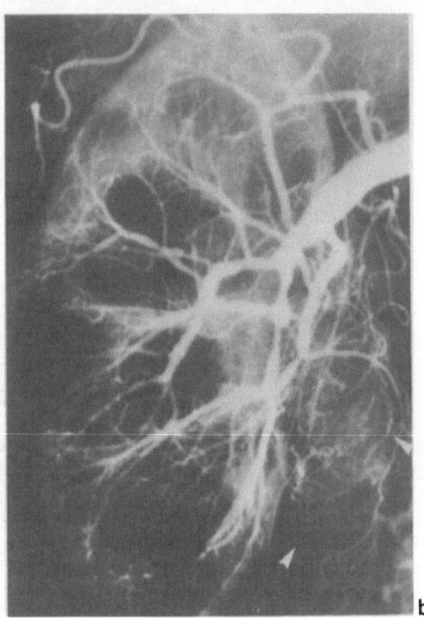

Fig. 17.13a,b. Solid mass of transitional cell carcinoma within hydronephrosis. Intravenous urography on this 86-year-old man with several episodes of gross hematuria showed no excretion of contrast medium by the right kidney. **a** CT with contrast enhancement shows marked right hydronephrosis with the contents of the dilated calyces being of water density (13 HU); the dilated renal pelvis contains a solid mass (59 HU). **b** Selective renal angiography shows encasement of renal pelvic vessels as well as neovascularity in a mass in the renal pelvis and upper segment of the ureter (*arrowheads*).

b

Stage A: Tumor confined to the pelvicalyceal system

Stage B: Tumor extending into the renal parenchyma but confined within the renal capsule

Stage C: Microscopic extension into the peripelvic fat, but without gross local extension, nodal metastases, or distant metastases

Stage D: Further local extension, nodal metastases, or distant metastases

Overall 5-year survival rate is about 35%, with about 60% for stage A, 40% for stage B, and only a few percent for stages C and D.

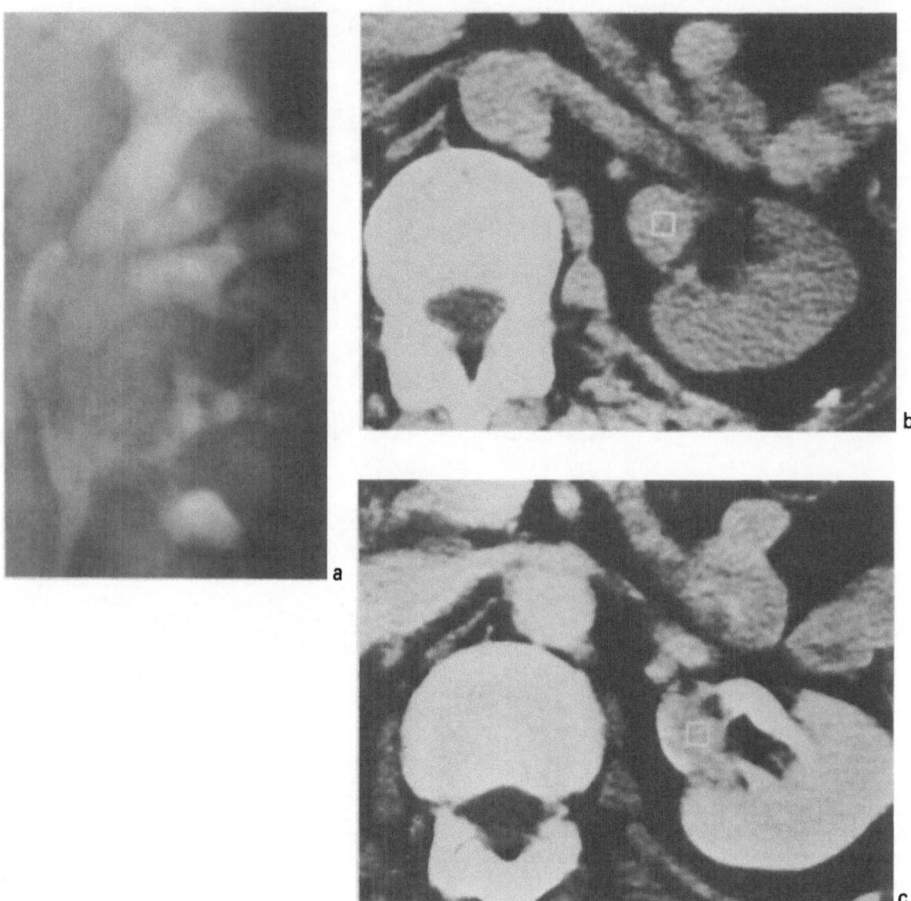

Fig. 17.14a–c. CT enhancement of transitional cell carcinoma. A 67-year-old woman who had total, gross hematuria for 2 days. **a** Intravenous urography shows dilatation of the left renal pelvis, containing a large filling defect. **b** Two days following urography, CT without contrast enhancement shows a soft-tissue mass in the pelvis (cursor), measuring 37 HU. **c** After contrast enhancement the mass measures 105 HU. Part of this increased attenuation is very likely related to partial volume averaging of contrast medium in the renal pelvis. Operation confirmed papillary transitional cell carcinoma measuring 3 cm in greatest diameter and confined to the pelvis of the kidney.

Computed tomographic findings in transitional cell carcinoma include three patterns: a focal intraluminal mass, ureteral wall thickening with luminal narrowing, and an infiltrating mass (Fig. 17.15). Attenuation is usually similar to that of normal renal parenchyma, and with careful technique enhancement can be demonstrated. Usually, transitional cell carcinoma infiltrating the renal parenchyma enhances to a lesser degree than the uninvolved renal parenchyma. Para-aortic adenopathy, if present, can usually be easily identified (Fig. 17.16). An isolated node greater than 1.5 cm in diameter or a large mass of matted nodes is considered evidence of metastasis. However, nodal enlargement is not necessarily due to tumor involvement; inflammation can enlarge nodes.

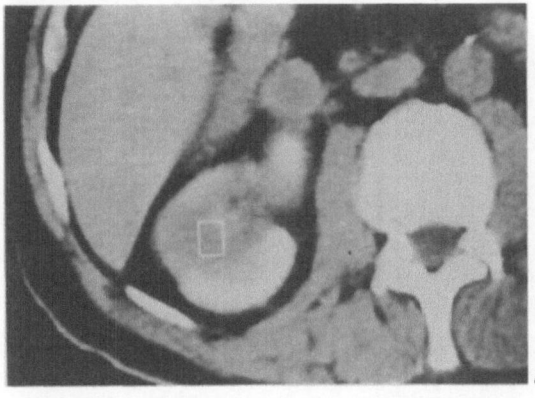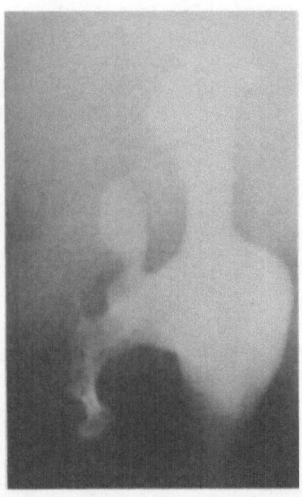

Fig. 17.15a,b. CT demonstration of parenchymal infiltration by transitional cell carcinoma. An 87-year-old man who had several episodes of gross hematuria during the past month, with right flank pain for the past several days. Admission urography and retrograde ureterography showed an obstructive nephrogram due to a blood clot in the lower segment of the right ureter. **a** Computed tomography on the following morning, without additional intravenous contrast medium, still shows the obstructive nephrogram but with a defect in the nephrogram (cursor) representing parenchymal infiltration by the transitional cell carcinoma (34 HU). **b** Retrograde pyelography after relief of the ureteral obstruction shows the transitional cell carcinoma arising in the mucosa of the lower calyces. Pathologic study of the nephrectomy specimen confirmed the parenchymal invasion, stage B.

Angiography

Not too long ago renal angiography was the critical examination for the diagnostic assessment of a renal mass. With the advent of the cross-sectional imaging techniques, ultrasonography and computed tomography, there is now only occasional need for angiography for diagnostic purposes. In many institutions, angiography is hardly ever part of the preoperative workup of renal malignancy, although there are still a few indications for its use [4, 54, 83]:

1. Study for extension of renal malignancy into the main renal vein or inferior vena cava, especially for a central tumor of the right kidney or a large tumor of the left kidney.
2. Occasionally ultrasonography and computed tomography provide equivocal or contradictory diagnostic findings and angiography may provide the clinching diagnostic evidence.
3. Despite the willingness to accept the diagnosis of renal malignancy from the cross-sectional imaging studies, some urologists insist on preoperative angiography for mapping of the vascular supply to the affected kidney and its neoplasm.
4. Vascular mapping is especially important if the patient has only a single kidney in which the neoplasm has grown, with the planned treatment being bench surgery or heminephrectomy. Preoperative angiography is also indicated in the presence of renal anomalies, e.g., horseshoe kidney.

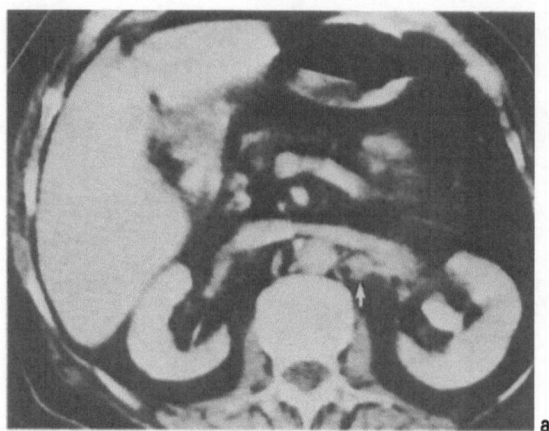

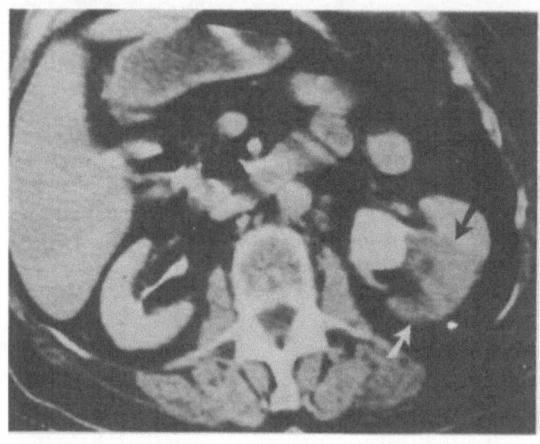

Fig. 17.16a,b. Nodal metastases from transitional cell carcinoma, stage D. A 78-year-old woman who had several episodes of gross hematuria over the past 2 years. Tomograms during intravenous urography showed a left renal mass obliterating the inferior calyces and impressing the lateral aspect of the renal pelvis. **a** CT with contrast enhancement shows an enlarged lymph node (*arrow*) posterior to the left renal vein. **b** A more caudal scan shows tumor infiltration (*arrows*) of the renal parenchyma. Radical nephrectomy and ureterectomy disclosed undifferentiated transitional cell carcinoma of the renal pelvis with infiltration of the renal parenchyma and positive lymph nodes at the renal hilum.

5. Angiography is also done when preoperative embolization of the neoplasm is part of the treatment protocol.

Selective study of the renal artery must be done. Magnification technique and the supplementary use of epinephrine-aided angiography can be helpful.

Renal Cell Carcinoma

The characteristic angiographic findings in renal cell carcinoma include enlargement of the main renal artery, and a network of irregular vessels of variable calibre in disorderly arrangement (Fig. 17.10c). Typically renal adenocarcinoma is

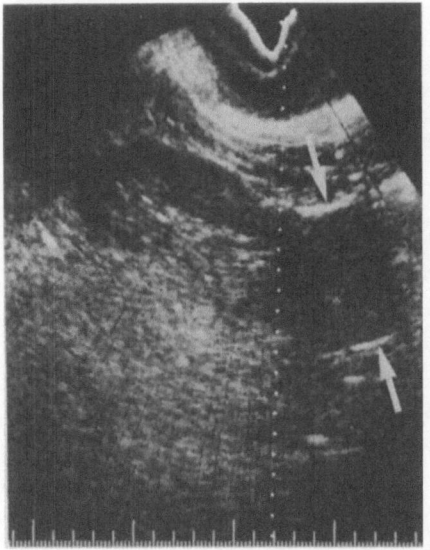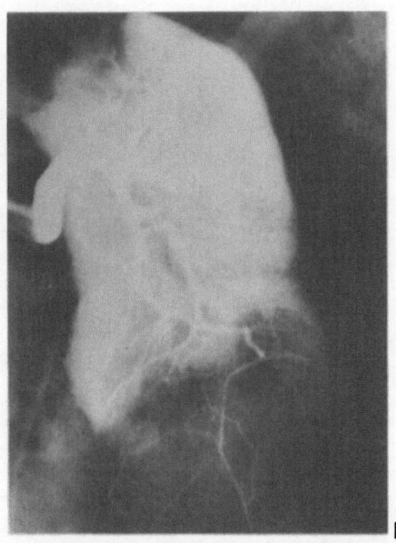

Fig. 17.17a,b. Papillary adenocarcinoma of the kidney. A 60-year-old man had a mass of the lower pole of the left kidney detected by intravenous urography done during the work-up of a urinary tract infection. **a** A coronal sonographic section of the left kidney shows a solid mass (*arrows*) of the lower pole. **b** Aortography demonstrated a small superior polar artery in addition to the main renal artery. Angiography, with injection into the major artery, shows the mass to be hypovascular, containing several narrowed, angled vessels. Pathologic study of the nephrectomy specimen disclosed papillary adenocarcinoma.

hypervascular, sometimes with numerous tumor arteriovenous shunts and early opacification of the main renal vein. The late phase of angiography shows mottled tumor staining, puddling of contrast medium, and venous lakes. Zones of necrosis within the tumor present as areas of avascularity, contributing to the mottling of the tumor staining [43].

Involvement of the renal vein can be assessed by high dose selective renal arteriography for opacification of the draining veins or by selective phlebography. A linear striated hypervascularity in the region of the renal vein and sometimes the inferior vena cava during the early phase of angiography is also a sign of extension of the neoplasm into the vein, representing arterial flow to the tumor in the vein [15, 20].

About 10%–15% of renal cell carcinomas are of papillary or tubular type histologically; these are usually hypovascular (Fig. 17.17), the angiographic appearance being quite different from that of the usual adenocarcinoma [51].

When the renal neoplasm extends outside the kidney to involve adjacent structures, e.g., the colon, part of the neoplasm can be shown to be fed by branches of vessels other than the renal artery, such as branches of the superior or inferior mesenteric artery. This is referred to as cannibalization of blood supply, and is considered a sign of an advanced lesion. However, highly vascular tumors still limited to the kidney can be fed by branches of preexisting collaterals from adrenal, ureteral, renal pelvic, gonadal, intercostal, lumbar, and even mesenteric

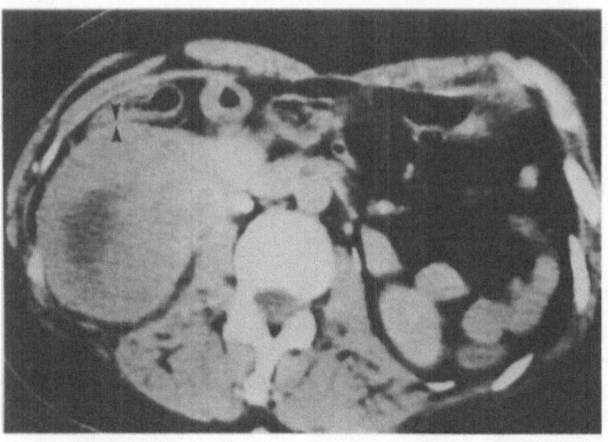

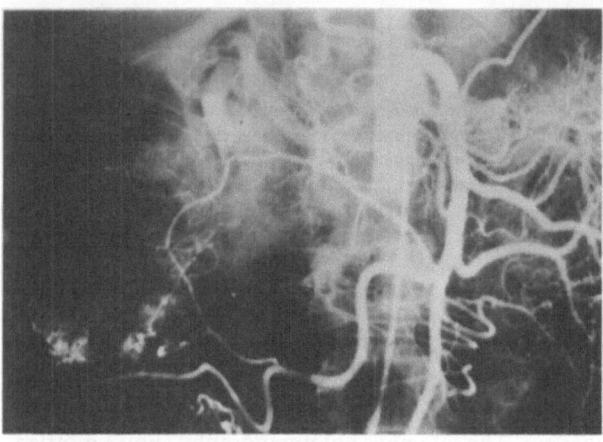

Fig. 17.18a,b. Renal cell carcinoma, stage 2, with apparent cannibalization of the superior mesenteric circulation. A 48-year-old woman who had gross hematuria for 3 days. Urography showed a large mass of the lower half of the right kidney with deformity of the pelvicalyceal system. **a** CT done immediately after the urography demonstrates the large neoplasm, with areas of necrosis, extending into the perirenal space. The ascending colon is deformed by the neoplasm but not infiltrated, as demonstrated by the preservation of a fat plane (*arrowheads*) between the colon and the tumor. **b** Selective superior mesenteric arteriography demonstrates that the caudal portion of the mass is perfused by SMA branches. Nephrectomy disclosed no invasion of the colon.

vessels (Fig. 17.18). Thus the use of the angiographic appearance of apparent cannibalization for staging the neoplasm can lead to inaccuracies [10].

In cystic carcinoma, most often owing to large central necrosis of the neoplasm, angiography usually shows an avascular or hypovascular center surrounded by a thick, usually hypervascular, wall—an appearance simulating that of a chronic renal abscess or even an atypical (infected or hemorrhagic) simple cyst.

Transitional Cell Carcinoma

Transitional cell carcinoma characteristically is hypovascular, with tumor vessels, when demonstrable, branching usually from renal pelvic arteries. As the mucosal neoplasm invades and infiltrates the renal parenchyma, it encases intrarenal arteries which on angiography appear straightened with localized rigid narrowings [24]. Vascular shunts, tumor staining, and contrast medium puddling are not usually seen. Extension of the neoplasm in the main renal vein can occur, although it does so less frequently than with renal cell carcinoma.

Lymphoma

Lymphoma is usually hypovascular without shunting or tumor staining. Palisading of vessels in the tumor is suggestive of lymphoma, angiography showing stretched, attenuated arteries lined up like fence posts. However, only a minority of renal lymphomas show palisading, and the appearance can occasionally be seen with other types of neoplasm [40, 41].

Metastasis

Metastases to the kidney, often bilateral, show no distinctive vascular pattern; they may be hypervascular or hypovascular. Capsular deposits or those in the peripheral cortex extending to the capsule show perfusion from branches of capsular arteries.

Capsular Sarcoma

Sarcoma of the renal capsule, an infrequent tumor, is usually large by the time of detection, enveloping and deforming as well as displacing the kidney but typically not infiltrating the renal parenchyma. It is fed by branches of capsular arteries, this being the typical angiographic finding. The neoplastic vessels are elongated and meandering, their sharp definition contrasting with the less well defined borders of the vessels of typical renal cell carcinoma. Since areas of necrosis or myxomatous degeneration are common in these very large neoplasms, the density in the late phases of angiography is apt to be markedly heterogeneous [19].

Oncocytoma

These well vascularized neoplasms have a variable angiographic appearance. Some have the disordered hypervascularity of the usual renal cell carcinoma, from which they cannot be differentiated. Others present with a characteristic spoke-wheel appearance, in which there are prominent curving arteries at the periphery of the tumor with branch vessels running toward the center of the mass in radial fashion [81]. Although the spoke-wheel appearance is highly suggestive of oncocytoma, some renal cell carcinomas have a similar appearance. Hence, the radiologic appearance of oncocytoma is not specific enough to preclude surgical exploration. Indeed, some pathologists consider oncocytoma to be a variant of renal cell carcinoma of low grade malignancy.

Simple Cyst

In the case of a simple renal cyst, angiography shows the mass to be avascular, with displacement of the normal vessels of adjacent parenchyma spread around the mass. The very thin wall of the cyst is not visualized by angiography. The "beak sign" represents normally opacified renal cortex rimming the cyst as it protrudes from the kidney through the cortex. The beak, when seen en face during angiography, appears as a thick rim of opacification around the cyst. The beak sign is not specific, being seen with benign solid masses and sometimes with malignant neoplasms.

Antegrade Pyelography

In antegrade pyelography, the renal collecting system is opacified for radiographic examination by direct instillation of contrast medium via a percutaneous route. The method is especially useful for investigating the possibility of a pelvicalyceal filling defect in a hydronephrotic kidney that is not adequately opacified by intravenous urography. Antegrade pyelography is not usually a primary modality in assessing renal tumors except when these are detected as an incidental finding in the evaluation of hydronephrosis.

Following percutaneous puncture of the renal collecting system, urine specimens are aspirated for cytology and culture and an equal or lesser volume of contrast medium injected. Radiographs may then be obtained in standard prone, supine, decubitus, and erect views or whatever obliquity demonstrates the finding to best advantage. Complications of antegrade pyelography include infection, urine leakage, hemorrhage, and bacteremia apparently resulting from overinjection into an obstructed and infected system [65].

Brush Biopsy of the Renal Collecting System

Retrograde brush biopsy of urothelial lesions was introduced in response to the low diagnostic accuracy of urine cytology. While the procedure has gained only limited acceptance, it has been recommended in specific instances in which extensive evaluation has failed to clarify the nature of a collecting system lesion or when confirmation of a low grade malignancy would permit a conservative approach in a patient with poor renal function or a single kidney.

The procedure is performed by cystoscopic introduction of a ureteral catheter through which nylon or steel bristle brushes are introduced on a long wire. Prior to actually brushing the lesion, contrast medium is flushed from the collecting system to avoid damage to the biopsy specimens. After brushing the lesion in a manner analogous to bronchoscopic biopsy, the biopsy brush is withdrawn, touched to a slide, and then soaked in a fixative for further cytologic or histologic specimens. At the conclusion of the procedure, the catheter is flushed to obtain any additional cells or tissue fragments [23, 33].

Despite the excellent results reported by Gill et al. [23], Blute et al. [8] found, in a survey of American urologists, an overall accuracy rate of only 78%. This survey also disclosed a significant complication rate, with major complications including severe bleeding, gram-negative sepsis, and ureteral perforation (a 7% incidence of major complications). A minor complication rate of 36% included transient hematuria and renal colic.

Gill et al. [23] were able to identify specifically causes of collecting system filling defect other than transitional carcinoma, including extension of renal cell carcinoma into the collecting system.

Lang et al. [44] used a percutaneous antegrade route to perform brush biopsy, with the help of a deflectable guide wire. In some of the patients examined, retrograde brush biopsy had been unsuccessful because of poor access to the lesions. Transitional cell carcinoma, metastatic tumors, and inflammatory lesions were diagnosed in the pelvicalyceal system and ureter.

Magnetic Resonance Imaging (MRI)

As this is written, it is still too early to assess the role of MRI in the specific diagnosis of renal malignancies. There are indications of significant potential of this new modality. Preliminary reports suggest that MRI is comparable to computed tomography in the accuracy of staging renal cell carcinoma [31]. The promise of the ability of MRI to study the vascular system without the need for injected foreign material may allow accurate, completely noninvasive studies for extension of renal neoplasm into the renal vein and inferior vena cava. Magnetic resonance may also offer the possibility of specific tissue identification. MRI has the advangage of providing not only cross-sectional studies, but also images in coronal, sagittal, and oblique projections.

Evaluation for Metastases

Having made the diagnosis of primary renal malignancy, how much of a radiologic search should be made for spread before deciding on definitive management of the patient?

The common sites for distant metastases from renal cell carcinoma are the lungs, lymph nodes, bones, liver, contralateral kidney, and adrenal glands. In the process of the initial workup for diagnosis or for staging of the renal neoplasm, computed tomography, particularly with a dynamic program, would have accurately evaluated local extension, renal vein and inferior vena cava involvement, localized adenopathy, liver, the contralateral kidney, and the adrenal glands. Abrams [1] has suggested radionuclide bone scan and chest film for further evaluation for metastases. Lang [45] has proposed computed tomography of the chest instead of or in addition to the chest film. If routine screening liver function tests (LDH, SGOT, SGPT, alkaline phosphatase) are abnormal, radionuclide liver scan would be indicated.

Transitional cell carcinoma metastasizes most commonly to regional lymph nodes, lungs, and liver, with a 30%–50% incidence to any of these sites in autopsy series. There is a 15% incidence of bone metastasis; the brain, heart, and adrenal glands are also infrequent sites of spread [79]. Computed tomography, possibly already done during the diagnostic workup, can evaluate renal hilar and lumbar lymph nodes as well as the liver. A chest radiograph and screening liver function tests should be done; if these show positive or suspicious findings, more detailed studies are indicated. One could also argue that a survey radionuclide bone scan should be done as part of the metastatic workup.

In some patients with demonstrated primary malignancy of the renal parenchyma or urothelium, the attending physician or urologist may determine that appropriate surgical excisional management should be done regardless of the presence or absence of metastases. In such cases there is less urgency for an extensive metastatic search with its attendant costs and time delay.

Patient Workup

The discussion of radiologic diagnostic evaluation has covered not only the most commonly used methodologies for investigating the possibility of renal neoplasm but also suggestions as to the indications and sequence of use of these methodologies. As a summary, algorithms are now offered as general guidelines for sequences of study following an initial finding, usually by urography. In the algorithms (Figs. 17.19–17.22), arrowed lines point to procedures or actions; unarrowed lines point to findings. Specific order and types of procedures will vary with available expertise and facilities, as well as with unique features of clinical presentation. Also, current recommendations for workup will change as new technologies are added to our diagnostic armamentarium.

Algorithm for Renal Mass (Fig. 17.19)

A renal mass demonstrated by intravenous urography is usually studied next by sonography. If a simple cyst is identified no further workup is necessary.

For the sonographic finding of atypical cyst, CT is done. Again the workup stops if a simple cyst is demonstrated. If CT shows an indeterminate cystic mass with increased attenuation after contrast enhancement, the presumptive diagnosis is cystic carcinoma and surgery is indicated. If CT shows an indeterminate cystic mass with no change in CT number after contrast enhancement, cyst puncture should be done, followed, if necessary, by double contrast (contrast medium and air) injection of the cystic mass. If cyst puncture demonstrates a simple cyst, the workup stops. If bloody fluid is found, with a smooth cyst wall and no evidence of fat or of elevated enzyme content, the presumptive diagnosis is hemorrhagic cyst, and the patient may be followed periodically by sonography or CT. However, if cyst puncture yields bloody fluid and the cyst wall is irregular or the fluid contains fat and elevated LDH, the presumptive diagnosis is cystic carcinoma and surgery is indicated. Aspiration of purulent fluid on cyst puncture warrants treatment for an abscess, i.e., drainage and appropriate antibiotic therapy, with the recognition, however, that occasionally a neoplasm may be secondarily infected. If cyst puncture yields no fluid, aspiration biopsy should be done with further workup or therapy dictated by the cytologic findings.

A complex or solid mass on sonography may next be evaluated by CT unless the patient already has evidence of metastatic disease at multiple sites, or has a single nonresectable metastatic lesion, or has a known primary neoplasm. In these instances a percutaneous biopsy of the renal mass is recommended. If CT demonstrates an indeterminate cystic mass, workup may proceed as detailed above for this finding. If CT shows evidence of a simple cyst, no further workup is needed. If CT demonstrates a solid mass containing fat, the presumptive diagnosis is angiomyolipoma and workup for neoplasm can stop. CT demonstration of a solid mass without fat content suggests the diagnosis of neoplasm and surgery is indicated.

If sonography indicates that the renal mass is very likely a pseudotumor, appropriate radionuclide studies may be next. If the mass functions as normal renal tissue, the diagnosis of pseudotumor is confirmed and the workup stops. If

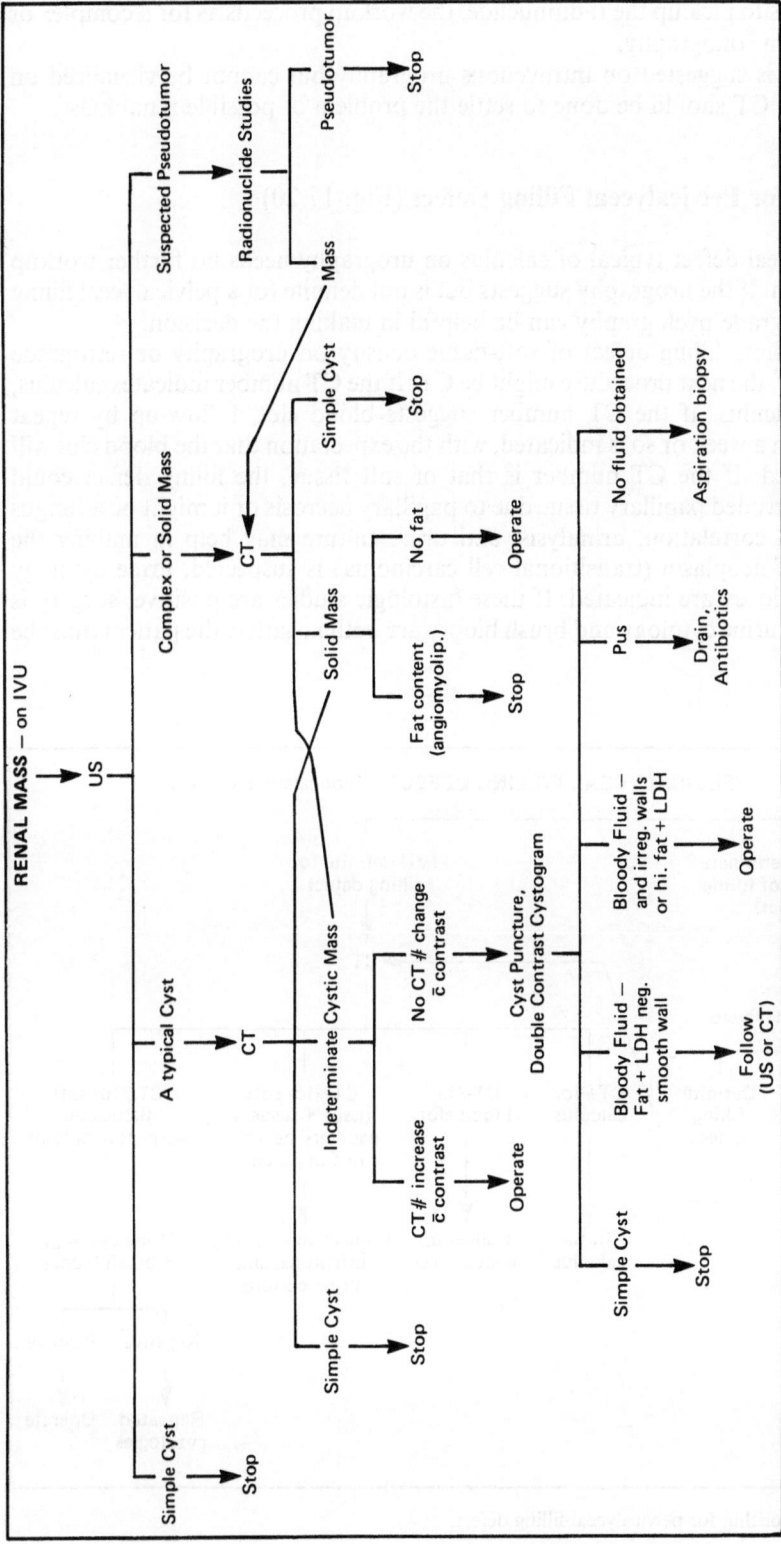

Fig. 17.19. Algorithm for renal mass. Here and in Figs. 17.20 and 17.21, where "Operate" is indicated, one may wish to perform angiography before surgery for reasons indicated in the text.

the mass fails to pick up the radionuclide, the workup proceeds as for a complex or solid mass on sonography.

If a mass is suggested on intravenous urography but cannot be visualized on sonography, CT should be done to settle the problem of possible renal mass.

Algorithm for Pelvicalyceal Filling Defect (Fig. 17.20)

A pelvicalyceal defect typical of calculus on urography needs no further workup for neoplasm. If the urography suggests but is not definite for a pelvicalyceal filling defect, retrograde pyelography can be helpful in making the decision.

For a definite filling defect of soft-tissue density on urography or retrograde pyelography, the next procedure might be CT. If the CT number indicates calculus, treat for calculus. If the CT number suggests blood clot, follow-up by repeat urography in a week or so is indicated, with the expectation that the blood clot will have resolved. If the CT number is that of soft tissue, the filling defect could represent extruded papillary tissue due to papillary necrosis or it might be a fungus ball; clinical correlation, urinalysis, and urine culture may help in making the diagnosis. If neoplasm (transitional cell carcinoma) is suspected, urine cytology and brush biopsy are indicated. If these histologic studies are positive, surgery is indicated. If urine cytology and brush biopsy are both negative, the patient must be

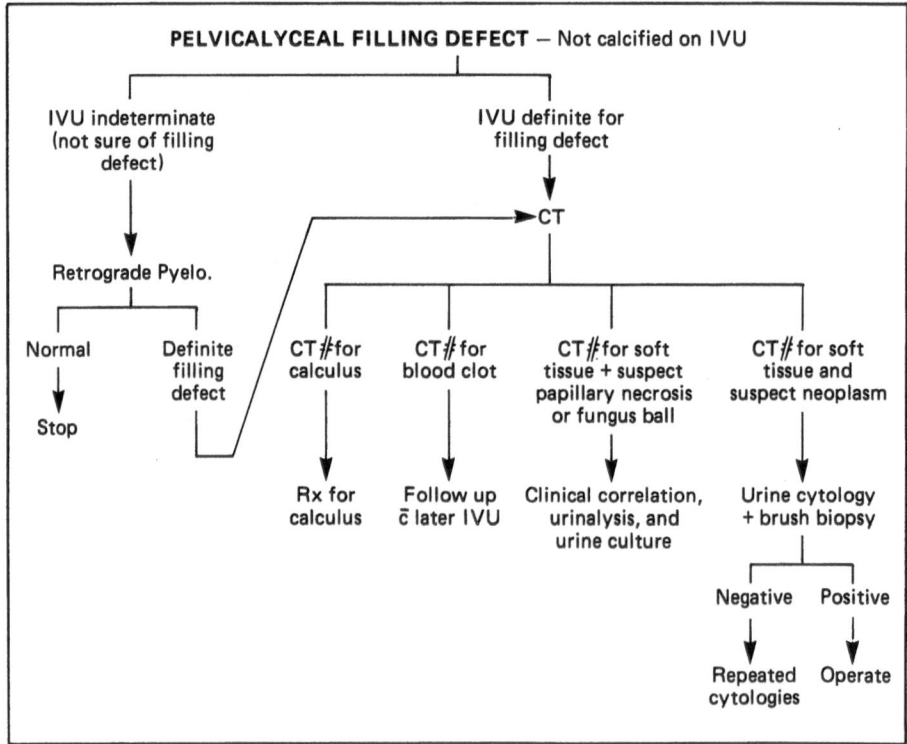

Fig. 17.20. Algorithm for pelvicalyceal filling defect.

followed closely, with repeat cytologic studies. Follow-up CT is also reasonable, looking for any increase in the size of the soft-tissue mass or evidence of contrast enhancement, either finding leading to the presumptive diagnosis of neoplasm. Because of the much greater likelihood of an intrapelvic soft-tissue mass being neoplastic rather than inflammatory, there is some justification for proceeding with surgical exploration once the initial CT study shows the filling defect to be of soft tissue density, especially if it manifests contrast enhancement.

Algorithm for Hydronephrosis (Fig. 17.21)

In a clinical situation suggesting the possibility of renal neoplasm, the finding of hydronephrosis on urography or sonography should be further evaluated with antegrade or retrograde pyelography, as well as urine cytology examination. If pyelography reveals the smooth narrowing typical for congenital ureteropelvic junction obstruction, there is no need of further workup for renal malignancy. Irregular narrowing at the region of the ureteropelvic junction may be due either to neoplasm or an inflammatory process. A positive brush biopsy indicates the need for surgery; CT may be done preoperatively for staging. If the brush biopsy is negative, CT or sonography (if not already done) would be the next step;

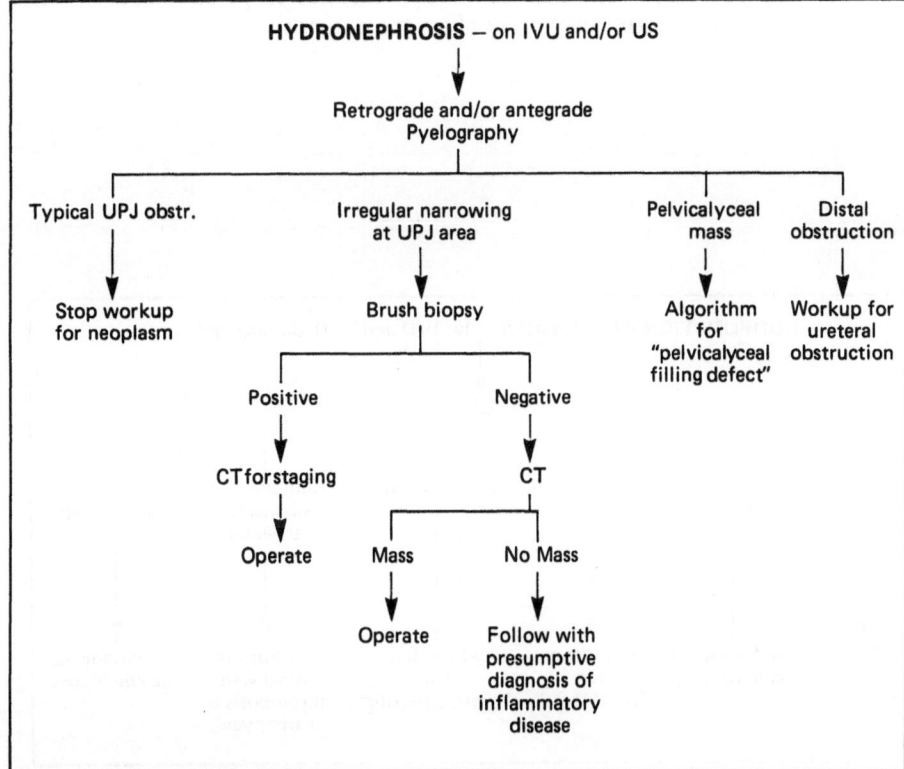

Fig. 17. 21. Algorithm for hydronephrosis.

demonstration of a soft-tissue mass in association with the irregular narrowing is an indication for surgery. In the absence of a mass, appropriate studies and careful follow-up are suggested for the presumptive diagnosis of inflammatory disease.

If antegrade or retrograde pyelography demonstrates a pelvicalyceal filling defect, the further workup proceeds along the course already discussed for such a finding. For hydronephrosis secondary to obstruction below the ureteropelvic junction, the workup is for ureteral obstruction rather than renal neoplasm.

Algorithm for Nonfunction of a Kidney (Fig. 17.22)

Nonfunction of a kidney on intravenous urography or renal scan is next evaluated by sonography. Possible sonographic findings include absence of the kidney (congenital or postoperative), medical renal disease (abnormal renal parenchyma or renal atrophy), normal appearance, replacement of the kidney by a mass, hydronephrosis, homogeneous enlargement as from edema or inflammation, and diffuse infiltration of the renal parenchyma by small focal lesions. With a normal appearance, further evaluation for renal arterial obstruction is warranted. For replacement of the kidney by a mass or for hydronephrosis, refer to the algorithms already discussed for those findings. Diffuse homogeneous enlargement of a nonfunctioning kidney with a sonographic appearance of edema suggests renal vein thrombosis or acute pyelonephritis, for both of which there are usually appropriate clinical signs. When diffuse infiltration of the kidney by neoplasm is suspected, e.g., lymphoma, leukemia, or multiple metastases, percutaneous needle biopsy is the most direct approach to confirm the diagnosis.

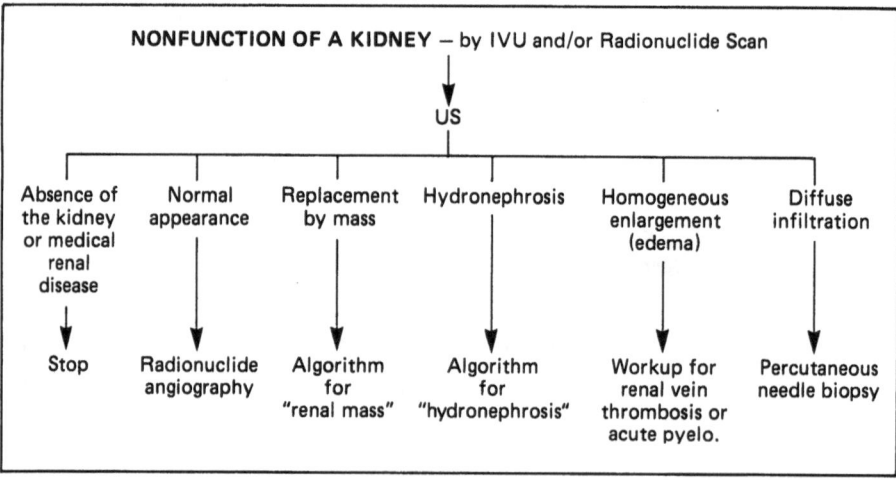

Fig. 17.22. Algorithm for nonfunction of a kidney.

References

1. Abrams HL (1978) Renal tumor versus renal cyst. Cardiovasc Radiol 1:59–75
2. Amis ES, Crenan JJ, Yader IC, Pfister RC, Newhouse JH (1982) Renal cysts: curios and caveats. Urol Radiol 4:199–209
3. Arger PH, Mulhern CB, Pollack HM, Banner MP, Wein AJ (1979) Ultrasonic assessment of renal transitional cell carcinoma: Preliminary report. AJR 132:407–411
4. Balfe DM, McClennan BL, Stanley RJ, Weyman PJ, Sagel SS (1982) Evaluation of renal masses considered indeterminate on computed tomography. Radiology 142:421–428
5. Baron RL, McClennan BL, Lee JKT, Lawson TL (1982) Computed tomography of transitional-cell carcinoma of the renal pelvis and ureter. Radiology 144:125–130
6. Behan M, Wixson D, Pitts WR, Kazam E (1980) Sonographic evaluation of renal masses. Correlations with angiography. Urol Radiol 1:137–145
7. Bhatt GM, Bernardino ME, Graham SD Jr (1983) CT diagnosis of renal metastases. J Comput Assist Tomogr 7:1032–1034
8. Blute RD, Gittes RR, Gittes RF (1981) Renal brush biopsy: Survey of indications, techniques, and results. J Urol 126: 146–149
9. Bosniak MA (1981) Angiomyolipoma (hamartoma) of the kidney: a preoperative diagnosis is possible in virtually every case. Urol Radiol 3:135–142
10. Bracken B, Jonsson K (1979) How accurate is angiographic staging of renal carcinoma? Urology 14:96–99
11. Branch CF (1929) Some observations on solitary cysts of the kidney. J Urol 21:451–453
12. Burstein J, Woodside JR (1977) Malignant hemorrhagic renal cyst with occult neoplasm. Radiology 123:599–600
13. Carlson DH, Carlson D, Simon H (1978) Benign multilocular cystic nephroma. AJR 131:621–625
14. Chilcote WA, Brokowski GP (1983) Computed tomography in renal lymphoma. J Comput Assist Tomogr 7:439–443
15. Clayman RV, Gonzalez R, Fraley EE (1980) Renal cell cancer invading the inferior vena cava: Clinical review and anatomic approach. J Urol 123:138–143
16. Coleman BG, Arger PH (1983) Sonography of renal adenocarcinomas. CRC Crit Rev Diagn Imaging 19:203–255
17. Coleman BG, Arger PH, Mulhern CB, Pollack HM, Banner MP, Arenson RL (1980) Gray-scale sonographic spectrum of hypernephromas. Radiology 137:757–765
18. Daniel WW, Hartman GW, Witten DM, Farrow GM, Kelalis PP (1972) Calcified renal masses: A review of ten years experience at the Mayo Clinic. Radiology 103:503–508
19. Elkin M (1980) Radiology of the urinary system. Little, Brown, & Co., Boston, p 297
20. Ferris EJ, Bosniak MA, O'Connor JF (1968) An angiographic sign demonstrating extension of renal carcinoma into the renal vein and vena cava. AJR 102:384–391
21. Frija J, Larde C, Belloir H, Botto H, Martin N, Vasile N (1980) Computed tomography diagnosis of renal angiomyolipoma. J Comput Assist Tomogr 4:843–846
22. Fishman MC, Pollack HM, Arger PH, Banner MP (1983) High protein content: another cause of CT hyperdense benign renal cyst. J Comput Assist Tomogr 6:1103–1106
23. Gill WB, Lu C, Bibba M (1979) Retrograde brush biopsy of the ureter and renal pelvis. Urol Clin North Am 6:573–587
24. Goldman SM, Meng C, White RI, Naraval RC, Siegelman SS, Diamond AB, Kaufman SL, Harrington DP (1977) Transitional cell tumors of the kidney: How diagnostic is the angiogram? AJR 129:99–105
25. Green WM, King DL, Casarella WJ (1976) A reappraisal of sonolucent renal masses. Radiology 121:163–171
26. Hata Y, Shimpei T, Kato Y, Onishi T, Masudo F, Machida T (1983) Staging of renal cell carcinoma by computed tomography. J Comput Assist Tomogr 7:828–832
27. Heiken JP, Gold RP, Schnur MG, King DL, Bashist B, Glazer HS (1983) Computed tomography of renal lymphoma with ultrasound correlation. J Comput Assist Tomogr 7:245–250
28. Hellsten S, Berge T, Linell F (1983) Clinically unrecognized renal carcinoma: aspects of tumour morphology, lymphatic, and haematogenous metastatic spread. Br J Urol 55:116–170
29. Hidalgo H, Dunnick NR, Rosenberg ER, Ram PC, Korobkin M (1982) Parapelvic cysts: appearance on CT and sonography. AJR 138:667–671
30. Hoddick W, Jeffrey RB, Goldberg HI, Federle MP, Laing FC (1983) CT and sonography of severe renal and perirenal infections. AJR 140:517–520
31. Hricak H, Williams RD, Moon KL, Moss AA, Alpers C, Crooks LE, Kaufman L (1983) Nuclear magnetic resonance imaging of the kidney: renal masses. Radiology 147:765–772

32. Jafri SZ, Bree RL, Amendola MA, Glazer GM, Schwab RE, Francis JR, Borlaza G (1982) CT of renal and perirenal non-Hodgkin lymphoma. AJR 138:1101–1105
33. Karlsen S (1981) Improved technique for retrograde brushing in diagnosis of urothelial tumors of the upper urinary tract. Urology 18:345–348
34. Kass DA, Hricak H, Davidson AJ (1983) Renal malignancies with normal excretory urograms. AJR 141:731–734
35. Kilton L, Matthews MJ, Cohen MH (1980) Adult Wilms' tumor: a report of prolonged survival and review of the literature. J Urol 124:1–5
36. Kissane JM (1976) The morphology of renal cystic disease. Perspect Nephrol Hypertension 4:31–63
37. Klein MJ, Valensi QJ (1976) Proximal tubular adenomas of kidney with so-called oncocytic features. A clinicopathologic study of 13 cases of a rarely reported neoplasm. Cancer 38:906–914
38. Kreel L, Bydder GM (1981) Evaluation of retroperitoneal liposarcoma with computed tomography. CT 5:111–117
39. Kremkau FW (1980) Diagnostic ultrasound. Physical principles and exercises. Grune and Stratton, New York
40. Kursh ED, Perskey L (1971) Selective renal arteriography in renal lymphoma. J Urol 105:772
41. Kyaw M, Koehler PR (1969) Renal and perirenal lymphoma: arteriographic findings. Radiology 93:1051–1053
42. Lang EK (1984) Angio-computed tomography and dynamic computed tomography in staging of renal cell carcinoma. Radiology 151:149–155
43. Lang EK (1973) Arteriography in the diagnosis and staging of hypernephromas. Cancer 32:1043–1052
44. Lang EK, Alexander R, Barnett T, Palomar J, Hemway S (1978) Brush biopsy of pyelocalyceal lesions via a percutaneous translumbar approach. Radiology 129:623–627
45. Lang EK, personal communication
46. Leekam RN, Matzinger MA, Brunelle M (1983) The sonography of renal columnar hypertrophy. JCU 11:491–494
47. Levine E, Huntrakoon M (1983) Computed tomography of renal oncocytoma. AJR 141:741–746
48. Lieber MM, Tomera FM, Taylor WF, Farrow GM (1981) Renal adenocarcinoma in young adults: survival and variables affecting prognosis. J Urol 125:164–168
49. Lingard DA, Lawson TL (1979) Accuracy of ultrasound in predicting the nature of renal masses. J Urol 122:724–727
50. McClennan BL, Stanley RJ, Melson GL, Levitt RG, Sagel SS (1979) CT of the renal cyst: is cyst aspiration necessary? AJR 133:671–675
51. McLaughlin AP III, Talner LB, Leopold GR, McCullough DL (1974) Avascular primary renal cell carcinoma: varied pathologic and angiographic features. J Urol 111:587–593
52. Madewell JR, Goldman SM, Davis JD Jr, Hartman DS, Feigin DS, Lichtenstein JE (1983) Multilocular cystic nephroma: a radiographic-pathologic correlation of 58 patients. Radiology 146:309–321
53. Mahony BS, Jeffrey RB, Laing FC (1983) Septa of Bertin: a sonographic pseudotumor. JCU 11:317–319
54. Mauro MA, Wadsworth DE, Stanley RJ, McClennan BL (1982) Renal cell carcinoma: angiography in the CT era. AJR 139:1135–1138
55. Morehouse HT, Weiner SN, Hoffman JC (1984) Imaging in inflammatory disease of the kidney. AJR 143:135–141
56. Pagani JJ, Bernardino ME (1982) Incidence and significance of serendipitous CT findings in the oncologic patient. J Comput Assist Tomogr 6:268–275
57. Pamilo M, Suramo I, Paivansala M (1983) Characteristics of hypernephromas as seen with ultrasound and computed tomography. JCU 11:245–249
58. Parienty RA, Ducellier R, Pradel J, Lubrano J-M, Coquille F, Richard F (1982) Diagnostic value of CT numbers in pelvocalyceal filling defects. Radiology 145:743–747
59. Parienty RA, Pradel J, Imbert M, Picard J-D, Savart P (1981) Computed tomography of multilocular cystic nephroma. Radiology 140: 135–139
60. Parienty RA, Pradel J, Picard J-D, Ducellier R, Lubrano JM, Smolarski N (1981) Visibility and thickening of the renal fascia on computed tomograms. Radiology 139:119–124
61. Parvey LS, Warner RM, Callihan TR, Magill HL (1981) CT demonstration of fat tissue in malignant renal neoplasms: atypical Wilms' tumors. J Comput Assist Tomogr 5:851–854
62. Plainfasse MC, Merran S (1982) How does ultrasound show renal cancer: diagnostic difficulties and reliability. Prog Clin Biol Res 100:369–375
63. Pollack HM, Arger PH, Banner MP, Mulhern CB, Coleman BG (1981) Computed tomography of renal pelvic filling defects. Radiology 138:645–651

64. Pollack HM, Banner MP, Arger PH, Peters J, Mulhern CB, Coleman BG (1982) The accuracy of gray scale renal ultrasonography in differentiating cystic neoplasms from benign cysts. Radiology 143:741–745
65. Pollack HM (1971) Radiologic examination of the urinary tract. Harper and Row, New York, pp 103–104
66. Pollack HM (1971) Radiologic examination of the urinary tract. Harper and Row, New York, pp 86–102
67. Raymond HW, Swiebel WJ (eds) (1983) Physics. Semin Ultrasound 4:3–62
68. Richie JP, Garnick MB, Seltzer S, Bettman M (1983) Computerized tomography scan for diagnosis and staging of renal cell carcinoma. J Urol 129:1114–1116
69. Richmond J, Sherman RS, Diamond HD, Craver LF (1962) Renal lesions associated with malignant lymphomas. Am J Med 32:184–207
70. Robson CJ, Churchill BM, Anderson W (1969) The results of radical nephrectomy for renal cell carcinoma. J Urol 101:297–301
71. Rubenstein MA, Walz BJ, Bucy JG (1978) Transitional cell carcinoma of the kidney: 25-year experience. J Urol 119:594–597
72. Segal AJ, Spitzer RM (1979) Pseudo thick-walled renal cyst by CT. AJR 132:827–828
73. Shirkoda A, Staab EV, Mittelstaedt CA (1980) Renal lymphoma imaged by ultrasound and gallium-67. Radiology 137:175–180
74. Siminovitch JMP, Montie JE, Straffon RA (1983) Prognostic indicators in renal adenocarcinoma. J Urol 130:20–23
75. Sniderman KW, Krieger JN, Seligson GR, Sos TA (1979) The radiologic and clinical aspects of calcified hypernephroma. Radiology 131:31–35
76. Subramanyam BR, Raghavendra BN, Madamba MR (1982) Renal transitional cell carcinoma: sonographic and pathologic correlation. JCU 10: 203–210
77. Sufrin G, Etra W, Gaeta J, Merrin CE (1975) Hypernephroma arising in the wall of a simple renal cyst. Urology 6:507–510
78. Sussman S, Cochran ST, Pagani JJ, McArdle C, Wong W, Austin R, Curry N, Kelly KM (1984) Hyperdense renal masses: a CT manifestation of hemorrhagic renal cysts. Radiology 150:207–211
79. Thackray AC (1964) Malignant tumors of the urothelium. In: Riches E (ed) Tumors of the kidney and ureter. Williams and Wilkins, Baltimore, pp 87–98
80. Wallace S, Chuang VP, Swanson D, Bracken B, Hersh EM, Ayala A, Johnson D (1981) Embolization of renal carcinoma. Experience with 100 patients. Radiology 138:563–570
81. Weiner SN, Bernstein RG (1977) Renal oncocytoma: angiographic features of two cases. Radiology 125:633–635
82. Weyman PJ, McClennan BL, Lee JKT, Stanley RJ (1982) CT of calcified renal masses. AJR 138: 1095–1099
83. Weyman PJ, McClennan BL, Stanley RJ, Levitt RG, Sagel SS (1980) Comparison of computed tomography and angiography in the evaluation of renal cell carcinoma. Radiology 137:417–424

Chapter 18

Radiological Diagnosis of Benign Renal Neoplasms

Stanford M. Goldman

Introduction

Many have attempted to develop an appropriate classification for the myriad benign tumors that are found within the kidney. Part of the difficulty lies in the multiplicity of different cells that arise normally in the kidney and its capsule. In addition, unusual cell types not normally present in the kidney can occur, giving rise to rare neoplasms. Most common classifications are based purely on the cell of origin (Table 18.1) [63]. Others have combined cell type with site of tumor origin as the basis for their classification (Table 18.2) [35]. We propose the use of a more clinically oriented approach. This classification is divided into the commonly seen and/or radiographically important neoplasms and those benign tumors which are both extremely rare and extremely difficult to diagnose preoperatively (Table 18.3). We hope this classification will be somewhat more useful to the practicing urologist and radiologist.

Table 18.1. Benign tumors (modified from Lakey [63])

Adenoma
Fibroma
Lipoma
Leiomyoma
Angiomyoma
Rhabdomyoma
Neurofibroma
Teratoma
Angiomyolipoma

Table 18.2. Classification of Deming and Harvard (modified) [35]

1. Tumors of the renal capsule
   a) Fibroma
   b) Leiomyoma
   c) Lipoma
   d) Mixed

2. Tumors of mature renal parenchyma
   a) Adenoma
   b) Papillary cystadenoma
   c) Oncocytoma

3. Epithelial tumors of the renal pelvis
   a) Transitional cell papilloma

4. Vascular tumors
   a) Hemangioma
   b) Hamartoma—angiomyolipoma
   c) Lymphangioma

5. Neurogenic tumors
   a) Neuroblastoma
   b) Sympathicoblastoma
   c) Schwannoma

6. Mesenchymal derivatives
   a) Connective tissues—fibroma
   b) Adipose tissue—lipoma
   c) Muscle tumors—leiomyomas

7. Perirenal tumors

Table 18.3. Benign renal tumors—present classification

A. *Common clinically seen and/or radiographically important tumors*
   1. Angiomyolipoma—isolated
   2. Angiomyolipoma in tuberous sclerosis and other overlapping syndromes
   3. Adenoma
   4. Oncocytoma
   5. Mesoblastic nephroma (fetal renal hamartoma)
   6. Multilocular cystic nephroma
   7. Diffuse nephroblastomatosis and nodular blastema
   8. Hemangioma
   9. Leiomyoma
   10. Juxtaglomerular tumors

B. *Rarely seen tumors*
   1. Lipoma
   2. Myelolipoma
   3. Lymphangioma
   4. Fibroma
   5. Hemangiopericytoma
   6. Ganglioneuroma
   7. Endometriosis
   8. Carcinoid tumors
   9. Teratoma

Common Benign Tumors

Angiomyolipomas

General Concepts

The angiomyolipoma (AML) is a benign renal tumor composed of varying amounts of blood vessels, fat, and smooth muscle [70]. The majority of AMLs are found as small asymptomatic lesions at autopsy. However, they do represent 1% of all renal tumors explored surgically. About 75% occur as an isolated solitary renal mass in middle-aged females. However, the tumor can be seen at any age [13]. An additional 20% are seen in tuberous sclerosis patients, but these are multiple and bilateral (see below). There is another 5% of patients with multiple bilateral AML without the stigmata of tuberous sclerosis. Whether this latter group should be considered in the spectrum of tuberous sclerosis remains to be determined.

As will be discussed below, many of these isolated tumors are now being identified by serendipity during routine CT and ultrasonic examinations. In the symptomatic group, 75% had flank pain, 41% noted a flank mass, 30% had hematuria, and 18% were admitted with hypotension [90]. The latter arises because of a definite tendency for hemorrhage to occur in AML, which can lead to a rapid demise. It is for this reason that the larger lesions should always be removed.

On gross examination, the masses are smooth, round, or oval, and well circumscribed but not encapsulated. The tumor tends to be located near the surface of the kidney and has a tendency to grow into the perirenal space rather than intrarenally. The intrarenal component of the tumor does not invade the parenchyma but tends to compress the renal tissue. The amounts of adipose tissue, smooth muscle, and blood vessels vary from tumor to tumor as well as from area to area within the individual tumor. Thus, grossly, the tumor may be yellow (predominantly fat) or tan or gray (predominantly smooth muscle). Hemorrhage and necrosis are often present [40, 90]. Characteristically the small arteries and most of the larger ones are devoid of elastica. The smooth muscle also tends to form a collar about the periphery of the vessel or show an intimate, perpendicular orientation in relation to it [90]. Although considered benign, local lymph nodes [22] and the inferior vena cava [61] may be involved, probably secondary to multicentric tumors.

Radiographic Findings

On plain film, fat is occasionally seen and is almost diagnostic of AML (less than 10%) (Fig. 18.1a). Rarely, calcification will be noted (Fig. 18.1b). On intravenous urogram (IVU), a smooth mass is seen which may occasionally distort but never invade the calyces. The nephrotomogram may demonstrate the fat that may not have been apparent on the plain film (Fig. 18.1c).

In the mid-1960s, the angiographic examination (Fig. 18.2) was being touted as virtually pathognomonic [104]. The AML was described as being hypervascular with large feeding vessels passing through the mass. In addition, one noted the following [9, 19, 30, 55, 104]:

1. Multisacculated aneurysmal dilatations (bunch of grapes)

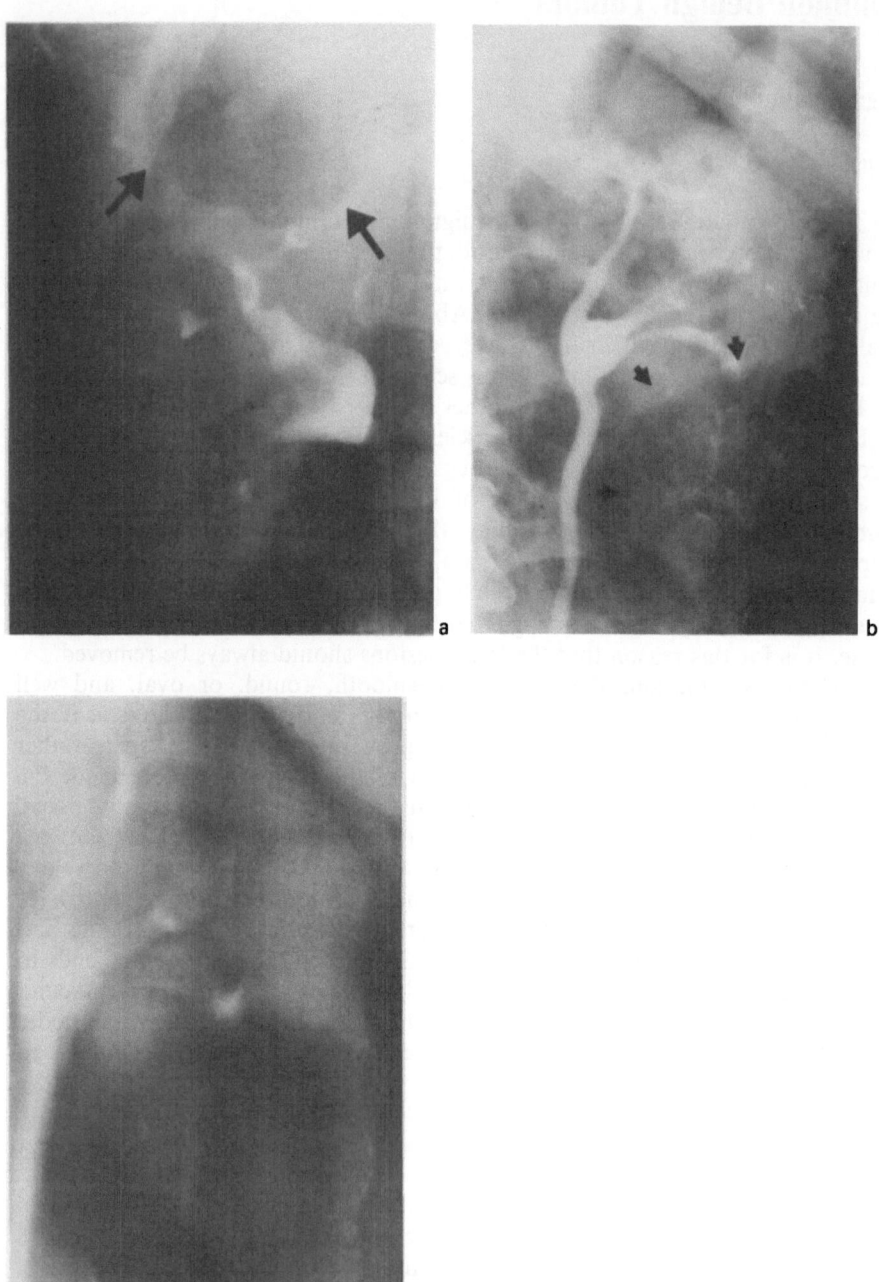

Fig. 18.1a–c. Plain film and IVU changes in angiomyolipomas. **a** Fatty tumor (*arrows*) clearly seen in upper pole of kidney. **b** Calcification and fat in lower pole mass (*arrows*). **c** Nephrotomogram in same patient as **b,** more clearly demonstrating the fat.

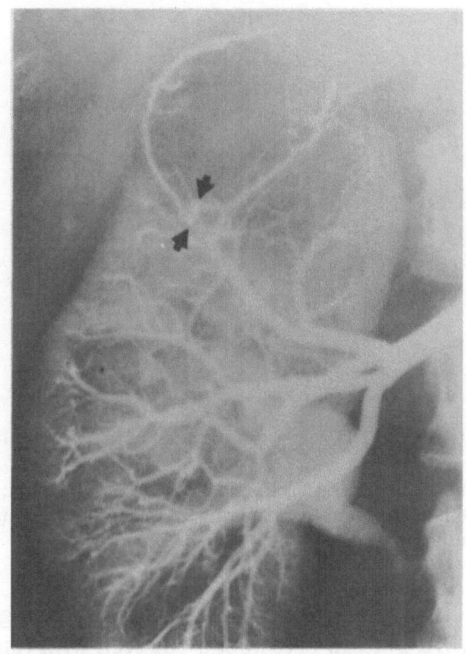

Fig. 18.2. Angiographic findings in angiomyolipomas. RU pole mass which is fatty. Note the mass to be quite vascular with a few microaneurysms (*arrows*).

2. Microaneurysms
3. Delicate, discrete neovascularity *without* AV shunting
4. "Onion peeling"
5. Whorled appearance in the venous phase

It soon became clear, however, that similar findings could be seen in hypernephroma as well [55]. Furthermore, these tumors could be avascular. Jander and Tonkin [55] have advocated the use of epinephrine. They believe that vasoconstriction will occur with an AML but not with a hypernephroma. We have serious doubts that this method need be invoked in the era of CT and ultrasound (to be described below), and we would expect some angiographic false-positives and false-negatives to occur.

With the advent of ultrasound (Fig. 18.3) it soon became obvious that lipomatous tumors show a distinctive pattern which is very suggestive of AML [10, 87], that of a highly echogenic tumor mass. Behan and Kazam [10] suggest that this pattern reflects a mixture of fat and water, rather than fat alone. It is the acoustic impedance mismatch of the interfaces of fat and soft tissues with "subsequent large differences in acoustic impedance that results in the high echogenicity." Although this pattern is characteristic [10, 77, 87, 88] and most common, variations can occur. In our series of ten cases, six demonstrated the typical pattern, but even these had some areas with lesser echogenicity representing nonfatty elements of the tumor, focal hemorrhage, and/or dilated calyces. In two, a mixed pattern was noted corresponding to areas of hemorrhage. The final two had low echogenicity representing areas of old organized hemorrhage, cavitation, a relative absence of fat, or a combination of all three. In addition, evidence of an associated perirenal hemorrhage was often demonstrated.

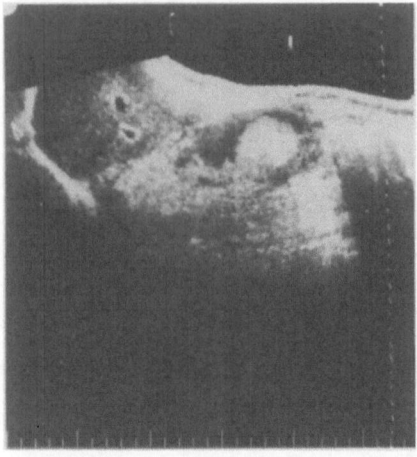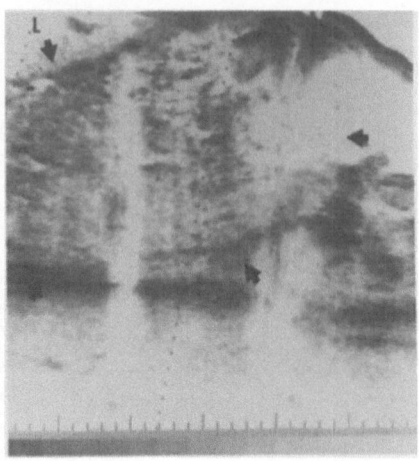

Fig. 18.3. a Classic ultrasound of an AML with typical, highly echogenic pattern. b A typical ultrasound with mixed ultrasonic pattern because the tumor is mostly nonfatty (*L*, liver; *arrows* delineate kidney outline).

However, it is clear that this highly echogenic pattern is not pathognomonic for AML but can occasionally be seen with renal carcinomas [50], cavernous hemangiomas, renal oncocytomas [23], and sclerosing metanephric hamartomas, a lesion somewhat similar to a Wilms tumor (personal experience). For this reason, we believe that the ultrasound alone should not be relied upon and that a CT should be performed in all these cases (including the small, less than 2 cm, serendipitously identified tumors).

In those cases of AML with significant fat content, CT can be diagnostic, requiring no further workup. The CT findings [49, 77, 88, 90, 101] are those of a well-circumscribed tumor whose predominant CT numbers are low, in the range of fat (−70 HU) (Fig. 18.4a). Intermixed within it, one can appreciate areas of varying size with CT numbers corresponding to tissue density (Fig. 18.4b). These areas represent portions of the tumor with predominantly leiomyomatous and/or hematogenous elements. Regions where recent hemorrhage or old hemorrhagic breakdown have occurred are also readily identified. Extension of the tumor into the perirenal space and perirenal hemorrhage are also easily recognized.

In the occasional case where the leiomyomatous and/or hematogenous elements predominate, the CT will not be characteristic as the CT numbers will be greater than fat [90]. In some cases there will be the stigmata of tuberous sclerosis that will suggest the proper diagnosis (see below). In one case, the highly echogenic ultrasound was suggestive even though the CT was totally nondiagnostic. On the pathological slides of this case, one noted that the fat and other elements were completely and uniformly intermixed, giving a CT number far above normal adipose tissue. A few isolated cases of AML will not be diagnosed preoperatively because of the relative absence of fat. Fortunately, these are rare.

Two other unusual manifestations of AML deserve to be mentioned. Regional lymph node involvement can occur [22] and may possibly be identified on CT. These are felt to be secondary to a multicentric origin of the AML and not metastases. Recently, extension of AML into inferior vena cava has been recognized by ultrasound and obviously will be confusing.

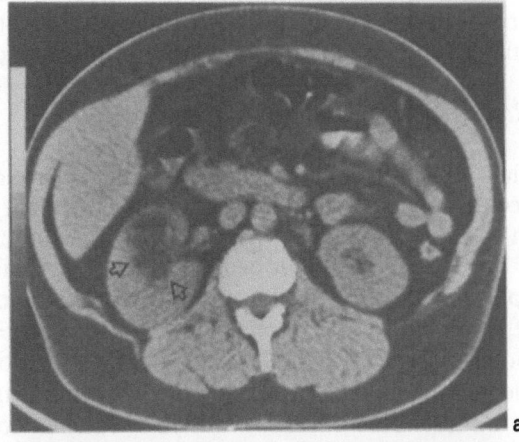

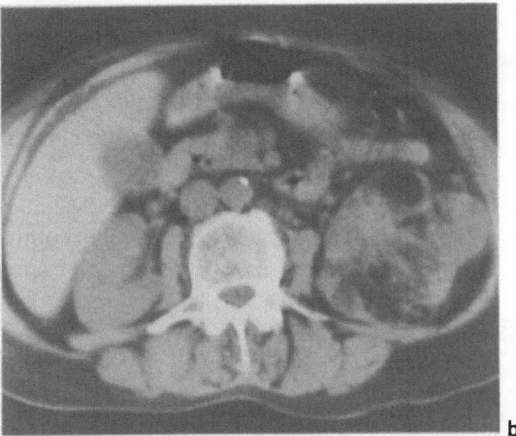

Fig. 18.4a,b. CT of angiomyolipomas. **a** Typical AML (*arrows*) on nonenhanced CT. **b** Less typical left renal AML composed of areas of both low (i.e., fat) and high (i.e., myelogenous and/or hematogenous fat) CT density.

Tuberous Sclerosis (Bourneville's Disease)

General Concepts

Tuberous sclerosis is an autosomal dominant disease with a classic clinical triad which consists of adenoma sebaceum, seizures, and mental retardation [14, 27]. This, however, hardly encompasses the many systems that can be and often are involved. The brain lesions represent hamartomas in the cerebral cortex and paraventricular regions. In addition, the cerebellum, medulla, and spinal cord may be affected. The lesions are of two types: cortical foci or tubules and subependymal nodules. The skin lesions include adenoma sebaceum, ungual fibromas, café au lait spots, fibroepithelial tags, shagreen patches, port-wine nevi, and/or achromic patches. Retinal phakomas, cardiac tumors (myxoma, rhabdomyoma), pulmonary lesions (spontaneous pneumothorax, cystic changes associated with hyperplasia of the surrounding pulmonary tissue, pulmonary involvement with lymphangiomyomatosis), bone abnormalities (bone sclerosis, cystic areas), kidney angiomyolipomas and/or cysts, and gastrointestinal tract, liver, and splenic tumors are also seen in tuberous sclerosis. Although the diagnosis may be obvious clinically, it is often first suspected during the uroradiological evaluation. Renal involvement is usually bilateral and occurs in 50%–80% of tuberous sclerosis patients.

Radiographic Findings

Plain films showing oval or flair-like, sclerotic patches in the pelvic bone or occasionally in the vertebra suggest the possibility of tuberous sclerosis (Fig. 18.5). In a small percentage of patients (10%) the fat can be identified on the plain film.

The IVU, CT, and ultrasound show the typical characteristics of the angiomyolipomas as described above. However, the lesions are usually bilateral and are often extensive in nature. On IVU, the changes can mimic those of polycystic kidneys [4] (Fig. 18.5). However, the CT and ultrasound will usually demonstrate the fatty component in the angiomyolipoma (Fig. 18.6).

In those cases where the muscle or vascular components predominate, the only clues to correct diagnosis of tuberous sclerosis would be:

1. Sclerotic bone changes as described above.
2. Periosteal new bone formation in the metatarsals and/or metacarpals, and/or cystic changes in the phalanges.
3. Signs of cardiac enlargement on the chest film. Echocardiographic or angiographic findings of cardiac tumors.
4. Evidence of a diffuse interstitial process in the lung. In the early phases, the pattern is reticulonodular; later, honeycombing develops. Lymphangiomatosis of the lung may cause cor pulmonale or spontaneous pneumothorax.

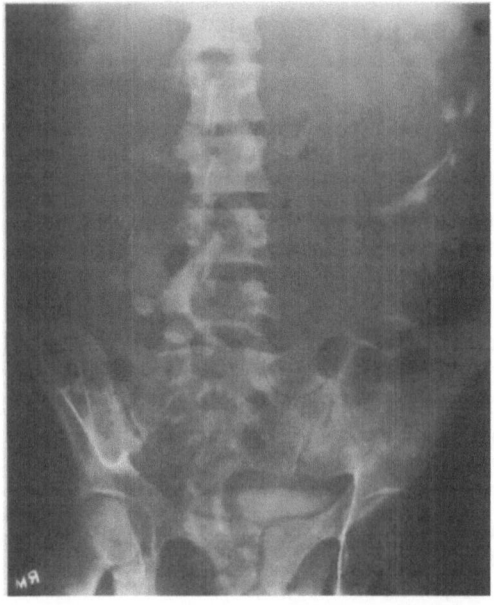

Fig. 18.5. IVU in patient with tuberous sclerosis. Note sclerotic areas in left iliac bone and in both pubic rami which suggest the diagnosis. Note the bilateral renal masses which alone would have suggested polycystic kidneys.

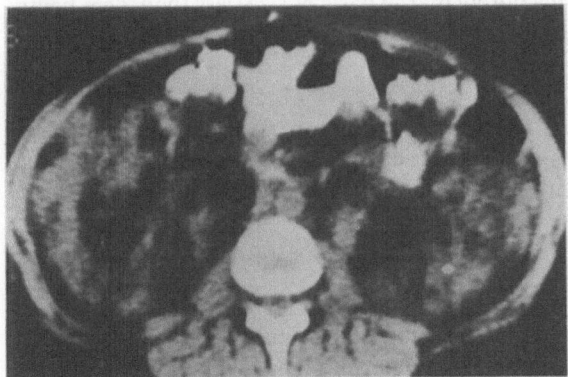

Fig. 18.6. CT findings in tuberous sclerosis. Typical bilateral AML with both fatty, myelogenous and hematogenous elements.

5. Calcification in singular or multiple paraventricular subependymal nodules.
6. Angiographic and/or CT demonstration of adrenal and hepatic hamartomas [30].

Overlapping Syndromes

There have been several reports of patients with tuberous sclerosis who have had other syndromes as well:

1. Polycystic kidney disease (Wenzel et al. [108]; Kissane [59]).
2. Renal cell carcinoma (Suslavich et al. [98]).
3. Lymphangiomatosis: This is believed to be a forme fruste of tuberous sclerosis, with 15% developing renal AML. In patients with lymphangiomatosis, a renal mass must be considered as an AML until proven otherwise even in the absence of fat [84].

Adenomas

General Concepts

Adenomas are the most common benign tumors and are found frequently (up to 22.4%) as incidental findings at autopsy [21]. There are three histological types [21]:

1. Papillary, a frond-like tumor with a single layer of small cells, often with cystic changes.
2. Tubular, with elevated irregular tubules composed of basophilic cells.
3. Alveolar, with large polyhedral cells with clear cytoplasm that are frankly difficult to distinguish from a clear-cell adenocarcinoma. The relationship between this lesion and renal cell carcinoma is subject to a great deal of controversy [72, 105]. Some believe the adenoma to be premalignant, others do

not. Some separate these lesions purely on the basis of size (less than 3 cm being considered benign), although there are clearly renal carcinomas that are smaller than 2 cm.

The papillary and tubular types are the most common, with the alveolar being seen infrequently (3%). The lesion is seen twice as often in males, usually occurring in those over 40. They present with hematuria (50%) and less frequently abdominal discomfort.

Radiographic Features

On plain film, a mass may be seen. Calcification has been reported in a few instances [21, 81]. The IVU will show a tumor which is either solid or cystic looking with a thick rim [89]. There is usually no tracer uptake on isotopic scans [25]; the ultrasound will have varying echogenicity, compatible with a solid mass.

The tubular adenoma is usually hypervascular (82%), with neovascularization being noted in about a quarter of the lesions [21, 25, 52, 56]. In the nephrographic phase the mass is dense (82%) and homogeneous (64%), without AV shunting. The tumor is well circumscribed without parenchymal invasion.

Papillary (nononcocytic) adenomas are hypo- to avascular with faint, usually homogeneous tumor blush, while the alveolar adenoma is hypervascular with a heterogeneous, though sharply circumscribed, nephrographic phase. No arteriovenous shunting is noted in these lesions. The response of these lesions to epinephrine is variable although usually positive.

The noncontrast CT tends to show either a solid, homogeneous, well-circumscribed mass or occasionally one with a necrotic center and a thick rim. The enhanced study tends to show homogeneous uptake of contrast in most of the small, solid lesions. Cystic tumors can have an enhancing wall with a center displaying CT numbers of water or slightly above. Although the small lesion with uniform enhancement may be suggestive in the asymptomatic patient, it is presently impossible to exclude a renal carcinoma.

Oncocytomas (Benign Oxyphil Adenomas, Proximal Tubular Adenomas)

General Concepts

In recent years a subgroup of renal adenomas have become of diagnostic significance to radiologists and urologists because of their occasionally characteristic angiographic pattern [1]. These tumors are felt to arise from proximal tubules which have been transformed into the oxyphil cell. The latter contain swollen mitochondria rich with eosinophilic oxydative enzymes (hence the appellation benign oxyphil adenoma). In the past they were often misdiagnosed as renal cell carcinomas. They have been reported to comprise about 5% of all renal tumors [94]. They have a characteristic tan color [1] without hemorrhage and are usually exophytic. The tumors are usually asymptomatic and rarely bleed or cause pain unless very large.

Radiographic Findings (Figs. 18.7, 18.8)

The plain films are nonspecific, usually showing a solid mass. A case of ring-shaped

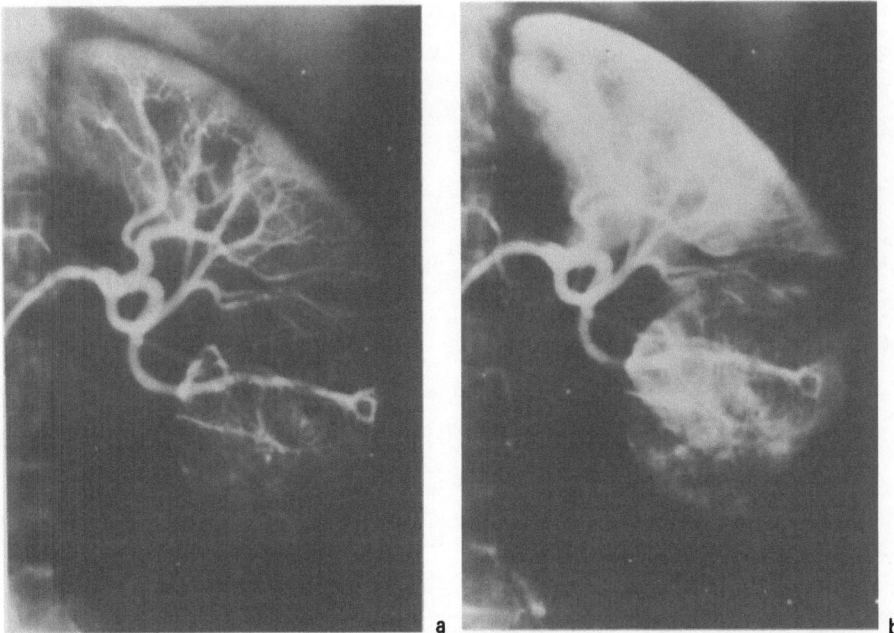

a   b

Fig. 18.7a,b. Typical spoked-wheel pattern of an oncocytoma. (By courtesy of E. K. Lang)

calcification has been reported [107]. The IVU shows a solid mass with well-defined borders. Although the tumor is made of proximal tubular cells, studies with ^{99m}Tc-glucoheptonate and ^{131}I-orthoidohippurate have shown no uptake by oncocytomas [16, 65].

The real interest in this tumor was spurred by the report [109] of a characteristic spoked-wheel angiographic pattern to the vasculature of this tumor. In addition, there is usually a homogeneous blush with sharp margination and no irregular vessels or AV *shunting*. Oncocytomas can also be hypovascular [95]. In the hypovascular tumors, the lesions are indistinguishable from other renal masses. Occasionally, aneurysms are noted within the tumor [94].

The ultrasonic picture is that of a uniform, solid, sharply circumscribed mass with moderate echogenicity. When exophytic, the echogenicity is similar to that of normal renal parenchyma [62]. A central stellate scar may be identified ultrasonically [80], which can be helpful.

The CT pattern reflects the uniform cell characteristics described above. On the unenhanced study, the tumor has a sharp margin with a uniform CT number slightly above that of normal renal tissue (20–30 HU) [67] to slightly below it [2]. No extra renal or intraparenchymal infiltration is present. With contrast there is uniform enhancement, and with dynamic scanning a spoked-wheel pattern has been reported [2]. Occasionally a central scar is noted, which is suggestive of the correct diagnosis [2, 29]. We have seen an oncocytoma without this uniform pattern and this is to be expected since necrosis, etc. can occur. The MRI pattern is that of a mass with signal characteristics of normal kidney but which is sharply defined [46]. We are in agreement with Levine [67] that, although ultrasound and CT may be helpful, angiography is much more suggestive.

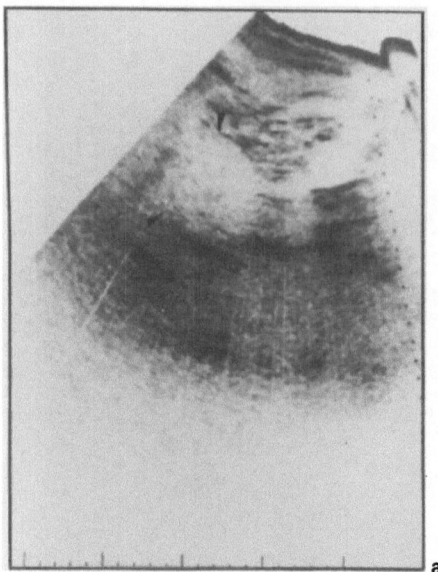

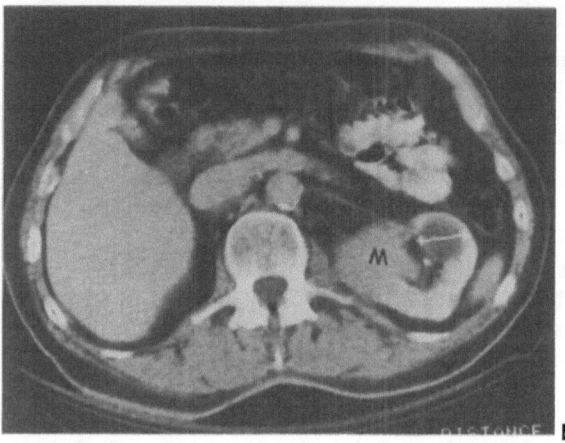

Fig. 18.8a,b. Another typical oncocytoma. **a** Ultrasound showing a moderately echogenic mass (*arrows*) which on its own is indistinguishable from a hypernephroma. **b** CT showing solid, homogeneous mass (*M*) consistent with oncocytoma. Benign cyst noted laterally.

Mesoblastic Nephromas (Fetal Renal Hamartomas)

General Concepts

In the past, this benign tumor of children under 1 year was mistaken for a Wilm's tumor. However, in the mid- and late-1960s, fetal renal hamartoma (FRH) became recognized as a distinct pathological entity [15, 51, 68, 71, 80]. Typically, the tumor is solid, whorl-like, unencapsulated, and replaces 60%–90% of the renal parenchyma. Hemorrhage and necrosis are uncommon but, when present, result in irregular areas of cystic degeneration. The tumor has a tendency to invade locally into the perirenal space and retroperitoneum but it does not metastasize. Occasionally, cysts are noted near the junction of the tumor and the uninvolved parenchyma. Microscopically, FRH consists of interlocking bundles of smooth muscle or mesenchymal cells. The tumor tends to grow between intact nephrons. This growth pattern may have significant diagnostic implications. In addition to the mesenchymal cells, a small number of dysplastic tubules and glomeruli are noted which may represent either trapped nephrons or benign neoplastic differentiation of the metanephric blastema [51].

These tumors are seen under 1 year of life, usually within the first 2 months postdelivery, and are the most common renal neoplasm in this age group. They usually present because of a palpable mass.

Radiographic Findings (Fig. 18.9)

The plain films demonstrate a soft tissue tumor usually without calcification [12, 15]. The IVU shows a kidney two to seven times larger than that on the opposite side, with a tumor distorting the calyces. There is often no evidence of hydronephrosis. Total body opacification techniques show a mixture of dense and lucent areas corresponding to compressed parenchyma as well as hypervascular and/or necrotic areas within the hamartoma [12]. Occasionally, small amounts of contrast are visualized within the tumor, representing dye in a distorted calyx. The tumor clearly arises within the kidneys and should not be confused with a neuroblastoma.

Recently, uptake of ^{99m}Tc-glucoheptonate by an FRH has been reported [97].

Angiographically, these tumors are usually quite vascular although they may appear hypovascular because of the cystic component. The vessels are irregular, bizarre, with a wandering, tortuous course [12]. There is an inhomogeneous blush without sharp margins consistent with its infiltrating nature.

The ultrasonic picture is that of a large mass with multiple areas of low level echoes interspersed with anechoic areas of varying size. The latter probably represent areas of hemorrhage and cystic degeneration within the tumor. It should not be confused with infantile polycystic kidneys, which is a bilateral disease. In hydronephrosis the dilated renal pelvis is usually readily identifiable on ultrasound, though the unilateral multicystic kidney may occasionally lead to confusion. However, in the latter, the entire kidney is involved and the "cystic" areas representing the abnormal calyces are usually larger than the anechoic areas seen in this tumor.

The CT findings suggest a solid or a mixed solid and cystic tumor.

Multilocular Cystic Nephromas (Multicystic Kidneys)

General Concepts

Multilocular cystic nephroma (MLCN) is an uncommon, nonfamilial, renal neoplasm being reported with increasing frequency. It is characterized by a well-circumscribed, encapsulated tumor that contains many noncommunicating fluid-filled locules. The tumor is usually contained by a thick, fibrous capsule. The locules are lined by thin, translucent septae. No functioning kidney elements are found in these septae. In children, microscopic foci of nephroblastoma may be seen

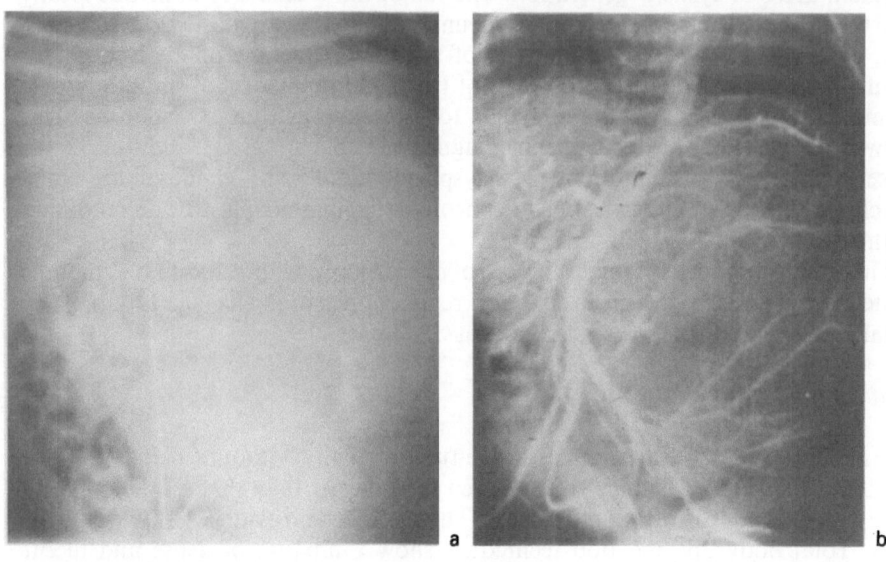

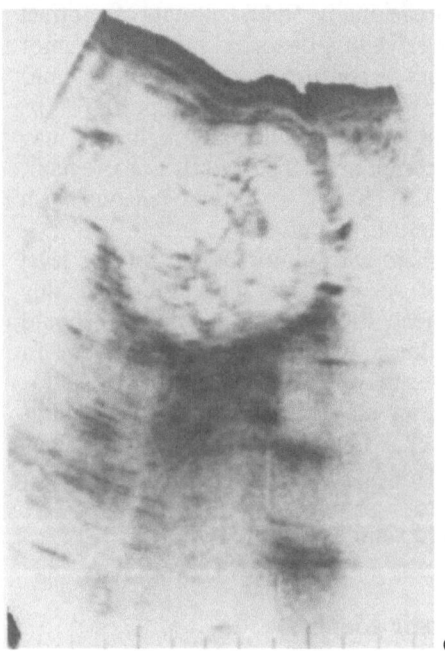

Fig. 18.9a–c. Renal hamartoma. **a** IVU demonstrating a nonspecific mass in the upper pole of left kidney. The LL pole calyx is noted to be functioning. **b** The angiogram shows a nonspecific vascular mass. Angiography is no longer recommended. **c** Ultrasound shows low level echoes interspersed with anechoic areas of varying size.

and occasionally a spindle cell pattern is identified in adults [69]. In a few adults, sarcomatous metastases occur [69]. According to the Armed Forces Institute of Pathology, the presence of renal carcinomatous tissue automatically means that one is dealing with a cystic renal carcinoma which should never be confused with MLCN.

The various synonyms for MLCN reflect the difficulty in diagnosing this lesion and the arguments as to its etiology. Other appellations include: multilocular cyst, multilocular renal cyst, cystic nephroma, cystic adenoma, Perlmann's tumor, cystadenoma, benign cystic differentiated nephroblastoma, polycystic Wilms tumor, cystic lymphangioma, partial polycystic kidney, etc. The more accepted theories as to its etiology are [6, 7, 59, 69, 79]:

1. A developmental, cystic enlargement of the collecting tubule. If the whole kidney is involved, then one is dealing with a multicystic kidney. If only a portion is affected, then an MLCN will develop.
2. A neoplasm, i.e., hamartoma, ripened Wilms tumor, etc. It is felt that MLCN and Wilms tumor have a common ancestor, the metanephric blastema, and thus there are occasional tumors with both cellular elements.

Children usually present with an incidental mass whereas adults present with pain and hematuria in addition. The sex distribution in children is about equal; however, in adults most MLCNs occur in females. Occasionally, hypertension appears to be associated with MLCN in adults.

Radiographic Findings

On plain films, a renal mass may be seen with only occasional calcification. On IVU, a well-defined nonfunctioning mass is noted, usually in a normally functioning kidney (Fig. 18.10a). Pelvic herniation of MLCN is the exception to the above and will often cause nonfunction secondary to obstruction. Occasionally, the septae can be identified on nephrotomography. The retrograde pyelogram will occasionally show the tumor herniating into the renal pelvis surrounded by contrast. Nuclear medicine will only demonstrate a nonfunctioning mass. On angiography, most are avascular or hypovascular; but highly vascular MLCN have been reported. The tumor is usually supplied by the renal artery; but, occasionally lumbar, intercostal, or other extrarenal arteries can feed the neoplasm [69] (Fig. 18.10b). Cyst puncture is unnecessary as the fluid is nondiagnostic and contrast will not fill the entire MLCN since the locules do not communicate.

On ultrasound, one usually demonstrates a cluster of echo free "cystic" masses separated by the intense echoes of the septae (Fig. 18.10c). Occasionally, if the cystic masses are extremely small, only a solid, nonspecific echogenic mass is identified. On CT, one notes a large, smooth, multiloculated mass (Fig. 18.10d). The septae may enhance but the fluid-filled locules (water density) should not demonstrate any contrast enhancement.

Based on the CT and ultrasound, Banner et al. [7] have suggested that the diagnosis can be made preoperatively in most cases; and they suggest a partial nephrectomy as the treatment of choice. If, on pathological examination, the diagnosis is incorrect or there are malignant changes, reexploration can then be undertaken. On the other hand, Feldberg and van Waes [41] have reported a multilocular renal carcinoma indistinguishable from MLCN by radiological techniques. In addition, an occasional Wilms tumor will be multilocular as well.

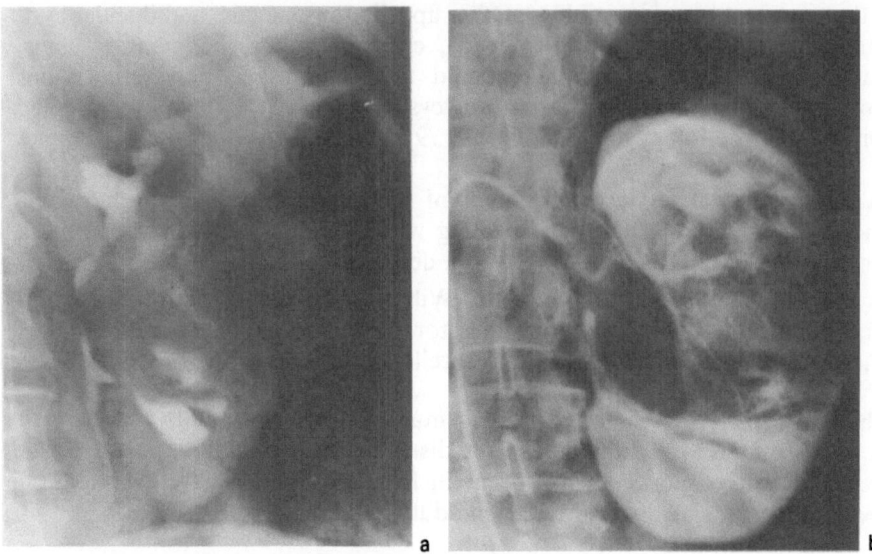

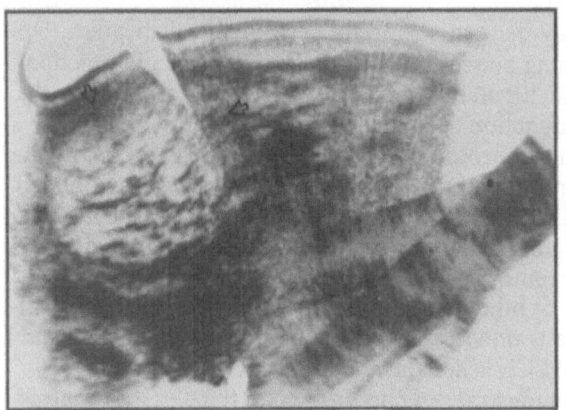

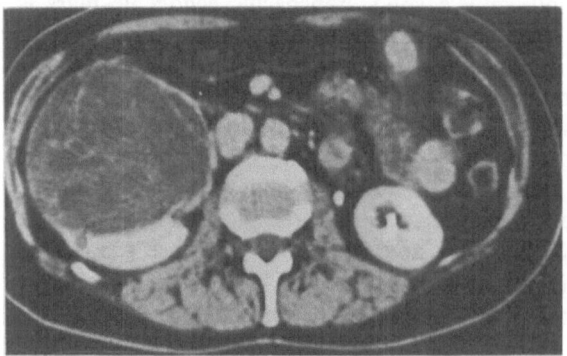

Fig. 18.10a–d. Multilocular cystic nephroma. **a** IVU showing mass in mid kidney. **b** Angiogram showing hypovascular mass. **c** Ultrasound showing multiple low density areas representing cysts (*arrows*). **d** CT showing typical septated cystic mass.

Diffuse Nephroblastomatosis and Nodular Blastema

General Concepts

These tumors are divided into diffuse and nodular forms. They can be inherited as an autosomal, dominant trait or develop as a spontaneous mutation [73]. In the nodular form (nodular blastema), foci of metanephric blastema are seen just beneath the capsule, in the peripelvic area and in the columns of Bertin [17, 53]. In the diffuse variety, the nephroblastomatosis involves the entire renal cortex, causing enlarged kidneys with prominent fetal lobulation. Usually, these lesions, which are extremely common in the newborn, being present in one in every 200–400 infant autopsies, regress; but they are often present in kidneys with Wilms tumor, especially in patients with bilateral tumors. It is for this reason that some believe Wilms tumor may develop from the metanephric blastema [18, 83]. There is also an association with hemihypertrophy, Beckwith-Wiedeman syndrome, and a few other chromosomal anomalies [42].

Radiological Findings

Radiologically, the nodular lesions are rarely recognized. In the diffuse form, the kidneys are also enlarged, with prominent fetal lobulation [8, 18, 83]. On IVU, a faint prolonged nephrographic effect with prompt function and calyceal distortion produce a picture similar to polycystic kidneys [8].

The aortogram demonstrates elongated cortical vessels, diminished cortical vascularity, and distorted and stretched interlobar and arcuate arteries. The nephrogram may mimic polycystic kidneys but there is a smooth outer rim [18, 42, 73, 83]. Bizarre puddles within the intervening renal parenchyma have been reported [83]. Ultrasonically, there is bilateral nephromegaly with hypoechoic or echogenic subcapsular and parenchymal regions [42, 73]. The CT can show marked nephromegaly with splaying and distortion of the pelvicalyceal system of the kidney. The cortex, especially, was enlarged [42]. Kuhn [60] also reported the presence of either an avascular rind or focal low density areas in one or both kidneys. On the other hand, Nordshy et al.'s [73] case demonstrated symmetric, well-demarcated tumor masses with homogeneous enhancement and displacement of the pelvic system.

The diagnosis can be difficult but, in the newborn, nephroblastomatosis is more common than adult polycystic kidney.

Hemangiomas

General Concepts

Hemangiomas are felt to be congenital in origin and composed of vessels which originate from vascular or lymphatic tissue [98]. These rare tumors can vary in size from being almost microscopic to 10 cm. They are most frequently found in the medulla, often adjacent to the collecting system, but they can be subcapsular and bleed into the perirenal space [32, 76]. They can be multiple (12%) and occasionally bilateral.

Although most feel the sex distribution is equal, Ekelund and Gothlin [38] reported a significant female predominance. The clinical presentation is usually gross intermittent hematuria.

Radiological Findings

With small, medullary lesions, the IVU and retrograde pyelogram may be completely normal. A small irregular defect of the wall of a calyx is sometimes demonstrated on retrograde pyelograms [32]. The angiogram may also be normal with small peripelvic lesions. With larger cortical lesions, the calyces may be displaced.

The angiogram is the preferred method of making the diagnosis [3, 38, 99]. Typically found are a group of coiled, overlapping, fine vascular loops or clusters of opacified vessels [3, 39]. In contrast, cavernous hemangiomas may show bowing and separation of the intrarenal arteries and a hypovascular mass with poor margins [39, 96]. Unlike an arteriovenous malformation, they do not demonstrate rapid shunting. In fact, focal collections of contrast are often seen early and stay late into the venous phase [39]. Because of the lack of contractile elements, there is no epinephrine response by the neoplastic vasculature [38], and this may make the small tumors more visible.

On ultrasound hemangiomas may be highly echogenic. Similarly, the CT may show a lesion which enhances significantly with contrast. Dynamic studies may be of value in showing early and persistent enhancement.

Leiomyomas

General Concepts

After adenomas, leiomyomas of the renal cortex are the most common benign renal tumors found at autopsy [111]. They are of little clinical significance [28, 31]. Rarely, leiomyomas may present as large solitary lesions arising in the renal pelvis [28]. The four or so large pelvic leiomyomas [103] have all been in women and have presented with colicky, flank pain.

Radiographic Findings

The plain film findings may rarely demonstrate calcification, but more often a large, nonspecific renal mass will be seen. The IVU and retrograde pyelogram may demonstrate a large homogeneous pelvic filling defect similar to a clot or transitional cell carcinoma [103], whereas the cortical lesions present as masses which compress but do not invade the calyces [111]. The larger tumors occasionally calcify.

Angiographically, the lesions most often have moderate to significantly increased vasculature [111]. The vessels are irregular; there is no AV shunting or renal vein invasion.

The ultrasonogram will show a large, homogeneous pelvic filling defect [103] or an intraparenchymal lesion with limited through transmission, low echogenicity, and no far wall enhancement [111]. The CT findings are often inconclusive.

Juxtaglomerular Tumors

General Concepts

Juxtaglomerular tumors are small solitary tumors usually 2–3 cm in size (occasionally somewhat larger). They are most often located just above the renal pelvis, but occasionally arise in the renal cortex or even the perinephric space. Microscopically, juxtaglomerular tumors consist of sheets and/or cords of cells with numerous blood vessels. The cells resemble smooth muscle of the juxtaglomerular apparatus. They contain cytoplasmic granules which take up PAS or Bowie stains. Tissue assays reveal markedly increased renin levels [37]. Immunofluorescent studies show intracytoplasmic fluorescence [64].

Clinically, the patients are often 20 years or younger (mean age 31) and present with headaches, polydypsia, polyuria, and neuromuscular complaints (hypokalemia) [20, 34, 37, 82, 86]. There is always moderate to severe hypertension with its accompanying retinopathy. The peripheral renin level is elevated, with secondary hyperaldosteronism.

Radiological Findings

The IVU is often normal [37]. On ultrasound, the tumor is often highly echogenic because of the small vascular channels within the neoplasm. Areas of decreased echogenicity correspond to focal hemorrhage and necrosis (Fig. 18.11a). On CT, small isodense tumors may be missed on the unenhanced study but since they enhance poorly, will stand out against the surrounding functioning normal renal parenchyma after contrast injection [37] (Fig. 18.11b). The renal scan will show no function in the area of the mass. Angiographically, these lesions are always hypovascular and may be missed without selective angiography [34, 37] (Fig. 18.11c). Renal vein renins were lateralizing in eight of nine cases [64].

Rarely Seen Tumors

Lipomas

Lipomas originate in the kidney cortex or from the perirenal space. Usually, they are quite small but can become any size [100]. On plain film or nephrotomography, fat may be discernible, and on IVU it may displace some calyces. Ultrasound and CT should be diagnostic of this entity.

Myelolipomas

More commonly seen in the adrenal, this tumor composed of fat and hematopoetic elements has been reported in the kidney. The IVU is nonspecific; however, based on the pattern seen with adrenal lesions, the tumor should be highly echogenic sonographically and be of predominantly fat density on CT. These patients always have an accompanying blood dyscrasia when the tumor arises in the kidney, and this should help differentiate an AML from a myelolipoma.

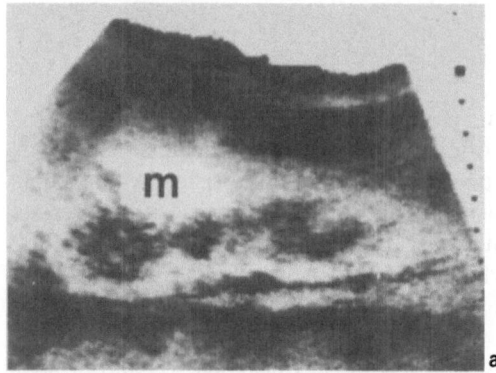

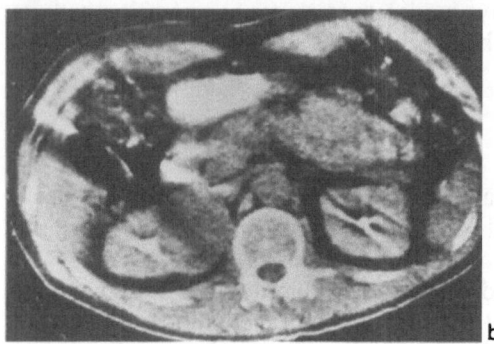

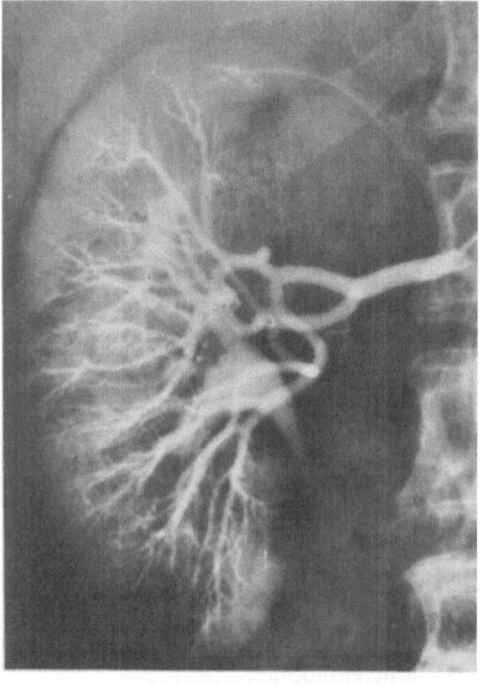

Fig. 18.11a–c. Juxtaglomerular tumors.
a Ultrasound. Usually these tumors
should be highly echogenic unless focal
hemorrhage has occurred (*m*, mass).
b CT—typical tumor. Usually
juxtaglomerular tumors are isodense
and may be missed on CT.
c Angiogram showing hypovascular
mass. (Reproduced from Dunnick NR
et al. [37]).

Lymphangiomas

Renal lymphangiomas are rare [58]. The average age at presentation is 33.7 years (six have been found in childhood). The patients present with a flank mass, hematuria, and/or colicky pain. The lesions are invariably benign. A mass may be seen on IVU. On angiograms they are hypo- or avascular.

Fibromas

These tumors can arise in the cortex, capsule, or perinephric tissue [26, 54, 66, 110], though more commonly they arise in the medullary portion without encapsulation. Only a few have been large enough to cause clinical symptoms. They are considered to be hamartomas because they contain "a non-growing and abnormal mixture of tissue native to an organ" [78].

Radiographically, they may present as a mass which can occasionally calcify on IVU [78]. Usually the tumors are avascular, but abnormal vascularity has been reported [78].

Hemangiopericytomas

Primary renal hemangiopericytomas arise in the renal capsule or extrarenally [5]. They are composed of numerous capillaries surrounded by a sheath of "pericytes." The latter should be diagnosed at electron microscopy, where a characteristic pattern is seen. Hemangiopericytomas can be benign or malignant, and it is often difficult to differentiate between them. In the clearly malignant variety, the tumor is not encapsulated and obviously invasive of the parenchyma, capsule, and the perirenal space. Metastases occur by hematogenous and lymphogenous routes.

The patients present with hematuria, a palpable mass, and/or hypoglycemia [93].

Radiographically, the tumors may be perirenal or intrarenal in location. The workup reveals a hypo- or hypervascular tumor, indistinguishable from a renal cell carcinoma [57, 99]. The only clue to diagnosis may be the presence of hypoglycemia.

Ganglioneuromas

These benign tumors usually arise from sympathetic ganglia. Only a few have been found in the kidney and they may be hormonally active, causing diarrhea, episodic hypertension, sweating, and flushing similar to that seen with pheochromocytomas [36]. The tumors are composed of Schwann cells in coarse interlocking fascicles. Mature ganglion cells are found in compact clusters or arranged in an irregular fashion.

Radiographically, the tumor can be hypo-, hyper-, or avascular. In the hypervascular tumors, the vessels are serpiginous and meandering but without evidence of puddling or shunting.

Endometriosis

Only a few cases of endometriosis involving the kidney have been reported, and these cases have presented with hematuria [48]. The cyclic pattern of symptoms so marked with endometriosis elsewhere is rarely seen with renal involvement. There are no distinctive radiographic findings.

Carcinoid Tumors

These rare tumors are composed of the Kulchitsky cell, which releases 5-hydroxytryptamine, a vasoconstrictive agent [43]. The clinical manifestations include vasomotor, cutaneous (sudden red flushing of the upper trunk), gastrointestinal (abdominal cramps, diarrhea), and cardiopulmonary symptoms (asthma) [43]. Later complaints include cardiac failure secondary to fibrous thickening of the endocardium and the valves. In one of the reported cases [43], an avascular solid mass in the lower pole of the kidney was noted.

Teratomas

As of 1980, only five renal teratomas had been reported [44]. The tumors can be cystic and solid.

On IVU, a mass possibly with a rim of normal tissue is seen. Teratomas are relatively avascular and can be mistaken for a cyst. The ultrasound and CT findings should be similar to those of teratomas elsewhere.

References

1. Ambos MA, Bosniak MA, Valensi QJ, et al. (1978) Angiographic patterns in renal oncocytoma. Radiology 129:615–622
2. Amendola MA, Jasinski RM, Glazer GM, Bree RL (1984) Computed tomography of renal oncocytomas (abstr). Program of the 84th American Roentgen Ray Society Annual Meeting. Las Vegas, 9–13 April 1984, p 55
3. Anderson LB, Rasmussen T (1964) Renal hemangioma diagnosed preoperatively by selective renal angiography. Acta Radiol Diagn 2:201–204
4. Anderson D, Tannen RL (1969) Tuberous sclerosis and chronic renal failure: Potential confusion with polycystic kidney disease. Am J Med 47:163–168
5. Backwinkel KD, Diddams JA (1970) Hemangiopericytoma: Report of a case and comprehensive review of the literature. Cancer 24:896–901
6. Baldauf MC, Shulz DM (1976) Multilocular cyst of the kidney: Report of three cases with review of the literature. Am J Clin Pathol 65:93–102
7. Banner MP, Pollack HM, Chatten J, Witzleben C (1981) Multilocular renal cysts: Radiological-pathologic correlation. AJR 136:239–247
8. Bar Ziv J, Hirsch M, Perlman M (1975) Bilateral nephroblastomatosis. Pediatr Radiol 3:85–88
9. Becker JA, Kinkhabwala M, Pollack H, et al. (1973) Angiomyolipoma (hamartoma) of the kidney. An angiographic review. Acta Radiol [Diagn] 14:561–568
10. Behan M, Kazam E (1978) The echographic characteristics of fatty tissues and tumors. Radiology 129:143–151
11. Beraha D, Block NL, Politano VA (1974) Myelolipomas of the kidney. J Urol 112:19–21

12. Berdon WE, Wigger HJ, Baker DH (1973) Fetal renal hamartoma—a benign tumor to be distinguished from Wilm's tumor. Report of a case. AJR 118:18–27
13. Bernie JE (1973) Renal angiomyolipoma in an adolescent: A case report. J Urol 109:492–494
14. Bissada NK, White HJ, Sun CN, et al. (1975) Tuberous sclerosis complex and renal angiomyolipoma: Collective review. Urology 6:105–113
15. Bolande RP (1973) Congenital mesoblastic nephroma of infancy. Perspect Pediatr Pathol 1:227–250
16. Bonavita JA, Pollack HM, Banner M (1981) Renal oncocytoma: Further observations and literature reviews. Urol Radiol 2:229–234
17. Bove KE, Koffler H, McAdam AJ (1969) Nodular renal blastema. Definition and possible significance. Cancer 24:323–332
18. Brantley RE, Simpson LR Jr (1976) Angiography and histopathology of nephroblastomatosis. Radiology 120:151–154
19. Brendler H, Maguire J, Mitty H (1971) Angiographic characteristics of renal hamartoma. Br J Urol 43:674–678
20. Brown JJ, Lever AF, Robertson JJ, Fraser R, Morton TJ, et al. (1973) Hypertension and secondary hyperaldosteronism associated with a renin-secreting renal juxtaglomerular tumour. Lancet II:1228–1231
21. Bruneton JN, Ballanger P, Ballanger R, DeLorme G (1979) Renal adenomas. Clin Radiol 30:343–352
22. Busch FM, Bark CJ, Clyde HR (1976) Benign renal angiomyolipoma with regional lymph node involvement. J Urol 116:715–717
23. Bush WH Jr, Freeny PC, Orme BM (1979) Angiomyolipoma characteristic images by ultrasound and computed tomography. Urology 14:531–535
24. Butt AJ, Perry JQ (1951) Hemangioma of the kidney. J Urol 65:15–19
25. Caplan GE, Hartman HR, Young R, et al. (1968) The "hot" renal tumor. Scanning and angiographic characteristics of a solid renal adenoma. Radiology 91:991–992
26. Cassimally KA (1971) Fibroma filling the renal pelvis: Report of a case. Can J Surg 14:350–352
27. Charlot-Charles J, Jones GW (1974) Renal angiomyolipoma associated with tuberous sclerosis. Review of the literature. Urology 3:465–469
28. Clinton-Thomas CL (1956) A giant leiomyoma of the kidney. Br J Surg 43:497–501
29. Cohan RH, Dunnick NR, Degesys GE, Korobkin M (1984) Computed tomography of renal oncocytoma. J Comput Assist Tomogr 8:284–287
30. Compton WR, Lester PD, Kyaw MM, Madsen JA (1976) The abdominal angiographic spectrum of tuberous sclerosis. AJR 126:807–813
31. Crabtree EG (1944) Leiomyoma of the kidney associated with hemorrhagic cyst. J Urol 52:480–488
32. Crissey MM, Kearney GP, Sos T, Levin DC (1980) Renal hemangioma: Diagnostic aspects and management techniques. Cardiovasc Intervent Radiol 3:170–173
33. Cubillo E, Hesker AE, Stanley RJ (1973) Cavernous hemangioma of the kidney: An angiographic-pathologic correlation. J Can Assoc Radiol 24:254–256
34. Davidson JK, Clark DL (1974) Renin secreting juxtaglomerular cell tumor. Br J Radiol 47:594–597
35. Deming CL, Harvard BM (1970) Tumors of the kidney. In: Campbell MF, Harrison JH (eds) Urology, vol 2, 3rd edn. W. B. Saunders, Philadelphia, pp 895–998
36. Dunnick NR, Castellino RA (1975) Arteriographic manifestations of ganglioneuromas. Radiology 115:323–328
37. Dunnick NR, Hartman DS, Ford KK, Davis CJ Jr, Amis ES Jr (1983) The radiology of juxtaglomerular tumors. Radiology 147:321–326
38. Ekelund L, Gothlin J (1975) Renal hemangioma: An analysis of 13 cases diagnosed by angiography. AJR 125:788–794
39. Evans JA, Bosniak MA (1971) Atlas of tumor radiology; the kidney. Yearbook Medical Publishers, Chicago, pp 278–289
40. Farrow GM, Harrison EG Jr, Utz DC, et al. (1968) Renal angiomyolipoma. A clinicopathologic study of 33 cases. Cancer 22:564–570
41. Feldberg MAM, van Waes PFGM (1982) Multilocular cystic renal cell carcinoma. AJR 138:953–955
42. Franken EA, Yiu-Chiu V, Smith WL, Chiu LC (1982) Nephroblastomatosis: clinicopathologic significance and imaging characteristics. AJR 138:950–952
43. Ghazi MR, Brown JS, Warner RS (1979) Carcinoid tumor of kidney. Urology 14:610–612
44. Glazier WB, Lytton B, Tronic B (1980) Renal teratomas: Case report and review of the literature. J Urol 123:98–99

45. Goldman SM, Meng CH, White RI, Naraval RC, Siegelman SS, Diamond AB, Kaufman SL, Harrington DP (1977) Transitional cell tumors of the kidney: How diagnostic is the angiogram? AJR 129:99–105
46. Grossman LB (1984) NMR of oncocytoma (abstr). Program of the 84th American Roentgen Ray Society Annual Meeting. Las Vegas, 9–13 April 1984, p 55
47. Gwinn JL, Lee FA, Grooms AM, et al. (1972) Fetal mesenchymal hamartoma of kidney (radiological case of the month). Am J Dis Child 123:585–586
48. Hajdu SI, Koss LG (1970) Endometriosis of the kidney. Am J Obstet Gynecol 106:314–315
49. Hansen GC, Hoffman RB, Sample WF, Becker R (1978) Computed tomography diagnosis of renal angiomyolipoma. Radiology 128:789–791
50. Hartman DS, Goldman SM, Friedman AC, Davis CJ Jr, Madewell JE, Sherman JL (1981) Angiomyolipoma: Ultrasonic-pathologic correlation. Radiology 139:451–458
51. Hartman DS, Lesar MSL, Madewell JE, Lichtenstein JE, Davis CJ Jr (1981) Mesoblastic nephronia: Radiologic-pathologic correlation of 20 cases. AJR 136:69–74
52. Holt RG, Neiman HL, Korsower JM, et al. (1975) Angiographic features of benign renal adenoma. Urology 6:764–767
53. Huff DS (1973) Nodular renal blastema, nephroblastomatosis and Wilms' tumor: A report of two cases. Am J Pathol 70:23a–24a
54. Immergut S, Cottler ZR (1951) Intrapelvic fibroma. J Urol 66:673–676
55. Jander HP, Tonkin IL (1979) Epinephrine enhanced renal angiography in the diagnosis of hamartoma (angiomyolipoma): a re-evaluation. Radiology 132:61–66
56. Jarman WO, Spence IJ (1971) Preoperative angiographic demonstration of renal adenoma. J Urol 105:24–26
57. Joffe N (1960) Hemangiopericytoma, angiographic findings. Br J Radiol 33:614–617
58. Joost J, Schafer R, Altwein JE, Renal lymphangioma. (1972) J Urol 118:22–24
59. Kissane JM (1944) In: Hepintall RH (ed) Pathology of the kidney, 2nd edn. Little, Brown & Co., Boston, pp 86–87
60. Kuhn JP (1984) CT of the body in children. In: Syllabus for the categorical course on computed body tomography with MRI correlation. American Roentgen Ray Society, pp 108–129
61. Kutcher R, Rosenblatt-Mitsudo SM, Goldman M, Kogan S (1982) Renal angiomyolipoma with sonographic demonstration of extension into the inferior vena cava. Radiology 143:755–756
62. Lafortune M, Breton G (1983) Echographic demonstration of an oncocytoma. J Can Assoc Radiol 34:144–146
63. Lakey WH (1975) Tumors of the kidney. In: Karafin L, Kendall AR (eds) Urology, vol 2. Harper & Row, Hagerstown, Md
64. Lam ASC, Bedard YC, Buckspan MB, Log AG, Steinhardt MI (1982) Surgically curable hypertension associated with reninoma. J Urol 128:572–575
65. Lautin EM, Gordon PM, Friedman AC, McCormick JF, Fromowitz FB, Goldman MJ, Sugarman LA (1981) Radionuclide imaging and computed tomography in renal oncocytoma. Radiology 138:185–190
66. Lennox KW, Clark RE (1975) Renal medullary fibroma: Report of a case presenting as a submucosal pelvic tumor. J Urol 113:288–290
67. Levine E, Huntrakoon M (1983) Computed tomography of renal oncocytoma. AJR 141:741–746
68. Lin F (1971) Congenital mesoblastic nephroma. Cancer Semin 4:184–187
69. Madewell JE, Goldman SM, Davis CJ Jr, Hartman DS, Feigin DS, Lichtenstein JE (1983) Multilocular cystic nephroma: A radiographic-pathologic correlation of 58 patients. Radiology 146:309–321
70. McCullough D, Scott R, Seybold H (1971) Renal angiomyolipoma (hamartoma): Review of the literature and report of seven cases. J Urol 105:32–44
71. Minielly JA, Tuttle RJ, Thompson GD (1974) Fetal hamartoma of the kidney—a benign tumor to be distinguished from Wilms' tumor. Can J Surg 17:235–238
72. Murphy GP, Mostofi FK (1970) Histologic assessment and clinical prognosis of renal adenoma. J Urol 103:31–36
73. Nordshy T, Stake G, Oppendal B, Knutrud O (1982) Nephroblastomatosis. Acta Radiol [Diagn] Fasc 3B, 23:279–284
74. Palmisano P (1967) Renal hamartoma (angiomyolipoma): Its angiographic appearance and its response to intra-arterial epinephrine. Radiology 88:249–254
75. Parienty RA, Pradel J, Imbert M, Picard JD, Savart P (1981) Computed tomography of multilocular cystic nephroma. Radiology 140:135–139
76. Peterson NE, Thompson HT (1971) Renal hemangioma. J Urol 105:27–31
77. Pitts WR Jr, Kazam E, Gray G, Vaughan ED (1980) Ultrasonographic, computerized transaxial tomography and pathology of angiomyolipoma of the kidney: Solution to a diagnostic dilemma.

J Urol 124:907–909

78. Polga JP (1976) Renal medullary fibroma presenting as a calcified mass with neovascularity. J Urol 116:105–106
79. Potter EL, Craig JM (1975) Pathology of the fetus and infant, 3rd edn. Yearbook Publications, Chicago, pp 456–478
80. Quinn MJ, Hartman DS, Friedman AC, Lautin EM, Pyatt RS, Sherman J (1984) Renal oncocytoma: Is a radiological diagnosis possible (abstr). Program of the 84th American Roentgen Ray Society Annual Meeting. Las Vegas, 9–13 April 1984, p 56
81. Rabinowitz JG, Wolf BS, Goldman RH (1968) Roentgen features of renal adenoma. Radiology 84:263–269
82. Robb-Smith AH (1971) Renin secreting kidney tumours. Lancet II:493
83. Rosenfield NS, Shimkin P, Berdon W, Barwick K, Glassman M, Siegel NJ (1980) Wilms tumor arising from spontaneously regressing nephroblastomatosis. AJR 135:381–384
84. Rumancik WM, Bosniak MA, Rosen RJ, Hulnick D (1984) Atypical renal and pararenal hematomas associated with lymphangiomatosis. AJR 142:971–972
85. Samellas W, Morphis LG (1976) Hemangioma of the kidney. J Urol 116:653
86. Schambelan M, Howes EL Jr, Stocki G, et al. (1973) Role of renin and aldosterone in hypertension due to a renin-secreting tumor. Am J Med 55:86–92
87. Scheible W, Ellenbogen PH, Leopold GR, Siao NT (1978) Lipomatous tumours of the kidney and adrenal. Apparent echographic specificity. Radiology 129:153–156
88. Shawker TH, Horvath KL, Dunnick NR, Javadpour N (1979) Renal angiomyolipoma: Diagnosis by combined ultrasound and computerized tomography. J Urol 121:675–676
89. Shelley HS (1953) Renal adenoma: Pyelogram showing growth over a 5 year period. J Urol 69:480–483
90. Sherman JL, Hartman DS, Friedman AC, Madewell JE, Davis CJ Jr, Goldman SM (1981) Angiomyolipoma: Computed tomographic-pathologic correlation of 17 cases. AJR 137:1221–1226
91. Shimshony Z, Merimysky E, Suprun H (1983) Adenoma of kidney. Br J Urol 35:256–260
92. Shucksmith HS (1963) Fibroma of the renal pelvis. Br J Urol 35:263–264
93. Simon R, Greene RC (1964) Perirenal hemangiopericytoma: A case associated with hypoglycemia JAMA 189:155–156
94. Slasky BS, Bron KM (1982) Aneurysms in renal oncocytoma. Urology 20:552–554
95. Sos T, Gray G Jr, Baltaxe HA (1976) The angiographic appearance of benign renal oxyphilic adenoma. AJR 127:717–722
96. Stanley RJ, Cubillo E, Mancilla-Jiminez R (1975) Cavernous hemangioma of the kidney. AJR 125:682–686
97. Sty JR, Oechler H (1980) Tc-99m glucoheptonate renal imaging: Congenital mesoblastic nephroma. J Nucl Med 21:809–810
98. Suslavich F, Older RA, Hinman CG (1976) Calcified renal carcinoma in a patient with tuberous sclerosis. AJR 133:524–526
99. Sutton D, Pratt AE (1967) Angiography of hemangiopericytoma. Clin Radiol 18:324–329
100. Tahara C, Hess E (1945) Massive renal fibrolipoma. Report of two cases. J Urol 54:107–115
101. Takeyama M, Arima M, Sagawa S, Sonoda T (1982) Preoperative diagnosis of coincident renal cell carcinoma and renal angiomyolipoma in non-tuberous sclerosis. J Urol 128:579–581
102. Telander RL, Gilchrist GS, Burgert EO Jr, et al. (1978) Bilateral massive nephroblastomatosis in infancy. J Pediatr Surg 13:163–166
103. Uchida M, Watanabe H, Mishina T, Shimada N (1981) Leiomyoma of the renal pelvis. J Urol 125:572–574
104. Viamonte M Jr, Ravel R, Politano V, et al. (1966) Angiographic findings in a patient with tuberous sclerosis. AJR 98:723–732
105. Wagner M, Kiselow M, Buffington G (1972) Renal cortical adenoma vs. adenocarcinoma. Tumor diameter is not a valid distinguishing criterion. Geriatrics 27:114–115
106. Waismann J, Cooper PH (1970) Renal neoplasms of newborn. J Pediatr Surg 5:407–412
107. Wasserman NF, Ewing SL (1983) Calcified renal oncocytoma. AJR 141:747–749
108. Wenzel JE, Lagos JC, Albers DD (1970) Tuberous sclerosis presenting as polycystic kidneys and seizures in an infant. J Pediatr 77:673–678
109. Wiener SN, Bernstein RG (1977) Renal oncocytoma: Angiographic features of two cases. Radiology 125:633–635
110. Xipell JM (1971) The incidence of benign renal nodules; a clinicopathologic study. J Urol 106:503–506
111. Zollikofer C, Castaneda-Zuniga W, Nath HP, Valasquez G, Formanek A, Feinberg SB, Amplatz K (1980) The angiographic appearance of intrarenal leiomyoma. Radiology 136:47–49

Chapter 19

Radiological Diagnosis and Assessment of Inflammatory Renal Diseases

Stanford M. Goldman

Introduction

A myriad of inflammatory processes may affect the renal parenchyma (Table 19.1). In spite of innumerable clinical and animal studies over the years, a great deal of controversy still exists as to the mechanisms by which renal involvement occurs. However, in recent years, significant progress has been made in resolving these conflicts and slowly the pieces of the jigsaw puzzle are beginning to fit together to make possible a more complete understanding of the processes involved. In the sections below, our approach to understanding the mechanisms of these renal infections will first be outlined, followed by our schema of radiologically evaluating these patients.

Acute Pyelonephritis and Its Variants

General Considerations

Theoretically, acute infections reach the kidney via one of three routes: (a) ascending, (b) hematogenous, and (c) lymphatic. In the preantibiotic era, hematogenous involvement of the kidney was a significant problem. Dental extractions and pustules on the skin sometimes led to kidney involvement with predominantly gram-positive organisms such as *Staphylococcus* or *Streptococcus*. Nowadays, the ascending route from the bladder is the predominant source of infection; the agents involved are gram-negative organisms such as *E. coli*, *Proteus*, *Pseudomonas*, etc. whose source is the anovulvar or anoscrotal area [39]. Another major source is the use of unsterile needles by drug addicts.

Table 19.1. Inflammatory processes that may affect the renal parenchyma

I.		Acute processes
	A.	Diffuse pyelonephritis
		1. Acute bacterial nephritis
	B.	Focal
		2. Lobar nephronia (focal bacterial nephritis)
	C.	Emphysematous pyelonephritis
	D.	Abscesses
		1. Intrarenal
		2. Perirenal and pararenal
II.		Chronic pyelonephritis
III.		Granulomatous disease
	A.	Tuberculosis
	B.	Xanthogranulomatous pyelonephritis
	C.	Malacoplakia (tumefactive megalocystic interstitial nephritis)
	D.	Schistosomiasis
	E.	Candidiasis
	F.	Echinococcus
	G.	Brucellosis
	H.	Actinomycosis
	I.	Other rare inflammatory lesions
IV.		Acute and chronic pyonephrosis
V.		Renal fistula
VI.		Renal papillary necrosis
VII.		Cholesteatoma, leukoplakia, squamous metaplasia
VIII.		Pyelitis cystica
IX.		Septic emboli
X.		Atrophic pyelonephritis
XI.		Pancreatitis

It is now generally accepted that the ascending infection is made possible by preexisting ureterovesical reflux and that the infection first spreads from the bladder. Females, because of their short urethra, are more susceptible to urinary tract infections (UTI), and there is some suggestion that there is a change in the pH of the vaginal secretions which allows for bacterial migration into the urethra.

One would expect that the constantly flowing urine would be able to flush out the bacteria from the ureter. However, it has been shown that many of these gram-negative organisms have mannase-resistant fimbriae which attach to the ureteral wall and preclude dislodgement. These organisms also often secrete an endotoxin which causes ureteral pseudo-obstruction and this allows for reflux into the papilla.

It is felt that because of the shape of the upper and low pole papilla (i.e., the compound calyx), the infecting organism tends to be located in these calyces.

Diffuse Acute Pyelonephritis

The radiographic picture on intravenous urogram (IVU) correlates well with the outpourings of fluid, polymorphic leukocytes, etc. in response to the bacterial infection. The kidney becomes swollen and the calyces are compressed with poor filling. There may be linear striations of the mucosa, pelvis, and ureter secondary to this edema [12, 49, 86, 91]. Because of endotoxin and the secondary loss of peristalsis, the calyces may be blurred and the ureter dilated. Rarely, a striated nephrogram (Fig. 19.1a) is seen—a finding that is also seen in hypotension, Tamm-

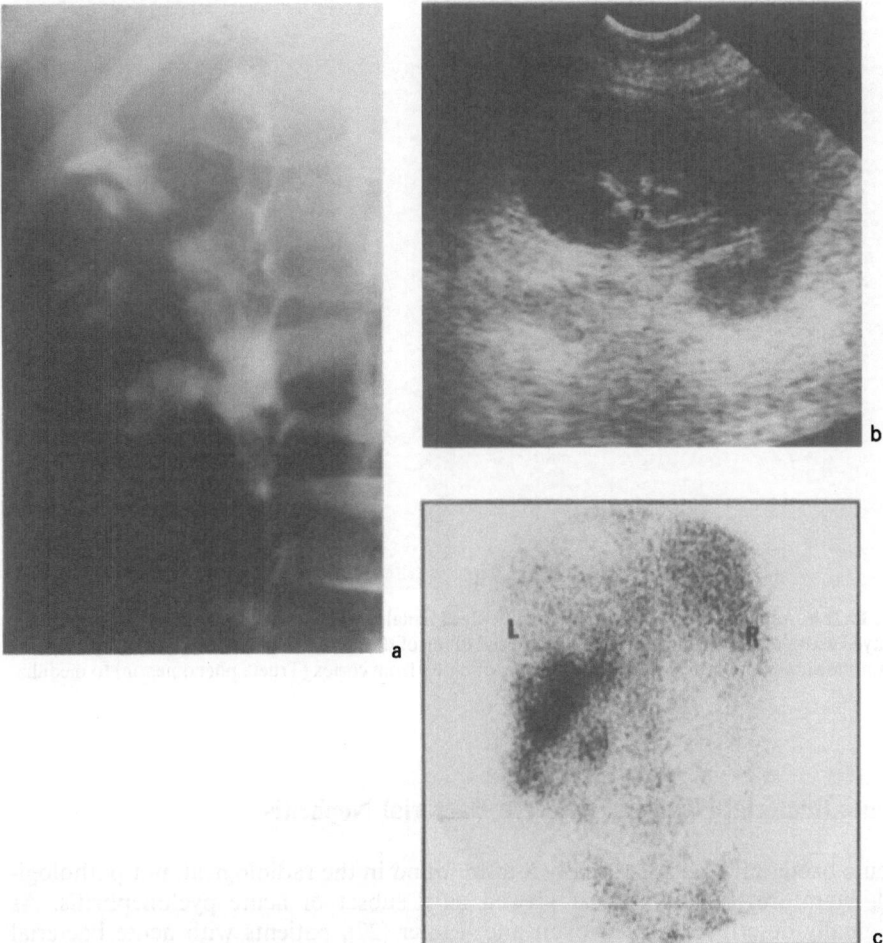

Fig. 19.1a–c. Acute pyelonephritis. **a** Striated pattern in acute pyelonephritis. **b** Ultrasound study showing a swollen cortex with some minimal decrease in echogenicity. Note renal pelvic structures (*P*) are not dilated, excluding obstruction (by courtesy of Dr. Sanford Minkin, Pikesville, Maryland). **c** Gallium scan showing marked uptake in left kidney.

Horsfall proteinuria, renal vein thrombosis, renal contusion, and ureteric obstruction [12]. It should, however, be noted that in a significant number of documented cases of pyelonephritis, the IVU is normal. Furthermore, in uncomplicated cases, an IVU is probably not indicated [34]. The ultrasonic pattern (Fig. 19.1b) is that of a swollen kidney with decreased cortical echogenicity without significant pelvocalyceal dilatation [30]. The latter finding excludes obstruction. The CT shows an edematous kidney occasionally with a striated nephrogram [43]. Tc-glucohepatonate scans demonstrate poor or delayed uptake while indium-labeled WBC or gallium (Fig. 19.1c) is notably positive in the affected kidney on delayed scans [18, 39, 74]. Care should be taken in interpreting bilateral uptake of gallium since increased accumulation can be seen normally. In order to diagnose bilateral acute infection, uptake should be definitely increased and nonrenal causes should be excluded [40].

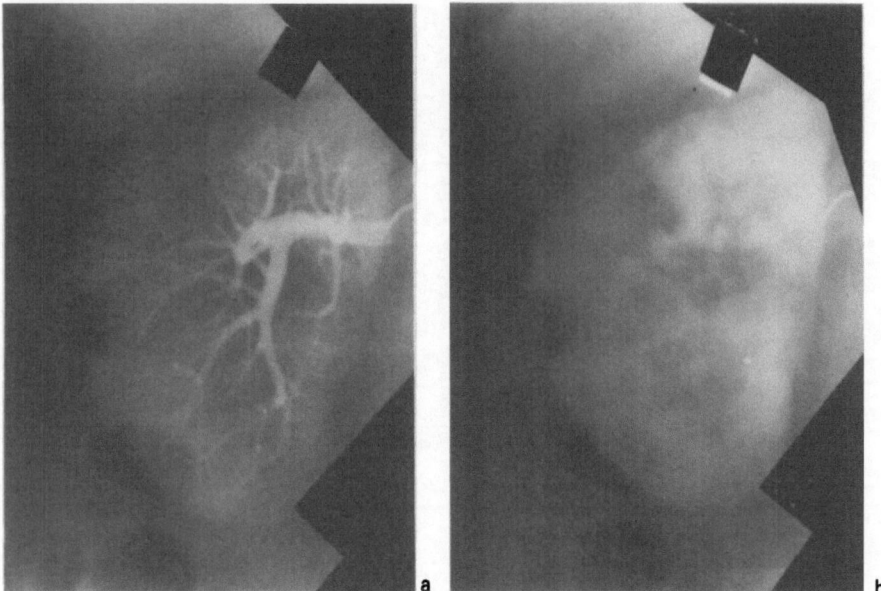

Fig. 19.2a,b. Acute bacterial nephritis in middle-aged female. **a** The angiographic phase was markedly delayed with slow flow and no evidence of arterial filling of the cortex. **b** Persistent nephrographic phase again showing poor cortical flow with shunting of blood from cortex (Trueta phenomenon) to medulla.

Acute Bacterial Nephritis—Severe Bacterial Nephritis

Acute bacterial nephritis is really a term found in the radiological, not pathological, literature. It can be best viewed as a subset of acute pyelonephritis. As originally described by Davidson and Talner [27], patients with acute bacterial nephritis were acutely ill, diabetic females who showed nonfunction on IVU. This reflected a severe, active pyelonephritis in a medically compromised patient. The reason for this nonfunction could be identified on angiograms (Fig. 19.2), where extremely slow arterial flow and a Trueta phenomenon with shunting of vascular flow away from the cortex into the medullary portion of the kidney were noted. Active antibiotic treatment rather than surgery can salvage these kidneys, although follow-up studies reveal the development of renal papillary necrosis [27].

Focal Pyelonephritis (Focal Lobar Nephronia, Focal Bacterial Nephritis)

Since the infection usually enters the kidney via reflux into upper or lower pole calyces, it would not be surprising to see an acute inflammatory reaction that is focal in nature. Failure to cure the infection leads to a focal indolent infection for which the term focal lobar nephronia or focal bacterial nephritis seems appropriate [96].

The IVU may be entirely normal; however, more often a localized mass is seen which on nephrotomography is of lower density than the surrounding normal

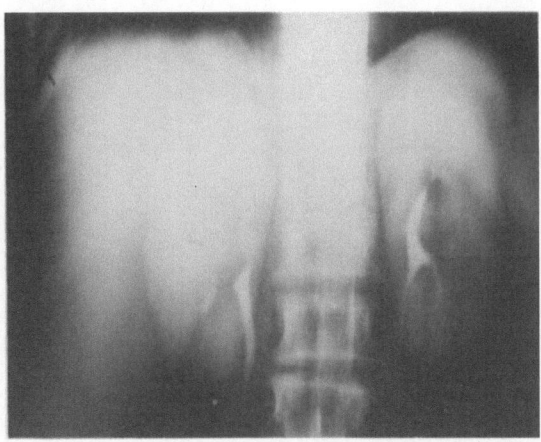

Fig. 19.3. Focal lobar nephronia. IVU showing mass in upper pole of right kidney.

kidney (Fig. 19.3). Tc-glucoheptonate scans (Fig. 19.4a) will show no accumulation in the affected area and the indium or gallium scan (Fig. 19.4b) will demonstrate marked focal uptake in the inflamed portions of the kidney. On ultrasound (Fig. 19.5a), a focal hypoechoic area will be noted without good through transmission that would be characteristic of an abscess [88]. On CT (Fig. 19.5b), a wedge-shaped or rounded defect with CT numbers slightly above those of water can be recognized. Occasionally, a few small focal areas will be identified in the affected area with CT numbers of water in it. The latter represent the beginnings of cavitation and abscess formation (Fig. 19.5b) [45, 58, 70].

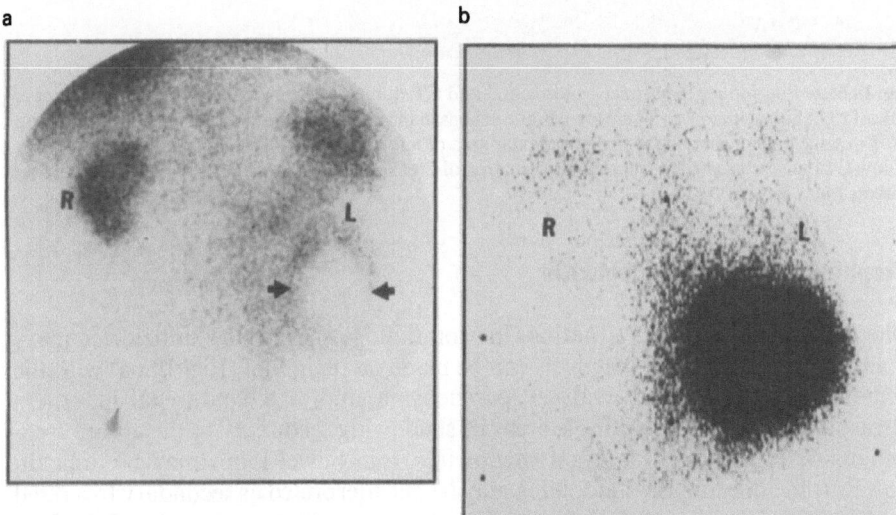

a   b

Fig. 19.4a,b. Focal lobar nephronia—isotopic studies. **a** Tc-glucoheptonate scan showing no uptake in lower pole of left kidney (*arrows*). **b** Gallium scan in same patient showing increased uptake in left kidney.

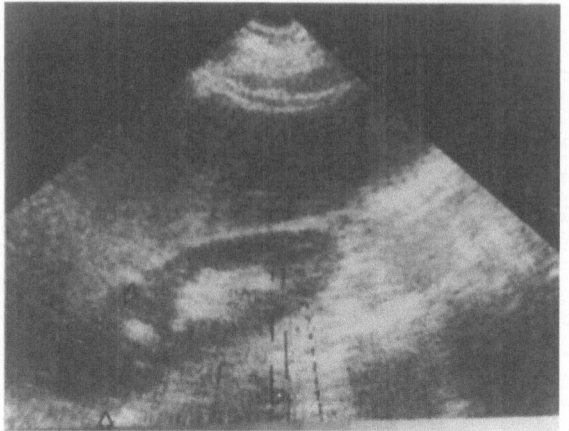

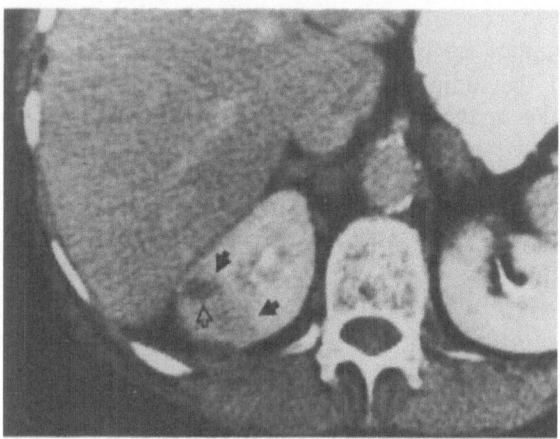

Fig. 19.5a,b. Focal lobar nephronia—ultrasound and CT studies. **a** Ultrasound showing mass in upper pole of right kidney (*arrows*). There are definite echoes in the mass, so a drainable abscess is not present. **b** CT in same patient showing typical, triangular area of infection posteriorly (*closed arrows*). Note area of low CT density within this, representing an area of breakdown which could be the beginnings of an abscess (*open arrow*).

Emphysematous Pyelonephritis

One of the true emergency situations in uroradiology is gas in the kidney secondary to infection [21, 69]. The diagnosis can be made on plain film (Fig. 19.6a) with the demonstration of air in the calyces, parenchyma, and/or the pararenal space. On ultrasound (Fig. 19.6b), multiple areas of shadowing secondary to the air are seen. Differentiation from the normal shadowing from bowel loops may be difficult, however. In addition, the shadowing may be misinterpreted as secondary to a renal calculus. On CT (Fig. 19.6c), the intrarenal air is readily recognized [63]. In fact, CT is extremely sensitive in demonstrating air, and, therefore, small amounts of air on CT probably do not have the dire consequences of the more advanced disease recognized on plain film. There are other causes of air in the kidney and these must be excluded:

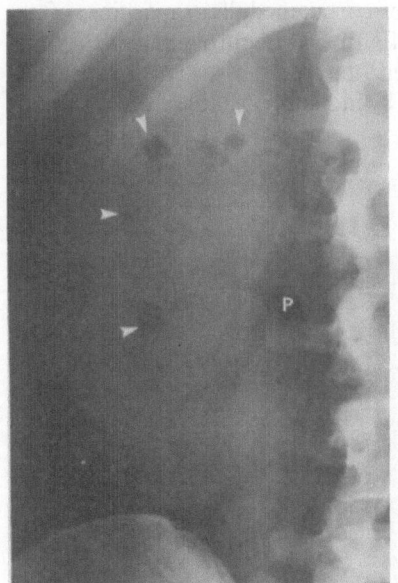
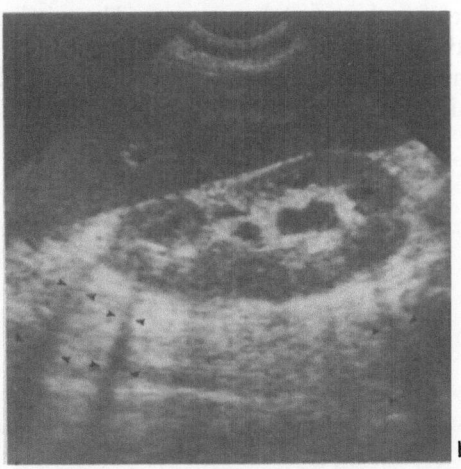
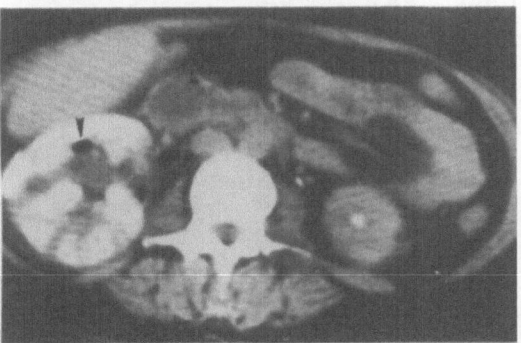

Fig. 19.6a–c Emphysematous pyelonephritis in diabetic female. a Plain film showing air in calyces (*arrows*) and pelvis (*P*). Smaller parenchymal air also noted. b Ultrasound in same patient demonstrating shadowing from calyces due to air (*arrows*). c CT showing nephrogram. Note air in calyx (*arrow*). (Case by courtesy of Dr. Sanford Minkin, Pikesville, Maryland)

1. An entero-, broncho-, or cutaneous renal fistula
2. Reflux from an ileal or colon conduit; this is a normal finding
3. Reflux of air from the bladder
4. Secondary to catheter placement

Abscesses

Intrarenal

Frank breakdown of focal lobar nephronia leads to the development of an abscess. On IVU (Fig. 19.7a), the abscess may mimic a cyst except the wall is usually thickened and there may be debris in it. Angiographically, the mass (Fig. 19.7b) stretches the intralobar arteries. There is loss of corticomedullary margins, often with hypervascularity in its periphery [19, 64]. In the nephrogenic phase, the central portion is usually lucent [38, 42]. There may be neovascularity present which does not respond to epinephrine and can be indistinguishable from a tumor.

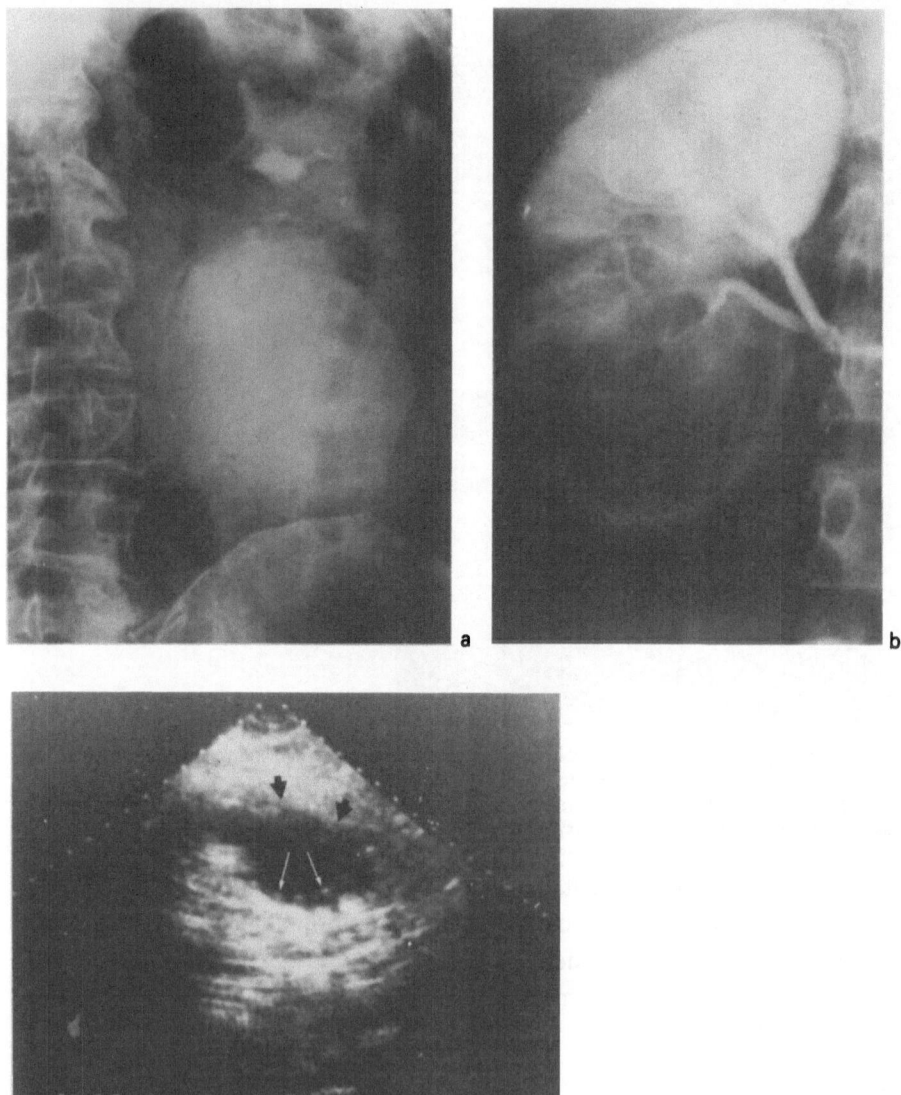

Fig. 19.7a–d. Intrarenal abscess. **a** Mass in left lower pole. Definitely not cyst. Some contrast noted in abscess. **b** Abscess in lower pole of right kidney. Increased vascularity around abscess (*arrows*) often mimics a tumor. **c** Intrarenal abscess in lower pole of right kidney (*black arrows*). Note debris in base (*white arrows*). **d** Intrarenal abscess in same patient as in **c** (*arrows*).

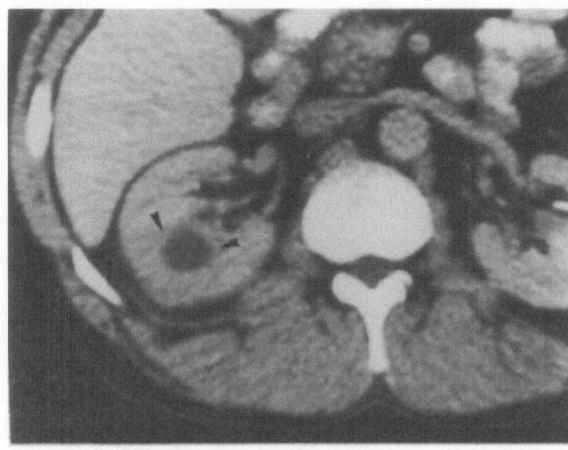

Fig. 19.7d

One cannot differentiate an abscess from focal pyelonephritis or even from a tumor by nuclear medicine techniques. The ultrasonic picture (Fig. 19.7c) is that of a predominantly anechoic "tumor" with a few internal echoes depending on the amount of intra-abscess debris. This debris will layer if the patient is turned on his side. Fairly good through transmission should be present in order to differentiate between an abscess and focal lobar nephronia [90]. CT (Fig. 19.7d) is ideal for demonstrating the fluid and debris-filled cavity and thus distinguishing it from the lobar nephronia. Once an abscess has been diagnosed, percutaneous drainage should be instituted. Although in the past abscesses were always treated surgically, it is now clear that many can be treated by percutaneous techniques [35, 46]. Use of Mucomyst in thick abscesses has been advocated by some [98] but disapproved of by others [28].

Perirenal and Pararenal

In most cases, perirenal inflammatory disease begins in the kidney with an intrarenal abscess. However, occasionally extrarenal sources such as diverticulitis, pancreatitis, etc. may be the source. Gallium 67 has been used [59] as well as angiography [64]. However, we prefer to use CT (Fig. 19.8a) to demonstrate perirenal disease, although ultrasound may occasionally be used [72, 77]. The perirenal fat is replaced by inflammatory disease that can usually be readily recognized on CT. Occasionally, on inspiratory and expiratory double exposure films one may note absence of movement of the kidney on the affected side. The kidney may be displaced by the process. It is most important to recognize gas bubbles in the peri- and/or pararenal space (Fig. 19.8b) on plain film and to differentiate this from normal colonic fecal material.

Involvement of the pararenal space may be due to intrarenal and extrarenal pathology. We have been impressed by the fact that some cases of xanthogranulomatous pyelonephritis or renal calculi have extensive pararenal but minimal perirenal involvement. We believe that in these somewhat indolent infections, Gerota's fascia becomes focally adherent to the inflamed kidney. Through this point of adherence, pus drains directly into the pararenal space, with relative sparing of the perirenal space.

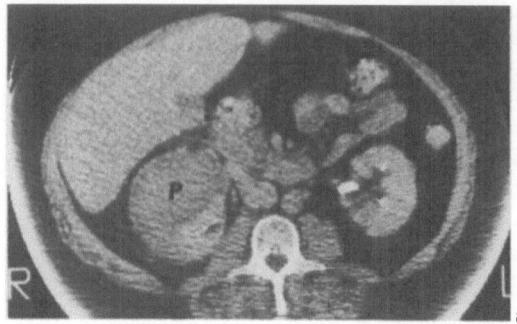

Fig. 19.8a,b. Perirenal and pararenal abscesses.
a Perirenal (*P*) spread of intrarenal abscess on CT.
b Air in perirenal space secondary to perforated
colonic cancer. One can see air around the ureter and
adrenal (*A*).

Chronic Pyelonephritis

General Considerations

Why scarring occurs is unclear. We do know that scarring is most severe with
reflux and infection. (Table 19.2). Scarring can occur without evidence of infection
and may then be due to a bacterial antigen or an autotoxicity factor from the
granulocyte [87]. For further information, see references 15, 33, 37, 55, 56, and 83.

Radiographic Findings

On IVU, we use the strict criteria of the presence of a renal scar overlying a blunted
calyx (Fig. 19.9a). This is due to the parenchymal scarring causing both calyceal
and cortical retraction. A cortical scar without an underlying calyceal change may
be seen with a vascular insult, while a blunt calyx without a cortical scar may be
due to past obstruction or reflux atrophy. The kidney may shrink focally or
globally. Focal compensatory hypertrophy may simulate a mass. In children,
careful routine follow-up studies should be performed using renal ultrasound and
voiding cystourethrography (with either contrast or, better, with isotopes). It is
important to identify yearly renal growth, paying particular attention to the

Table 19.2. The relationship of ureterovesical reflux and bacterial nephritis

```
                        UV reflux and bacteria


    +Diabetes


    Acute                   Acute diffuse        Focal pyelonephritis
    bacterial               pyelonephritis
    nephritis
                                                                    Return to
                                                                     normal


                                                    Focal lobar nephronia


                         Return to
    Renal                normal
    papillary                                             Abscess
    necrosis


                         Focal scarring
```

interpapillary line and the renal poles (Fig. 19.9b). The amount of cortex in the upper pole should be approximately equal to the volume in the lower pole. Similarly, the distance between papilla (medially) and the renal surface (laterally) should be roughly equal from side to side. Any deviation from this suggests scarring. Failure to demonstrate growth, even with an apparently normal IVU, carries a poor prognosis. Angiography is no longer a useful tool in diagnosing chronic pyelonephritis. On aortograms an end-stage kidney shows atrophy of the main renal artery after its normal-sized origin from the aorta (Fig. 19.9c). The interlobar arteries are widened proximally and are tortuous as they pass peripherally, giving a "pruned tree configuration." In the parenchyma, there is a sharp cutoff of peripheral vessels, crowding of vessels, neovascularity, and even early filling of veins [71]. Often the nephrogram appears "mottled." On ultrasound, the cortical scars are readily identified as highly echogenic (Fig. 19.9d) [61]. On CT, there is irregular loss of cortical tissue, shrinkage of the kidneys, evidence of

Table 19.3. Granulomatous disease

I.	Infections
	A. Tuberculosis
	B. Xanthogranulomatous pyelonephritis
	C. Malacoplakia (tumefactive megalocystic interstitial nephritis)
	D. Schistosomiasis
	E. Fungal and other chronic diseases, i.e., actinomycosis, moniliasis, candidiasis, brucellosis
II.	Foreign body reaction
III.	Other—including some possible autoimmune diseases
	1. Sarcoidosis
	2. Chronic granulomatous disease of infancy
	3. Wegener's granulomatosis

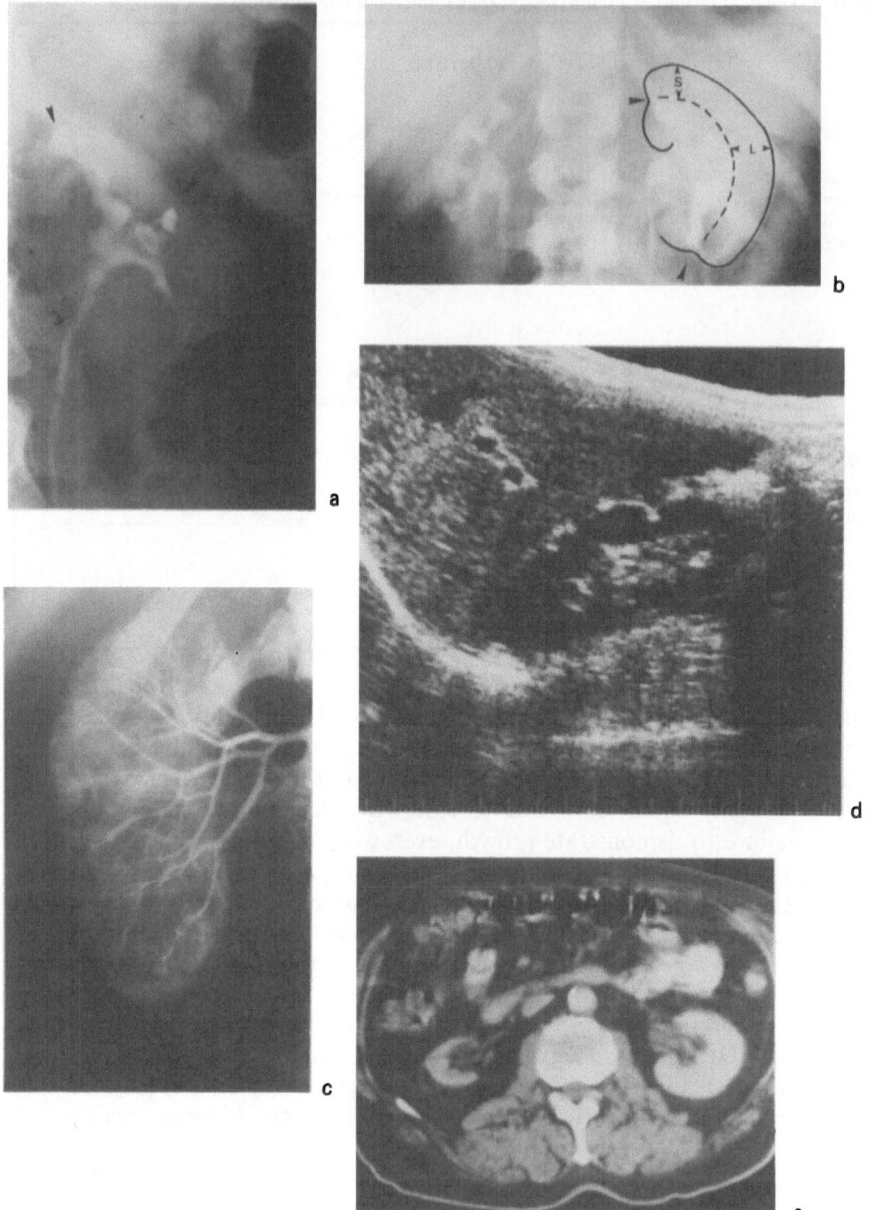

Fig. 19.9a–e. Chronic pyelonephritis. **a** Classic IVU; note thinning of kidney in upper half of kidney overlying blunt calyces (*arrows*). **b** Bilateral pyelonephritis. Right kidney is end-stage with most of the cortex destroyed. On the left there is focal scarring in the lower and upper poles (*arrows*). The interpapillary line (*broken line*) and kidney outline (*solid line*) are drawn in. *S* represents measurement of superior pole parenchyma, which normally should be equal to the inferior pole cortex. *L* represents measurements of lateral cortex on left and should normally be approximately equal to a similar measurement on the opposite kidney. **c** Angiogram in end-stage, pyelonephritic kidney (measuring 5 cm). Distal interlobar arteries are narrowed, irregular, and "corkscrew," giving a pruned tree appearance. **d** Ultrasound showing typical, highly echogenic scar (*arrow*). **e** CT demonstrating a small atrophic right kidney.

cortical scarring, and blunt calyces without evidence of obstruction (Fig. 19.9e). Radionuclide studies (i.e., radioisotopic renograms) are of value in determining renal function, which can be of importance in surgical and/or nonsurgical management.

Granulomatous Diseases of the Kidney

General Considerations

The previous sections have dealt with one type of defense mechanism, the acute defense system, which utilizes the polymorphic nucleocyte. This is the body's primary defense, and, when successful, rids the body of all residual disease. However, in certain instances this defense is unsuccessful either because the causative agent prevents the usual defense mechanisms from working and/or because the host's defenses are abnormal or inadequate in the first place. In this situation, the body makes use of its secondary defenses in an effort to contain the insult. This results in granuloma formation. In general, a granuloma is a somewhat abnormal response to a variety of noxious stimulae (Table 19.3) [16]. In the strict sense, a granuloma implies a tumor-like mass of granulation tissue, actively growing fibroblasts, and capillary buds. Histologically, a granuloma consists of a microscopic, focal, vascularized aggregation of histiocytes or macrophages and hypertrophic fibroblasts that assume a round or oval shape with abundant ground glass cytoplasm. The multinucleated giant cells of Langhans probably just represent a fusion of several histiocytes. The xanthoma cell is a histiocyte which has ingested fat cells. The Michaelis-Gutmann body results from engulfment of an infecting organism such as *E. coli* within the lysosome of the macrophage. All these mechanisms attempt to isolate the infecting organism.

Tuberculosis

General Considerations

Tuberculosis (TB) remains the example par-excellence of a granulomatous disease [48]. With progression, pulmonary TB is a cavitary process with a marked fibrotic reaction. Although the incidence of pulmonary TB has been decreasing in the United States, renal TB continues to remain a serious clinical problem. Urinary TB almost invariably begins from a small focus in the lungs and spreads hematogenously to the kidneys. From its introduction into the kidney via the bloodstream, the tubercle bacillus localizes in the glomerular and cortical arteries. These necrotize into the nephrons and advance to the loop of Henle. Thus, the first X-ray sign is a necrotizing papillitis. The marked fibrotic host response leads to cicatrization at the infundibulae, renal pelvis, ureteropelvic junction, and at other more distal locations in the urinary drainage system [8]. Such narrowing may lead to focal or global nonfunction.

Radiographic Findings

On plain films one may note a small kidney or a focal mass filled with caseous material [66]. Calcification which is irregular, indefinite, indistinct or ground glass in nature is seen (Fig. 19.10). One should carefully look for paraspinal, psoas ("cold") abscesses and hip changes that are suggestive of TB.

In early TB, one may see large kidneys and changes indistinguishable from an acute pyelonephritis of any origin. The earliest radiographic change which might suggest the diagnosis is that of an ulcerating papillitis leading to focal erosion in the papilla. The resultant fibrotic response will lead to an infundibular stricture and a blunt calyx (or group of calyces) secondary to either obstruction or a sloughed papilla secondary to renal papillary necrosis (Fig. 19.11) [17]. Cortical abscesses and dilated calyces often filled with caseous material will be identified. Strictures at the ureteropelvic junction will lead to a pyonephrosis, and fistulas to the colon and/or skin can occur. Typical changes in the ureter (corkscrew, pipe stem, or string of bead appearance with ureterovesical scarring) and/or in the bladder (a fibrosed small bladder with unilateral reflux) should be looked for and can be a clue to proper diagnosis.

Retrograde pyelography will demonstrate an obstructed pelvis and/or calyx (Fig. 19.12a).

The angiogram may be confusing, suggesting a solid or cystic mass or pyonephrosis [44]. Radionuclide techniques are far superior and safer for determining the functional status of the kidney. We, however, advocate the use of Tc-DTPA after an adequate period of antibiotic therapy since some return of function may occur after treatment. Thus, the kidney may become salvageable.

Recently, Schaefer et al. have described the ultrasonic picture in TB [89]. They described two patterns: (a) a hydronephrotic collecting system, and (b) an infiltrating pattern. In the former, dependent debris can be seen (i.e., a pyonephrosis pattern). The second pattern was more common (9/11), with the masses always

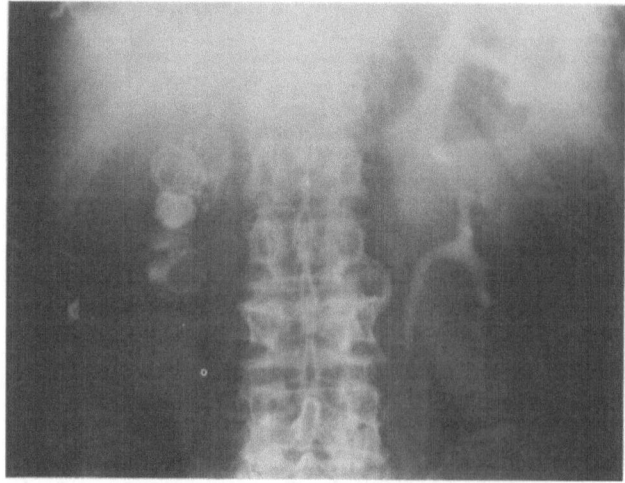

Fig. 19.10. Tuberculosis. Calcified, nonfunctioning right kidney.

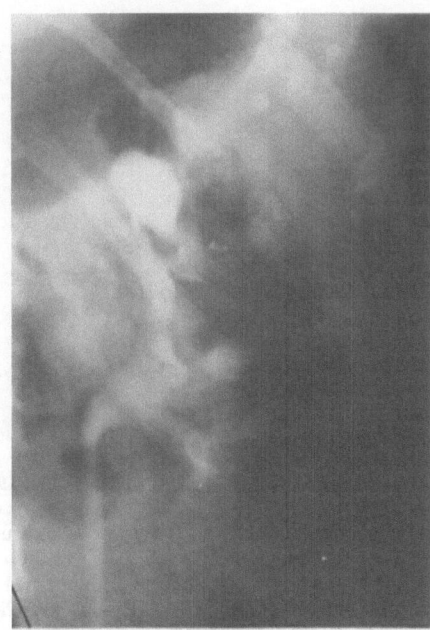

Fig. 19.11. Tuberculosis—early findings. Infundibular narrowing and dilated upper pole calyx.

showing some degree of echogenicity. However, the changes are nonspecific, reflecting the degree of calcification, pyonephrosis, and/or abscess formation present. The CT findings also may be confusing and represent an entire spectrum of disease. At one end of the spectrum is the small calcified kidney (Fig. 19.12b). Other patterns we have seen range from two or three obstructed calyces to a completely hydronephrotic kidney with the cortex markedly thinned and with fluid-filled calyces sometimes containing debris. Perirenal and psoas involvement are ideally demonstrated by CT (Fig. 19.13). The latter may be a clue to the diagnosis.

The development of nonfunction soon after treatment may not mean progression of disease but merely a healing stricture secondary to chemotherapy. The latter may even require surgical intervention.

The differential diagnosis unfortunately is long, including pyelonephritis, xanthogranulomatous pyelonephritis, pyonephrosis, tumor and tumor-like lesions, calculous disease, and renal papillary necrosis just to name a few.

Xanthogranulomatous Pyelonephritis

General Considerations

Xanthogranulomatous pyelonephritis (XGP) is an infection of the renal parenchyma and surrounding tissues characterized by the presence of large lipid-laden macrophages (xanthoma cells) [47]. It is the sequela of a severe, chronic, obstructing parenchymal inflammation. The process begins in the obstructed pelvis or

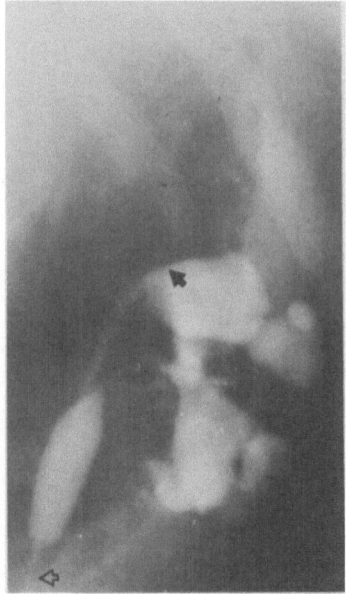

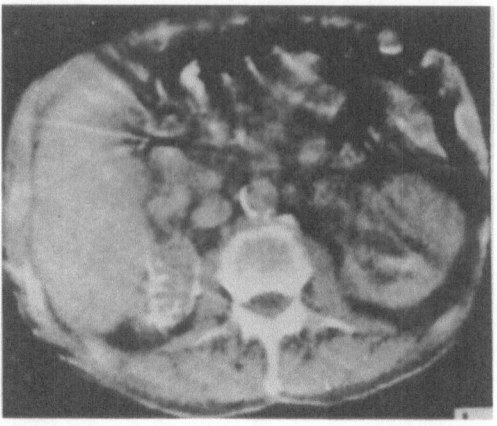

Fig. 19.12a,b. Tuberculosis—advanced cases. **a** Renal pelvis completely fibrosed. Entrance to upper pole obstructed (*closed arrow*). Portion of upper ureter also fibrosed (*open arrow*). **b** CT of calcified autonephrectomized kidney on right. (Case by courtesy of Dr. Ivan Gorelick, Columbia, Maryland)

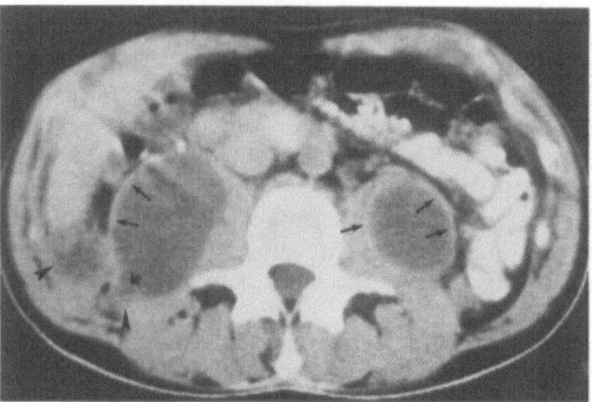

Fig. 19.13. Computed tomograms demonstrate well-demarcated low density masses extending into the psoas. The appearance is characteristic for a psoas abscess. The well-defined wall suggests considerable age and duration (*arrow*). A dehiscence in the wall (*arrowhead*) suggests communication to a daughter abscess. (By courtesy of E. K. Lang and Journal of Urology)

calyx and then extends and destroys first the medullary portion and finally the cortex of the kidney. In the diffuse form, the reniform shape is maintained although the kidney is enlarged. A staghorn calculus is present in a small encased pelvis. Other small calculi and scattered calcific flecks are also often noted in the calyces and residual cortex. The calyces, in contradistinction to the pelvis, are usually dilated with the surrounding parenchyma converted to a yellowish-orangish tissue. Both the calyces and the cortical abscesses are lined by xanthoma cells in solid sheets often admixed with lymphocytes and plasma cells. A diagnosis of XGP should be reserved for those cases where the xanthoma cell is predominant and not when only a few such cells are present. Extension into the perirenal and pararenal spaces is common. In the focal form, a calyx rather than the pelvis is obstructed.

Xanthogranulomatous pyelonephritis is usually found in women (4:1) in their middle decades. The complaints are often nonspecific, including malaise, back and flank pain, low grade fevers, chills, weight loss, and/or dysuria. Besides infection, neoplasia is often considered clinically. Many of the patients are diabetics. Urinalysis reveals pyuria, and often proteinuria, and/or microhematuria. Urine cultures usually grow *E. coli*, *Proteus*, *Pseudomonas*, and/or *Aerobacter*. Not infrequently, the organism found in the urine is not that grown from the pathological specimen.

Radiographic Findings

The plain film classically will show a staghorn calculus (70%–80%) or an obstructed calyx with a stone [9]. If, in addition, nonfunction is present (70%–90%) on IVU, one should suggest the possibility of XGP being present (Fig. 19.14). However, some function with hydronephrosis is present in 10%–30%. Occasionally, with the focal form, a mass lesion mimicking a tumor (either solid or necrotic) or abscess is seen.

On retrograde pyelography, complete obstruction at the pelvis is recognized in some. In others, the contrast may enter a small constricted pelvis lined with irregular granulomatous tissues and similarly lined, dilated calyces and/or communicating abscesses.

On angiography, one notes marked stretching of the segmental and/or interlobar arteries surrounding the calyces in a pattern similar to that of hydronephrosis (Fig. 19.15) [43]. The vascularity is usually increased.

In the proper clinical setting, the ultrasound is quite characteristic (Fig. 19.16a) [54, 97]. One notes renal enlargement, replacement of the normal architecture by multiple fluid-filled masses representing calyces, and/or abscesses with a small

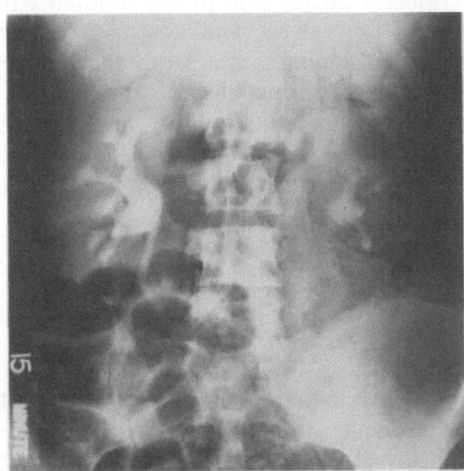

Fig. 19.14. Xanthogranulomatous pyelonephritis. IVU study showing enlarged, nonfunctioning kidney with staghorn calculus.

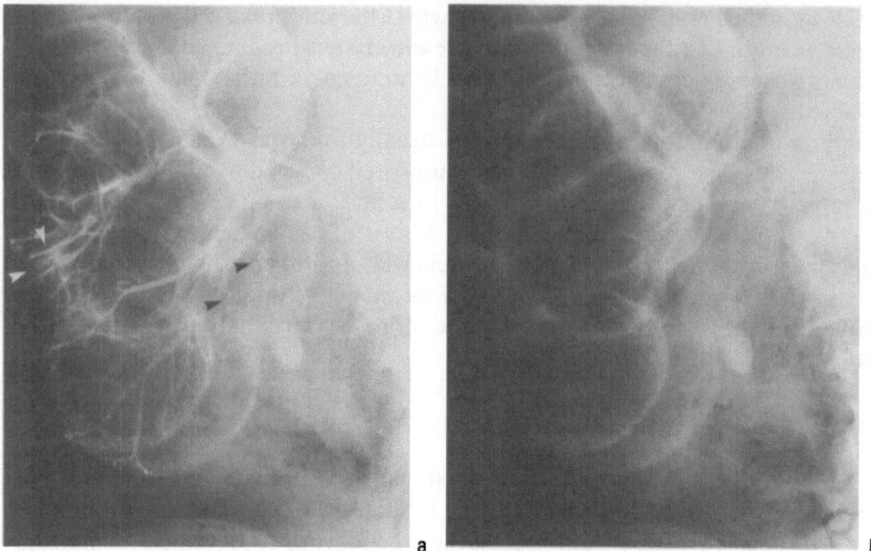

Fig. 19.15a,b. Xanthogranulomatous pyelonephritis. Angiographic findings demonstrating an enlarged kidney which, at first glance, is quite similar to those of hydronephrosis. However, an obstructing stone is present as well as inflammatory neovasculature (*arrows*). **a** late arterial phase; **b** nephrographic phase.

contracted renal pelvis. Depending on the amount of peripelvic fibrosis, shadowing from the staghorn calculus may or may not be seen. Even more impressive are the CT findings (Fig. 19.16b) [47, 94]. The kidney is usually enlarged with the parenchyma replaced by multiple, rounded, low density areas on CT that correspond to dilated calyces and/or abscesses pathologically. The CT numbers in these areas are of fluid density and not fat. (Although we are dealing with the lipid-laden macrophage, this is not pure fat and one should not expect CT numbers in fat ranges.) A staghorn calculus and other scattered calcifications are noted in both peripheral calyces and in the residual parenchyma. In our experience, the rims around the calyces and abscesses usually do enhance on dynamic CT. One important finding in our series was the frequent extension of the disease into the perirenal and pararenal space as well as the psoas in this disease. In many cases the pararenal and psoas muscle were extensively involved, with minimal perirenal involvement—a reflection, we believe, of a chronic indolent infection (Fig. 19.16c).

This extrarenal spread is seen in both focal and nonfocal forms.

Malacoplakia

General Considerations

Malacoplakia literally means soft plaque. It is an inflammatory process in which the histiocytes contain basophilic inclusion bodies (Michaelis-Gutmann bodies) as compared with fat inclusions in xanthogranulomatous pyelonephritis [22, 53, 92].

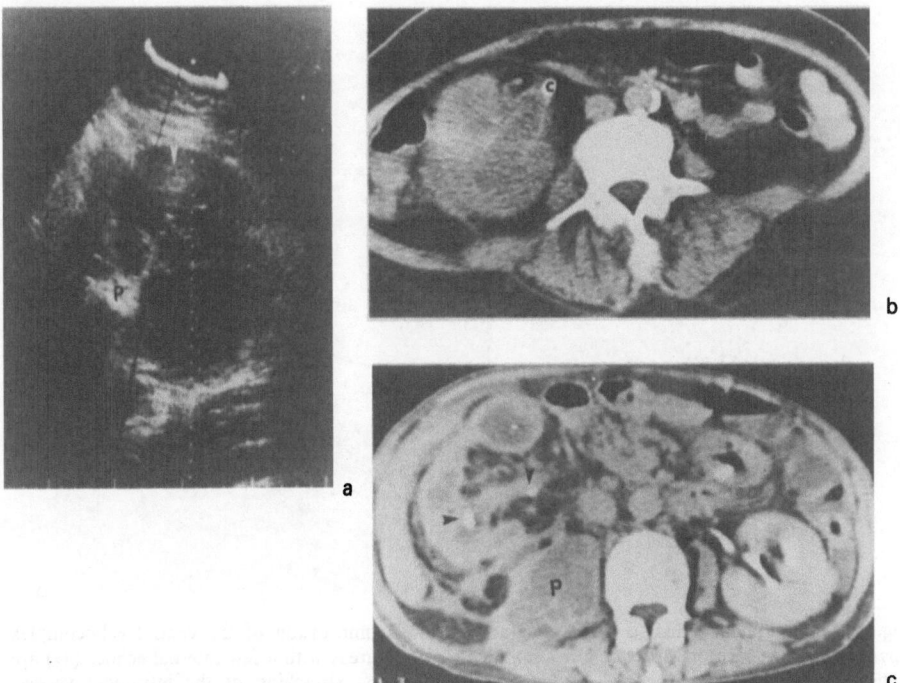

Fig. 19.16a–c. Xanthogranulomatous pyelonephritis. **a** Typical ultrasound showing smooth enlarged kidney with small renal pelvis (*P*). Note debris (*white arrow*) in the many cortical anechoic areas. The latter represent cortical abscesses and dilated calyces. **b** CT showing typical findings of a central obstructing calculus (*C*) with areas of low density representing calyces and cortical abscesses filled with fluid and xanthomatous material. The CT numbers in these are never those of fat. **c** CT showing marked involvement of psoas (*P*) with only minimal perirenal disease. The changes in the kidney are typical for XGP, with stones (*arrows*) and multiple lower density areas representing abscesses or obstructed calyces.

It is often seen in diabetics and in patients who are immunosuppressed. It is usually multifocal and often bilateral (50%). The kidney is usually enlarged, with multiple masses varying from millimeters to several centimeters in size. The smaller masses coalesce to form larger nodules. If limited to the medulla, malacoplakia may mimic renal papillary necrosis. Occasionally, the mass may be solitary, measuring 2.5–8 cm in diameter. The "tumor" is usually smooth and well margined with sharp demarcation from uninvaded parenchyma. Central necrosis or cyst formation may be present, usually without calcification.

Radiographic Findings (Fig. 19.17)

In the multifocal form, a large smooth kidney is seen without hydronephrosis [53]. If primarily cortical in nature, individual lesions may be seen by nephrotomography. If the medulla is involved, nonfunction is seen secondary to obstructive uropathy. A dominant mass with some echogenicity may be seen ultrasonically, which distorts the calyces. On angiography, the vessels are stretched, with a patchy nephrogram. The lesions may be hypo- or avascular.

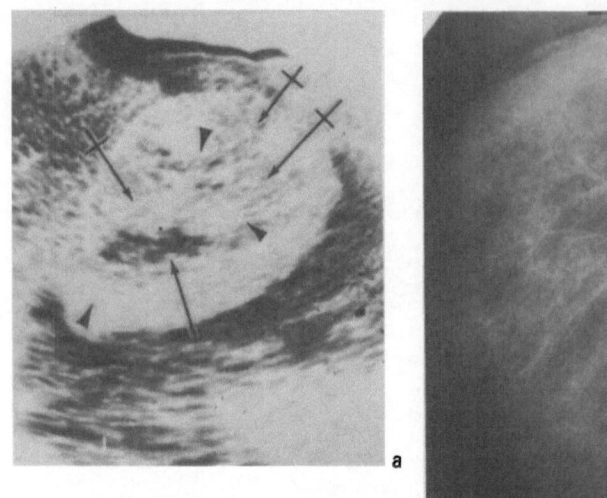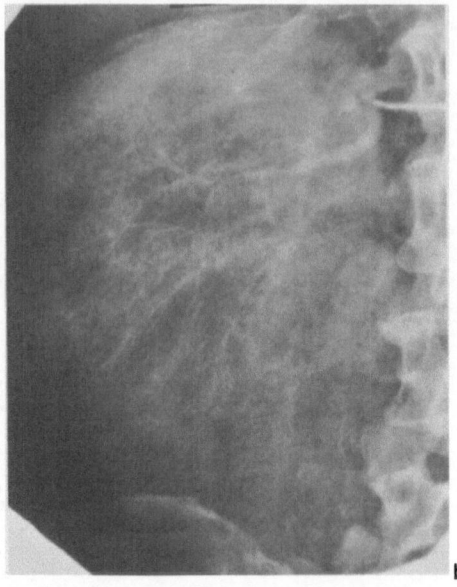

Fig. 19.17a,b. Malacoplakia. **a** Ultrasonogram showing compression of the central echocomplex (*arrowheads*). In addition, areas of low amplitude (→) and areas with a few internal echoes (↦) are noted throughout the kidney. **b** Angiogram demonstrating stretching of the intrarenal vessels, particularly in the lower half of the kidney, with areas of inhomogeneity and multiple irregular filling defects. (From Hartman et al. [53], with permission)

With the unifocal form, a mass may be seen which is indistinguishable from a tumor and may show neovascularity [53]. Thrombosis of the IVC or renal vein may be present [24]. Concomitant bladder lesions may also be helpful in suggesting the diagnosis.

Schistosomiasis

General Considerations

Schistosoma haematobium reaches the kidney through reflux from an infected bladder. There is a propensity for these patients to develop renal calculi and also squamous cell carcinomas. A history of possible exposure in those countries (the Middle East) where the disease is endemic is important for proper diagnosis [73].

Radiographic Findings

A critical diagnostic finding is calcification of the bladder and/or ureter on plain film [2]. This results from deposition of ova by the female parasite with secondary dystrophic calcification. Although mural calcification can be seen with other entities (i.e., TB, tumor, cystitis cystica, alkalinizing encrusting cystitis, etc.), significant, dense, wall calcification is most often secondary to schistosomiasis. However, such calcification need not be present. The IVU may show a mass and/or an obstructive hydro- or pyonephrosis.

Candidiasis

General Considerations

Involvement of the kidney usually occurs when host resistance is altered secondary to malignant diabetes, antibiotic or steroid therapy, and/or chronic debilitating diseases. When the kidney is involved because of disseminated systemic disease, the course is fulminant. The kidney can also be affected via the ascending route, usually with less serious consequences. In four-fifths of the latter cases, the disease is unilateral with flank pain. Hematuria is rare.

Radiographic Findings

The plain films are usually nonspecific unless the bladder is involved. In the latter, air surrounding the ribbon-like mycelia may be noted [13, 41, 67]. Varying patterns will be seen on the IVU, including acute pyelonephritis, a swollen kidney with multiple parenchymal abscesses, renal failure, and/or nonvisualization. In another form, renal papillary necrosis may develop. In the ascending form, irregular filling defects (fungus balls) in the calyces, renal pelvis, and/or bladder will be noted. The retrograde study will also demonstrate the mycetoma, while an echogenic non-shadowing renal pelvic mass will be identified on ultrasound [93]. The CT pattern should be that of a pelvic filling defect, possibly with a perinephric abscess. The fungus balls can occasionally be diagnosed and treated by antegrade techniques [68].

Echinococcus

General Considerations

Renal involvement is rare and is usually a primary infestation by the organisms which reach the kidney via the arterial system. Less commonly, secondary involvement occurs from adjacent organs. Positive intradermal (Cassoni) precipitin tests are used to aid in the diagnosis. Classically, the echinococcal cyst is surrounded by three layers.

Radiographic Findings

On plain films, the walls of the cysts may calcify. If a singular mass is present, a hypernephroma or other malignancy must be considered. In the presence of multiple masses, polycystic kidneys have to be excluded. Whether calcified or not, the walls are thick. Central necrosis and occasional air-fluid levels may be noted. The mass may compress the calyx, giving it a crescentic shape [43]. Angiographically, the masses are usually avascular [50]. A cyst puncture may be diagnostic but is extremely dangerous since spillage of a cyst's contents would lead to the development of peritoneal daughter cysts. Thick-walled, cystic masses which are often calcified have been described on CT. Sometimes air and debris have been noted within the masses. One should also search for liver involvement as a possible clue to the diagnosis [6]. Appearances on both ultrasound and CT can mimic a multilocular cystic nephroma (i.e., multicystic kidney) [6].

Brucellosis

General Considerations

Brucellosis is an amicrobic urinary tract infection associated with cystitis that is refractory to the usual forms of treatment. A positive agglutination test is available. Cystoscopy reveals an ulcerating cystitis much like that seen in tuberculosis.

Radiographic Findings

On plain films, large, gross calcifications are seen, as if splashed over the kidney by a paint brush [62]. The IVU will show cicatricial deformity of the calyces indistinguishable from that seen in TB. The differential diagnosis includes TB and tumor.

Actinomycosis

General Considerations

Normally actinomycosis is a saprophytic gram-positive anaerobe found in the mouth, tonsils, and GI tract. The kidney is secondarily involved from the GI tract or through the diaphragm from the lung [32, 100]. In Patel et al.'s case [82], the angiogram revealed neovascularity and areas of hypovascularity. CT and sonography merely suggested a solid mass. Actinomycosis occurs in three forms: (a) carbuncle, (b) pyelonephritis, and (c) pyonephrosis [Patel et al.]. Without evidence of sinus tracts, the diagnosis is impossible.

Radiographic Findings

Three radiographic forms have been noted. These are: (a) a pyelonephritis, (b) a pyonephrosis, and (c) a chronic suppurative pattern with cortical abscesses. Perinephric involvement is commonly present, probably being best identified on CT. An actinomycosis fistula tract injection may show communication with the kidney. When this diagnosis is being considered, "sulfur" granules should be looked for on the smear obtained from such tracts. The differential diagnosis includes tumor, TB, and abscess. When diagnosed, penicillin is an effective drug.

Other Rare Inflammatory Lesions

Blastomycosis and other rare infections of the kidney have been reported [26, 31].

Acute and Chronic Pyonephrosis

The term pyonephrosis is used to describe an infected hydronephrosis. This infection may be primary and cause the obstruction or secondary since the urine in

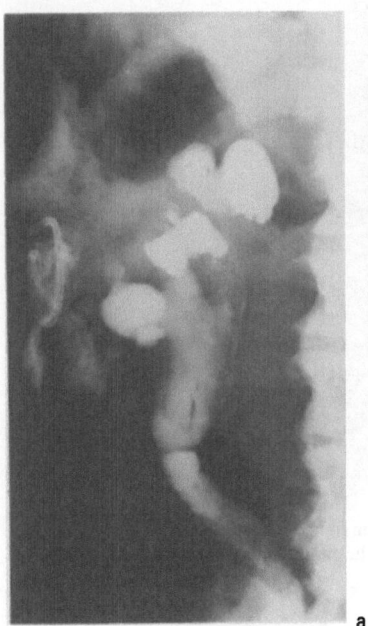
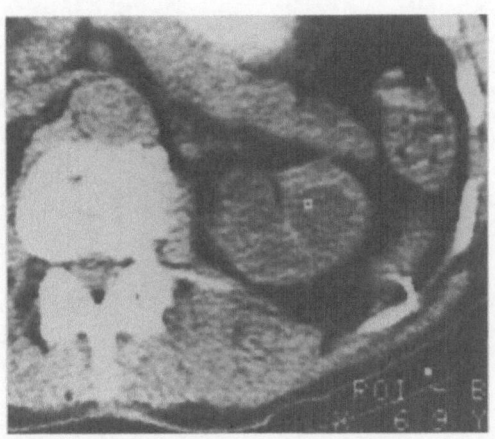

Fig. 19.18a,b. Pyonephrosis. **a** Antegrade pyelogram showing dilated calyces and pelvis as seen in hydronephrosis, except that one notes infected debris and irregularities of the wall which preclude a simple hydronephrosis. **b** CT demonstrating hydropelvis and hydrocalyces in same case.

an obstructed system is prone to infection. There is usually marked destruction and thinning of the cortex from the obstruction and the infection.

On plain film, a large or small kidney outline will be seen. The IVU will show the typical findings of hydronephrosis with poor and/or nonfunction, with dilated calyces being noted on tomography. An antegrade pyelogram will show the dilated calyces possibly with irregular walls and filling defects (Fig. 19.18a) [68]. A retrograde study will demonstrate similar findings or just define an obstruction. The angiogram will show diminished arterial flow with stretched vessels over the dilated calyces (i.e., a pattern of hydronephrosis) and possibly some neovascularity in areas of active infection. Ultrasound will exhibit the changes typical of hydronephrosis, with a dilated renal pelvis. Fluid levels seen as persistent, dependent echoes [25, 95] will be noted, representing layering of debris and infected material. The CT will also manifest the findings typical of an obstructive hydronephrosis but the CT numbers may be slightly above those of pure fluid (Fig. 19.18b). Debris will also often be displayed in the dilated calyces and/or pelvis. Without a history of infection, one cannot differentiate between a hydronephrosis and a pyonephrosis unless debris is identified in the calyces or the pelvis. CT will also provide evidence of perirenal extension if it is present.

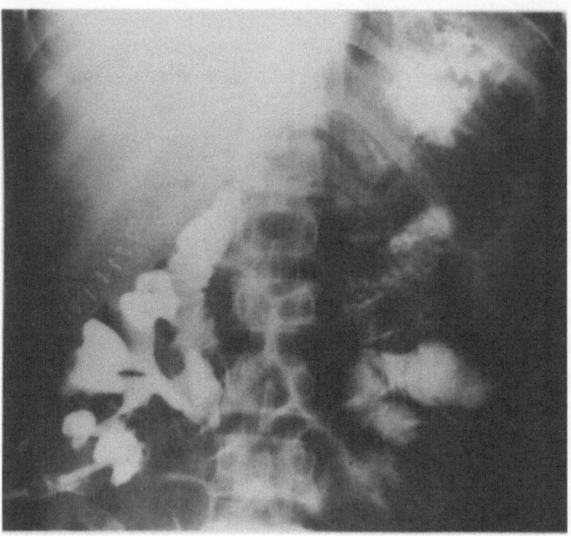

Fig. 19.19. Pyeloduodenal fistulas in postoperative patient after right renal stone removal. The kidney was ultimately removed and the diagnosis of XGP made. The fistulas may have actually predated surgery.

Renal Fistula

With infection, fistulas first develop to the perinephric and pararenal spaces. From there, nephrointestinal (Fig. 19.19), nephrocutaneous, and/or nephrobronchial fistula can occur [3, 14]. Other causes of fistulas include trauma, tumors primary in the kidney or elsewhere (i.e., GI tract), and surgery. The fistulas may be demonstrated by barium or Gastrografin GI studies, bronchography, and/or sinus tract injection. Only CT will identify the extent of the accompanying mass, and we strongly advocate the use of CT prior to surgical intervention.

Renal Papillary Necrosis

General Considerations

Renal papillary necrosis has many causes. One pneumonic commonly used by our residents is POSTCARD (pyelonephritis, obstruction, sickle cell disease, tuberculosis, cirrhosis, analgesic abuse, renal vein thrombosis, diabetes) [29, 51, 76]. Other causes include renal transplantation [60]. Of these, careful exclusion of analgesic abuse must be made, especially in the female population.

Whatever the underlying cause, the common denominator is an ischemic necrosis of the renal pyramid due to spasm or sludging within the small arterioles or venules supplying the pyramid. Two forms of necrosis have been described:

medullary and papillary. In the medullary form, multiple irregular linear cavities develop within the tip of the papilla. In the papillary form, fistulas develop from the fornices of the affected calyx and may ultimately result in a complete slough of the papilla. The latter may calcify and/or obstruct the calyx, pelvis, or ureter. The presenting systems include hematuria, pyuria, and/or renal colic. Careful analyses of the strained urine may demonstrate papillary fragments.

Radiographic Findings

The earliest finding in which the diagnosis should be suggested is the demonstration of one to three linear streaks of contrast within a single pyramid (Fig. 19.20a) [52]. Sometimes these streaks are irregular. Subsequent involvement of several calyces and/or both kidneys occurs. The pattern just described is the medullary form and must be differentiated from medullary sponge kidney or tubular ectasia [23, 29, 51].

In the papillary forms, contrast is noted extending from one fornix to the opposite one. With time the contrast is noted to be connecting both fornyces, and the papilla is, in fact, sloughed (Fig. 19.20b). Then the sloughed papilla, which may or may not be calcified, may be demonstrated floating in a blunt calyx. On

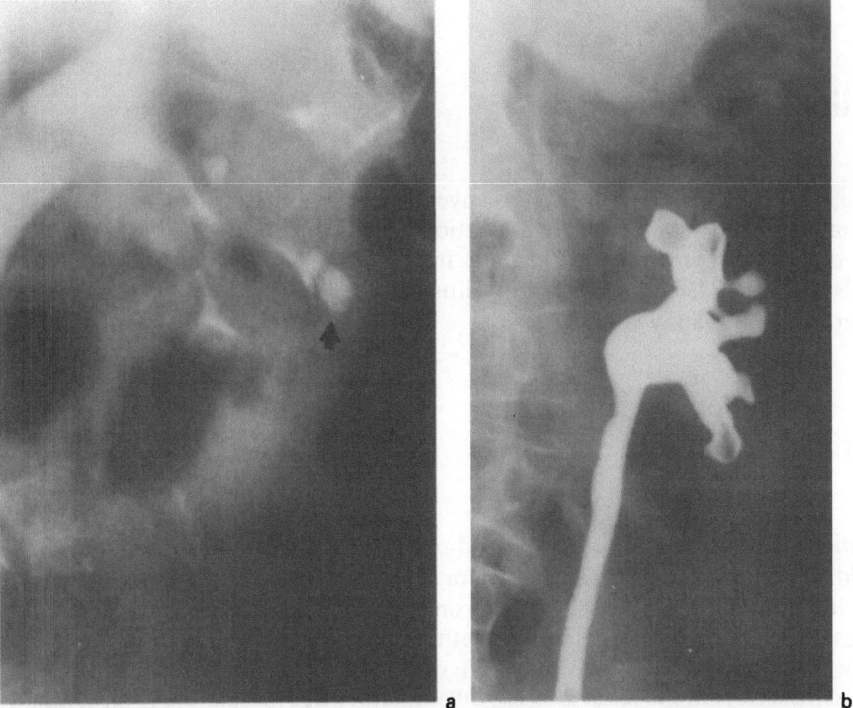

a   b

Fig. 19.20a,b. Renal papillary necrosis. **a** Medullary form; note cavity in medulla (*arrow*). **b** Papillary form; sloughed material noted in upper and lower pole calyces.

ultrasound, the sloughed papilla may be displayed within a calyx which, if calcified, will demonstrate shadowing. Similarly on CT one can see a sloughed papilla within its calyx.

Cholesteatoma, Leukoplakia, Squamous Metaplasia

General Considerations

Classic teaching classifies leukoplakia as a premalignant process although others disagree [4, 85]. Cholesteatoma represents a keratinizing process, while squamous metaplasia is without keratinization. Cholesteatoma is considered an inflammatory process.

Radiographic Findings

Both squamous metaplasia and cholesteatoma involving the renal pelvis will show irregularity of the involved calyx or the renal pelvis which can be indistinguishable from a transitional cell carcinoma on IVU, ultrasound, and CT [36, 99].

Pyelitis Cystica

In the local form of ureteritis cystica, pyelitis cystica is associated with chronic, focal mucosal and submucosal inflammation usually due to *E. coli* [75]. It is felt by some that these represent cystic changes in von Brunn's nests much like those of cystitis cystica. The diagnosis of pyelitis cystica is made on intravenous or retrograde pyelography (Fig. 19.21).

Septic Emboli

In patients with cardiac murmurs and abnormalities in the kidney, septic emboli should be considered. Renal scans and/or renal abscesses will be noted. Nuclear medicine studies will show filling defects on 2, 3-dimercaptosuccinic acid (DMSA) studies and hot spots with gallium or with indium-labeled white blood cells (Fig. 19.22a). The definitive study may, on occasion, be angiography, which will demonstrate clots in the renal arteries, inflammatory neovasculature (Fig. 19.22b), and possibly vegetations on the cardiac valves. The clots and vegetations may possibly also be identifiable on ultrasound.

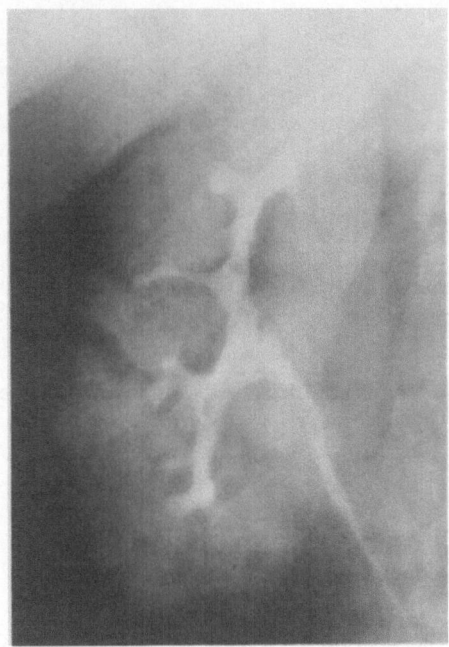

Fig. 19.21. Classic case of pyelitis cystica; note multiple filling defects.

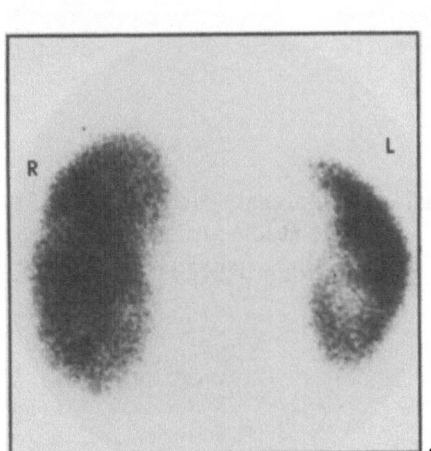

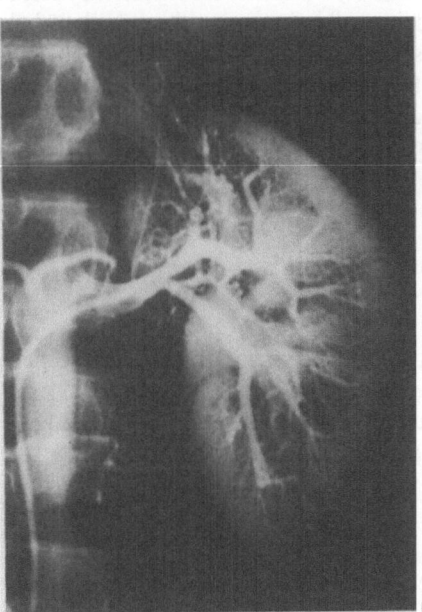

Fig. 19.22a,b. Septic emboli in 12-year-old with verrucae on diseased mitral valve secondary to rheumatic fever. **a** Tc-glucoheptonate scan. Note defect in LU pole and other defects. Scan reversed but properly labeled. **b** Angiogram showing embolic scars in upper pole with persistent collateral and inflammatory vessels seen in nephrographic phase. A mycotic aneurysm was present on the opposite side.

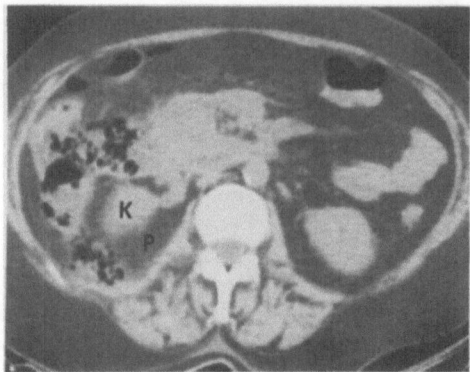

Fig. 19.23. Pancreatitis involving pararenal spaces (note fluid and gas) but not involving perirenal space (*P*) or kidney (*K*).

Atrophic Pyelonephritis

Hodson et al. described the development of pyelonephritic changes secondary to reflux in pigs [57]. This reflux ultimately led to small atrophic changes in the kidney indistinguishable from those seen in humans with chronic pyelonephritis. They also describe a few cases where they felt such scarring to occur in humans without evidence of infection, although they believe that ascending infection and reflux causes most renal damage. The problem of extrapolating this theory to humans is the fact that many females have asymptomatic intermittent bacteruria. Thus, it will be almost impossible to document a pure case of atrophic pyelonephritis in humans.

Pancreatitis

Not only can pancreatitis affect the perirenal and pararenal spaces (Fig. 19.23) [80], it can also mimic an intrarenal mass [7, 84]. Fine needle aspiration of these pseudocysts can confirm the diagnosis. In some of these patients, no definite history of pancreatitis is obtained.

References

1. Acton CM, Drew JH (1979) Vesicoureteric reflux in the neonatal period. In: Hodson CJ, Smith PK (eds) Reflux nephropathy. Masson, New York
2. Al-Ghorab MM (1968) Radiological manifestation of genito-urinary bilharziasis. Clin Radiol 19:100–111

3. Alvi AA, Goel TG, Dubey PC (1973) Reno-broncho-pyelocutaneous fistula. Br J Urol 45:233
4. Armstrong CP Jr, Harlin HC, Fort CA (1950) Leukoplakia of the renal pelvis. J Urol 63:208–213
5. Asscher AW et al. (Cardiff-Oxford Bacteriuria Study Group) (1978) Sequelae of covert bacteriuria in schoolgirls. A four-year follow-up study. Lancet II:889
6. Babcock DS, Kaufman L, Cosnow I (1978) Ultrasound diagnosis of hydatid disease (echinococcosis) in two cases. AJR 131:895–897
7. Baker MK, Kopecky KK (1983) Perirenal pancreatic pseudocysts: Diagnostic management. AJR 140:729–732
8. Barrie HJ, Kerr WK, Gale GL (1967) The incidence and pathogenesis of tuberculous strictures of renal pyelus. J Urol 98:584–589
9. Beachley MC, Ranniger K, Roth FJ (1974) Xanthogranulomatous pyelonephritis. AJR 121:500–507
10. Ben-Amni T (1984) The sonographic evaluation of urinary tract infections in children. Semin Ultrasound CT & MR 5:19–33
11. Bergner DM, Roth JK Jr, Lang EK (1982) The role of computerized tomography in the management of bilateral tubercular psoas abscess. J Urol 128:1020–1022
12. Berliner L, Bosniak MA (1982) The striated nephrogram in acute pyelonephritis. Urol Radiol 4:41–44
13. Biggers R, Edwards J (1980) Anuria secondary to bilateral ureteropelvic fungus balls. Urology 15:161–163
14. Bissada NK, Cole AT, Fried FA (1973) Reno-alimentary fistula: An unusual urological problem. J Urol 110:273–276
15. Bourne HH, Condon VR, Hoyt TS, Nixon GW (1976) Intrarenal reflux and renal damage. J Urol 115:304–306
16. Boyd W (1970) A textbook of pathology, 8th edn. Lea & Febiger, Philadelphia, pp 111–113
17. Bruce AW, Awad SA, Challis TW (1969) The recognition and treatment of tuberculous pyocalyx of the kidney. J Urol 101:127–131
18. Brugh R III, Gooneratne NS, Rous SN (1979) Gallium-67 scanning and conservative treatment in acute inflammatory lesions of the renal cortex. J Urol 121:232–235
19. Caplan LH, Siegelman SS, Bosniak MA (1967) Angiography in inflammatory space occupying lesions of the kidney. Radiology 88:14–23
20. Cardiff-Oxford Study Group (1979) Long term effects of bacteriuria on the urinary tract in schoolgirls. Radiology 132:343–350
21. Carris CK, Schmidt JE (1977) Emphysematous pyelonephritis. J Urol 118:457–459
22. Cavins JA, Goldstein AMB (1977) Renal malakoplakia. Urology 10:155–158
23. Christofferson JC, Andersen K (1967) Renal papillary necrosis. AJR 101:703–707
24. Clark RA, Weiss MA, Colley DP, Wyatt GM (1979) Renal malakoplakia with renal vein thrombosis. AJR 133:1170–1173
25. Coleman BG, Arger PH, Mulhern CB Jr, Pollack HM, Banner MP (1981) Pyonephrosis: Sonography in the diagnosis and management. AJR 137:939–943
26. Dansky AS, Lynne CM, Politano VA (1978) Disseminated mucormycosis with renal involvement. J Urol 119:275–277
27. Davidson AJ, Talner LB (1978) Late sequelae of adult-onset acute bacterial nephritis. Radiology 127:367–371
28. Dawson SL, Mueller PR, Ferucci JJ Jr (1984) Mucomyst for abscesses: A clinical comment. Radiology 151:342
29. Eckert DE, Jonutis AJ, Davidson AJ (1976) The incidence and manifestation of urographic papillary abnormalities in patients with S hemoglobinopathies. Radiology 113:59–63
30. Edell SL, Bonavita JA (1979) The sonographic appearance of acute pyelonephritis. Radiology 132:683–685
31. Eickenberg HV, Amin M, Lich R Jr (1975) Blastomycosis of the genitourinary tract. J Urol 113:650–652
32. Ellis LR, Kenny GM, Nellans RE (1979) Urogenital aspects of actinomycosis. J Urol 122:132–133
33. Elo J, Tallgren LG, Alfthan O, Sarna S (1983) Character of urinary tract infections and pyelonephritic renal scanning after antireflux surgery. J Urol 129:343–346
34. Fair WR, McClennan BL, Jost RG (1979) Are excretory urograms necessary in evaluating women with urinary tract infection. J Urol 121:313–315
35. Finn DJ, Palestrant AM, De Wolf WC (1982) Successful percutaneous management of renal abscess. J Urol 127:425–426
36. Freedberg LE, Stables DP, Blousten PA, Donoh R (1977) Cholesteatoma of renal pelvis. Urology 10:263–265

37. Friedland GW (1977) Long term effects of urinary tract infections. Radiology 124:263–264
38. Frimann-Dahl J (1966) Angiography in renal inflammatory disease. In: Kincaid OW (ed) Renal angiography. Year Book Medical Publishers, Chicago, pp 230–252
39. Froelich JW, Swanson D (1984) Imaging of inflammatory processes with labeled cells. Semin Nucl Med 14:128–139
40. Garcia JE, Van Nostrand D, Howard WH III, Kyle RW (1984) The spectrum of gallium-67 renal activity in patients with no evidence of renal disease. J Nucl Med 25:575–580
41. Gerle RD (1973) Roentgenographic features of primary renal candidiasis. AJR 119:731–738
42. Gilbert PG, Shirley SW (1973) The use of angiography in the diagnosis of space-occupying renal and perirenal inflammatory lesions. J Urol 110:11–15
43. Gilsanz V, Lozanot, Jiminez J (1980) Renal hydatid cysts: Communicating with collecting system. AJR 135:357–361
44. Giustra PE, Watson RC, Shulman H (1971) Arteriographic findings in the various stages of renal tuberculosis. Radiology 100:587–602
45. Gold RP, McClennan BL, Rottenberg RR (1983) CT appearance of acute inflammatory disease of the renal interstitium. AJR 141:343–349
46. Goldman SM, Minkin SD, Naraval DC, Diamond AB, Pion SJ, Meringoff BN, Sidh SM, Sanders RC, Cohen SP (1977) Renal carbuncle: The use of ultrasound in its diagnosis and treatment. J Urol 118:525–528
47. Goldman SM, Hartman DS, Fishman EK, Finizio JP, Gatewood OMB, Siegelman SS (1984) CT of xanthogranulomatous pyelonephritis: Radiologic-pathologic correlation. AJR 143:963–969
48. Gow JG (1963) Genitourinary tuberculosis: A study of 700 cases. Lancet II:261–265
49. Gwinn JL, Barnes GR Jr (1964) Striated ureters and renal pelvis. AJR 91:666–668
50. Haines JG, Mayo ME, Allan NA, Ansell JS (1977) Echinococcal cyst of the kidney. J Urol 117:788–789
51. Hare WSC, Poynter JD (1974) The radiology of renal papillary necrosis as seen in analgesic nephropathy. Clin Radiol 25:423–443
52. Harrow BR (1965) Early forms of renal papillary necrosis. AJR 95:335–343
53. Hartman DS, Davis CJ Jr, Lichtenstein JE, Goldman SM (1980) Renal parenchymal malako-plakia. Radiology 136:33–42
54. Hartman DS, Sanders RS, Davis CJ Jr, Goldman SM, Isbister SS (1984) Xanthogranulomatous pyelonephritis: Sonographic-pathologic correlation of 16 cases. J Clin Ultrasound Med 3:481–488
55. Hodson CJ, Edward D (1960) Chronic pyelonephritis and vesico-ureteric reflux. Clin Radiol 11:219–231
56. Hodson CJ, Davies Z, Prescod A (1975) Renal parenchymal radiographic measurement in infants and children. Pediatr Radiol 3:16–19
57. Hodson CJ, Maling TMJ, McManamon PJ (1975) The pathogenesis of reflux nephropathy (chronic atrophic pyelonephritis). Br J Radiol (Suppl) 13:1–26
58. Hoffman EP, Mindelzun RE, Anderson RU (1980) Computed tomography in acute pyelonepthri-tis associated with diabetes. Radiology 135:691–695
59. Hopkins GB, Hall RL, Mende CW (1976) Gallium-67 scintigraphy for the diagnosis and localization of perinephric abscess. J Urol 115:126–128
60. Kaude JV, Stone M, Fuller TJ, et al. (1976) Papillary necrosis in kidney transplant patients. Radiology 120:69–74
61. Kay CJ, Rosenfield AT, Taylor KJW, Rosenberg MA (1979) Ultrasonic characteristics of chronic atrophic pyelonephritis. AJR 132:47–49
62. Kelalis PP, Greene LF, Weed LA (1962) Brucellosis of the urogenital tract: A mimic of tuberculosis. J Urol 88:347–353
63. Kim DS, Woesner ME, Howard TF, Olson LK (1979) Emphysematous pyelonephritis demon-strated by computed tomography. AJR 132:287–288
64. Koehler PR (1974) The roentgen diagnosis of renal inflammatory masses—special emphasis on angiographic changes. Radiology 112:257–266
65. Koehler PR (1978) The roentgen diagnosis of renal inflammatory masses, special emphasis on angiographic changes. Radiology 112:257–266
66. Kollins SA, Hartman GW, Carr DT, Segura JW, Hattery RR (1974) Roentgenologic findings in urinary tract tuberculosis: A 10 year investigation. AJR 121:487–500
67. Kozinn PJ, Taschdjian CL, Goldberg PK, Wise GJ, Toni EF, Seelig MS (1978) Advances in the diagnosis of renal candidiasis. J Urol 119:184–187
68. Lang EK, Price EW (1983) Redefinition of indications for percutaneous nephrostomy. Radiology 147:419–426
69. Lautin EM, Gordon PM, Friedman AC, Dourmashkin L, Fromowitz F (1979) Emphysematous

pyelonephritis: Optimal diagnosis and treatment. Urol Radiol 1:93–96
70. Lee JKT, McClennan BL, Melson GL, Stanley RJ (1980) Acute bacterial nephritis. AJR 135:87–92
71. Levin DC, Gordon D, Kinkhabwala MN, et al. (1976) Reticular neovascularity in malignant and inflammatory renal masses. Radiology 120:61–68
72. Love L, Myers MA, Churchill RJ (1981) Computed tomography of extraperitoneal spaces. AJR 136:781–789
73. Mahmoud AA (1977) Schistosomiasis. N Engl J Med 297:1329–1331
74. McDougall IR, Baumert JE, Lanteri RL (1979) Evaluation of indium 111 in leukocyte whole body scanning. AJR 133:849–854
75. McNulty M (1957) Pyeloureteritis cystica. Br J Radiol 30:648–652
76. Mellins HZ (1971) Chronic pyelonephritis and medullary necrosis. Semin Roentgenol 6:292–308
77. Mendez G Jr, Isikoff MB, Morillo G (1979) The role of computed tomography in the diagnosis of renal and perirenal abscesses. J Urol 122:582–586
78. Mogle JM, Perlberg S, Heiman S, Caine M (1984) Emphysematous pyelonephritis. J Urol 131:203–208
79. Newcastle Asymptomatic Bacteriuria Research Group (1975) Asymptomatic bacteriuria in school children in Newcastle-upon-Tyne. Arch Dis Child 50:90–102
80. Nicholson RC (1981) Abnormalities of the perinephric fascia and fat in pancreatitis. Radiology 139:125–127
81. Nogrady MB, Lesk DM (1972) Renal papillary necrosis in the newborn: A case report with roentgenologic documentation of late sequelae. AJR 116:661–667
82. Patel BJ, Moskowitz, Hashmat A (1983) Unilateral renal actinomycosis. Urology 21:172–174
83. Ransley PG, Risdon RA (1979) The renal papilla, intrarenal reflux and chronic pyelonephritis. In: Hodson CJ, Smith PK (eds) Reflux nephropathy. Masson, New York, pp 126–133
84. Rauch RF, Korobkin M, Silverman PM, Dunnick NR (1983) Subcapsular pancreatic pseudocyst of the kidney. JCAT 7:536–538
85. Reece RW, Koontz WW Jr (1975) Leukoplakia of the urinary tract. A review. J Urol 114:165–171
86. Richie JP, Nicholson TC, Hunting D, et al. (1978) Radiographic abnormalities in acute pyelonephritis. J Urol 114:832–835
87. Roberts JA (1983) Pathogenesis of pyelonephritis. J Urol 129:1102–1106
88. Rosenfield AJ, Glickman MG, Taylor KJW. Crade M, Hodson J (1979) Acute focal bacterial nephritis (acute lobar nephronia). Radiology 132:553–561
89. Schaefer R, Becker JA, Goodman J (1983) Sonography of tuberculous kidney. Urology 21:209–211
90. Schneider M, Becker JA, Staiano S, Campos E (1975) Sonographic-radiographic correlation of renal and perirenal infections. AJR 127:1007–1014
91. Silver TM, Kass EJ, Thornbury JR (1976) The radiological spectrum of acute pyelonephritis in adults and adolescents. Radiology 118:67–71
92. Stanton MJ, Maxted W (1981) Malacoplakia: A study of the literature and current concepts of pathogenesis, diagnosis and treatment. J Urol 125:139–146
93. Stuck KJ, Silver TM, Jaffe MH, Bowerman RA (1981) Sonographic demonstration of renal fungus ball. Radiology 142:473–474
94. Subramanyam BR, Megibow AJ, Raghavendra BN, Bosniak MA (1982) Diffuse xanthogranulomatous pyelonephritis: Analysis by computed tomography and sonography. Urol Radiol 4:5–9
95. Subramanyam BR, Raghavendra BN, Bosniak MA, Lefleur RS, Rosen RJ, Horii SC (1983) Sonography of pyonephrosis: A prospective study. AJR 140:991–993
96. Thornbury JR (1979) Perirenal anatomy: Normal and abnormal. Radiol Clin North Am 17:321–331
97. Van Kirk OC, Go RT, Wedel VJ (1980) Sonographic features of xanthogranulomatous pyelonephritis. AJR 134:1035–1039
98. Van Waes PFG (1983) Management of loculated abscesses that are difficult to drain: A new approach. Radiology 147:57–63
99. Wills JS, Pollack HM, Curtis JA (1981) Cholesteatoma of the upper urinary tract. AJR 136:941–944
100. Yu HHY, Yim CM, Leong CH (1978) Primary actinomycosis of kidney presenting with renocolic fistula. Br J Urol 50:140

Subject Index

Clinical Practice in Urology

Series Editor: **G. D. Chisholm**, Edinburgh

Clinical Practice in Urology is an authoritative source of information and guidance for continuing professional education. The series combines a review of background material and advances in basic science with a critical evaulation of new techniques for clinical application. Each volume is written by recognized experts in their field and is carefully edited to ensure a clear, concise, practice-oriented presentation.

Bladder Cancer

Editors: **E. J. Zingg**, Berne; **D. M. A. Wallace**, London

1985. 50 figures. XII, 301 pages.
ISBN 3-540-13239-2

Contents: The Epidemiology and Aetiology of Bladder Cancer. - The Histopathology of Bladder Cancer. - Immunological Aspects of Bladder Cancer. - Symptomatology. - Diagnostic Procedures. - Classification of Bladder Tumours. - Carcinoma In Situ. - The Treatment of Superficial Bladder Tumours. - The Treatment of Muscle Invasive Bladder Cancer. - Chemotherapy of Bladder Cancer. - Palliative Treatment. - Subject Index.

The Pharmacology of the Urinary Tract

Editor: **M. Caine**, Jerusalem
1984. 27 figures. XII, 167 pages. ISBN 3-540-13238-4

This book gives an up-to-date account of the use of pharmacological agents in the management of urinary tract disorders. The emphasis is on the clinical and practical aspects of the subject, but it also includes an account of the underlying mechanisms of the models of action of the various groups of drugs.

Male Infertility

Editor: **T. B. Hargreave**, Edinburgh
1983. 56 figures. XII, 326 pages.
ISBN 3-540-12055-6

"This remarkable monograph distinguishes what is known from what is merely wishful guesswork... we are provided with clear guidelines for the investigations that are appropriate for each type of infertility, and a comprehensive account of their scientific background and sources of error..."
British Medical Journal

Urodynamics

by **P. Abrams, R. Feneley, M. Torrens**, Bristol
1983. 95 figures. XII, 229 pages.
ISBN 3-540-11903-5

"It is the only book I have seen which has managed very successfully to combine the detailed practical working knowledge of the subject together with an extensive review of earlier works. For those of us performing urodynamics, or thinking of setting up such a service, this book has admirably crystallized all aspects and knowledge of the subject."
Journal of the Royal Society of Medicine

Chemotherapy and Urological Malignancy

Editor: **A. S. D. Spiers**, Albany
1982. XVII, 163 pages. ISBN 3-540-11543-9

"The role of chemotherapy in the management of malignant disease of the urogenital tract is presented in this multiauthor volume according to anatomical site.. All chapters are well written and make up a well-balanced book."
The Lancet

Urinary Diversion

Editor: **M. H. Ashken**, Norwich
1982. 53 figures. XIII, 143 pages.
ISBN 3-540-11273-1

"The editor of this excellent little book has produced a work that must be read be every urologist and general surgeon who practices urology."
British Journal of Surgery

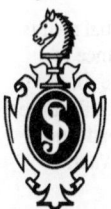

Springer-Verlag Berlin Heidelberg New York Tokyo

of further interest

Obstructive Uropathy

Editor: **P.H. O'Reilly,** Stockport

1985. 303 figures. Approx. 340 pages.
ISBN 3-540-15509-0

Contents: Upper Urinary Tract Obstruction: Introduction and General Considerations. - Laboratory Investigations. - Radiology. - Nuclear Medicine. - Antegrade Percutaneous Studies. - Urinary Stone Disease. - Idiopathic Hydronephrosis (Pelviureteric Junction Obstruction). - Ureteric Obstruction. - Percutaneous Renal Surgery in Obstructive Uropathy. - Lower Urinary Tract Obstruction: Basic Considerations. - Obstructive and Functional Abnormalities I. - Obstructive and Functional Abnormalities II. - Practical Aspects of the Management of Lower Urinary Tract Obstruction. - Subject Index.

This is the first work to distill and update the subject of obstructive uropathy in one volume. It covers the investigation of all types of urinary tract obstruction by means of laboratory tests, radiology, ultrasound, CT scanning, antegrade pyelography and perfusion pressure flow studies, and the management of conditions encountered in clinical practice.
Emphasis is laid on physiology, pathophysiology, function and dynamics as the consideration of these aspects determines diagnosis and management and forms the basis for the necessary practical approach.
Obstructive Uropathy will be of great value to all urologists, radiologists, surgeons, and pediatricians dealing with this common clinical condition, and will also provide a lucid and comprehensive guide for trainees and residents.

World Journal of

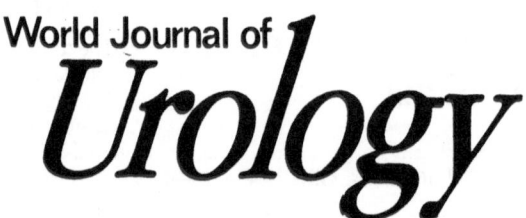

Urology

Official Journal of the Urological Research Society

ISSN 0724-4983   Title No. 345

Editors-in-Chief: U. Jonas, Leiden; **R. J. Krane,** Boston

The **World Journal of Urology** conveys regularly the essential results of urological research and their practical and clinical relevance to a broad audience of urologist in research and clinical practice. In order to guarantee a balanced program, articles are published to reflect the developments in all fields of urology on an internationally advanced level. Each issue treats a main topic in review articles of invited international experts.

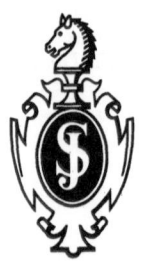

Springer-Verlag
Berlin
Heidelberg
New York
Tokyo